POWER AGING

POWER AGING

STAYING YOUNG AT ANY AGE

DR. GAYLE OLINEKOVA

Thunder's Mouth Press
New York

Published by
Thunder's Mouth Press
632 Broadway, Seventh Floor
New York NY 10012

Library of Congress Card Catalog Number on file with the publisher

ISBN 1-56025-123-9

Manufactured in the United States of America

CONTENTS

To Dennis, thank you for your loving strength, wisdom, and inspiration. For all the times I woke you up in the wee hours of the morning to blurt out the latest chapter, I give you my affectionate appreciation for your tenderness and sense of humor. It was a wonderful sharing. Your love is a great blessing to me.

ACKNOWLEDGMENTS

*T*here is a common, golden thread woven invisibly through this book by the love and energy of the people who have helped me finish the manuscript. Many gave hours of work with their only compensation in the intensity of their giving. I had an unofficial clipping service for years as I did the research for the book as my parents, sister, and brother read up to half a dozen newspapers a day to help ferret out

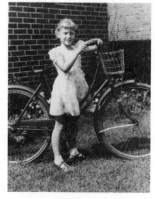

any scientific announcements that could lead to a phone interview, further information searches on the Net, or a different perspective. Patients, friends, and colleagues shared their stories, opinions, photographs, and their enthusiasm. One photo subject was born just as the book was going into final production. The death of some close friends during the long months of writing made me live the words I once heard Dr. Bernie Siegel say in an interview: " . . . We must learn to take that pain and to love others with it." I scribbled that phrase on a piece of paper I carry around in my wallet.

Even though writing a book can feel like a never ending, lonely endurance event, I am blessed by the special people in my life who have made it better. To you all, I am grateful for all understanding and generosity you have given to me. Thank you for your commitment and energy:

To my grandparents and great-grandmother, gratitude for your influence and enthusiasm.

To my mom and dad, and my sister Susan and brother Gary, thank you for being my family.

Director of Research: Eugene M. Linhart, B.S.M.E., M.S.A., M.B.A.

Gene, your good spirits and hard work toward this project were a major help to me.

Artist: Sylvia Lopez B.F.A. (Illustration). Thank you for your skill and understanding.

Photographer: Suzonne Stirling. I appreciate your artist's eye.

Maura Barraza
Michael Bober
Edith Butler
Joanne Du Bois
Gloria Frias
Bob Girvetz
Phyllis Girvetz

Nina Girvetz-White
Chaplain Bill Glaser
Sandy Glaser
Dr. Sanford Grossman
Jim Kupcho
Terri Loewy
Joan Long

PHOTO CREDITS

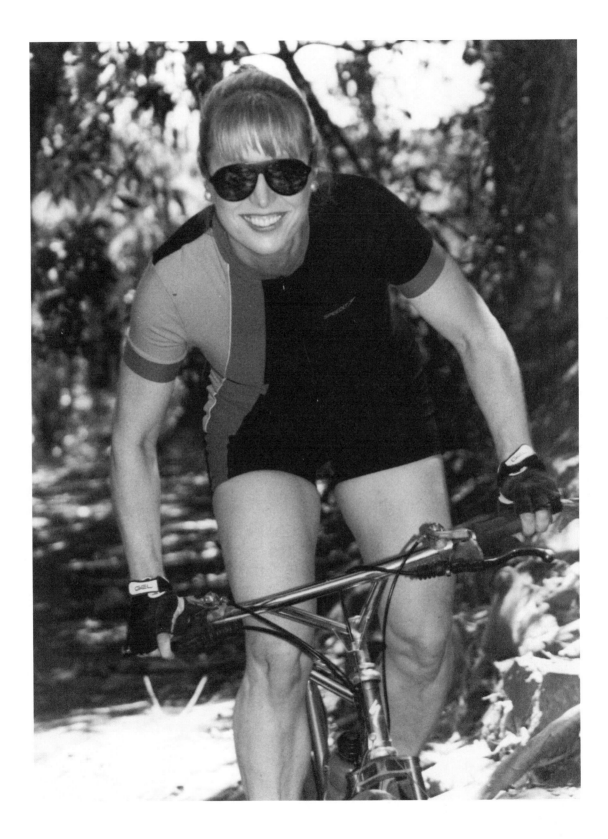

1 IT'S EARLIER THAN YOU THINK

Even in our sleep
and against our will
drop by drop
the pain of the day
falls on our hearts
Until comes wisdom . . .

—Pablo Picasso (1881–1973)

One day you're an ordinary boy or girl. You read an adventure book or see a movie, and you have the most wonderful time imagining that you are dangling off a cliff fighting pirates and saving the village. Yet afterward, you must go back to being a boy or girl again. But, when you dream and never give up that dream until you turn it into a goal that you can touch and feel and smell and taste, why then you will never be the same, because day by day, you can *become that dream* and make it come true. You give yourself a gift that no one else can give you.

That's how I became a long distance runner. Growing up in Toronto, I dreamed of how it would be to get stronger every day and become a champion athlete—one of the best in the world. And every night before I went to bed, I asked myself, What did you do today to make that dream come true? I would count up all the miles run and sit-ups done and fall asleep full of plans for another day.

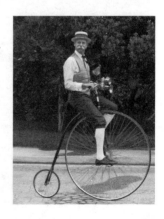

I adopted this goal the night before my sixteenth birthday. Six months later, I was on a plane to Japan, representing my country in an international track meet as national champion in the 400 meters.

But tragedy stuck a couple of years later when I felt the

first searing pain of a hamstring injury that left me hobbling around for nine frustrating months of inactivity. After following the traditional route of prescription drugs
and painful cortisone injections, I gave away all my possessions (there weren't many)
and bought a one-way standby ticket to Europe, thinking that in the great sport centers of Europe I could find somebody who would know a better way of healing.

The night before I left, I met Dr. Adrian Grice, a chiropractor, who examined me,
told me the biomechanical reason for the hamstring injury, and explained how he was
going to treat it through spinal manipulation. I was very skeptical, in the way that
teenagers can be. But somehow it was all so logical that I also half believed him. He
treated me and I was shocked at how much better I felt, how the pain just disap-
peared. My mind said, Maybe it's a trick. So I dashed outside in my bare feet to see if

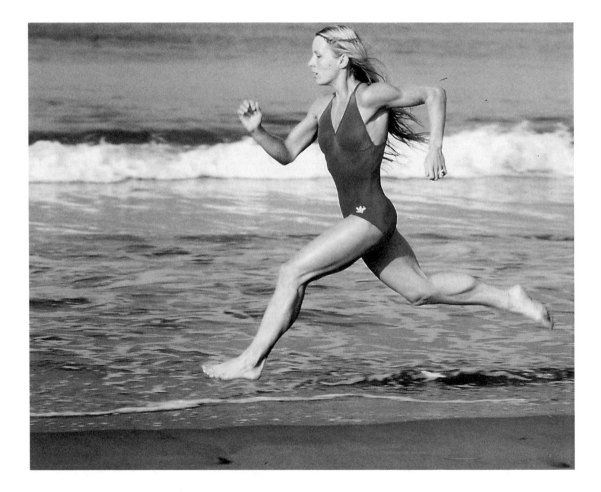

I could really raise my leg and run again—oblivious to the four inches of new snow on the ground. It worked. I *sprinted* across the parking lot, leaving wide-spaced, perfectly matched footprints. To the surprise of a number of waiting patients, I did a little celebration dance.

I still left for Europe the next day. Dr. Grice set me up with a colleague of his in Switzerland, a Dr. Illi, who, I would learn later, is considered "the grandfather of chiropractic." But before leaving, I told Dr. Grice "If what you have taught me will help me make my dreams come true and give me a career as a champion athlete, then I promise that someday I will do something to help."

GREEN MEDICINE

After twenty years as a world-class athlete, I began to fulfill that promise. Going back to school after such a long hiatus was a real eye-opener. Initially, I worried about whether or not I could get the grades, since I had avoided science classes like the plague my first time in college. Nobody was more shocked than I when I scored 100 percent in one of the early courses. "Go to medical school," encouraged my professors. I audited a lot of medical classes and it became apparent that I would be studying conventional, drug-based therapies that I didn't believe in. And, in my years as an athlete, it was the hands-on therapy of chiropractic, not the traditional drug-based therapies, that saved my career time and time again. I doubt that my body could have withstood all the surgeries that were proposed to correct the wear and tear injuries of a marathon runner. It was when I learned more about the human body that I came to know the biomechanical basis for preventing the injuries in the first place. So I became a doctor of chiropractic instead of a doctor of medicine.

Incidentally, twenty-four years after meeting Dr. Grice, I called him up. He was still at the same telephone number! "Do you remember me?" I asked. "Remember my promise? I'm graduating from chiropractic college today and it's all your fault." He remembered. And then two people, several thousand miles apart, laughed and cried at the same time.

Don't get me wrong—I've also been saved on a few occasions by antibiotics for pneumonia and surgery for a hot appendix, and I have a lot of respect for the doctors who helped me. I am a firm believer in calling the fire department when your house is on fire, but the most powerful therapies of all are surely based in *prevention*. Hotels, houses, and apartments are required by law to have smoke detectors and sprinkler systems to prevent disasters or catch them before they destroy the structure. Are our bodies not at least as important as buildings made of wood and cement?

Therefore, in the book that follows, I have concentrated on the therapies that deal with the "green medicine" of prevention. Presented are the foods, herbs, and supplements to your diet; the exercises and lifestyle changes; physical, mental, and even financial planning that can help you achieve your goal of power aging. These are the elements of the equation that allow you to maximize the biochemistry of living.

OLD AIN'T WHAT IT USED TO BE

When I started this book many years ago, I thought about calling it *The Secrets of Youth*. However, as I watched some teenagers hanging out by the local mall and eavesdropped on some of their conversations, I thought to myself, What secrets could they possibly have? What did I know at that age? (Well, okay, I *thought* I knew everything—all you had to do was ask me!) Our elderly are the ones who have the secrets. Before the sixties—the "don't trust anyone over thirty era"—it was called wisdom. At any rate, after that realization I changed the title of the book to *Power Aging* and things rapidly started to fall into place. It was like pressing a magic button as patients, friends, and colleagues were talking to me about their own experiences and turning me on to some incredible research.

The generation that was born in the ten years after World War II is reinventing the rules and roles of aging, making it sexy to go gray and get older with power and increased intellectual and physical prowess.

We are living longer. According to census data, there are more than 52,000 people alive over the age of one hundred right now. That's three times the number of centenarians in 1980. We're approaching a time when sixty or seventy will be considered middle age. When I was a teenager, my parents were over forty and they were, by my definition, definitely middle aged. However, since I turned forty, I have noticed that middle age always seems to be about fifteen years older than whatever my age is at the time.

We are staying active longer. And while some of us grow old gracefully, few of us manage to grow old gratefully. The physical changes that occur over the years seem to happen with sometimes alarming speed. One day you're looking in the mirror and wondering how to treat your unsightly teenage blemishes; the next day you're looking in the mirror and wondering if it's worth saving up for a face-lift.

This book is not so much about what time is doing to you—although we will discuss the issues of your health as you age — but what we can do on a daily basis to keep ourselves mentally, physically, and even financially fit so that we can age with grace and power.

Let's face it, nobody gets out of this life alive. But every health- and heart-building thing that you can do now—in your forties, fifties, and sixties—is an investment in

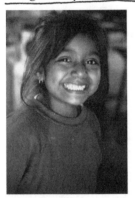

your future, like money in the bank for your seventies, eighties, and nineties.

I've seen patients who learn how to build health from the inside out, who learned how to love themselves from the inside out. Then, when they look in the mirror, with each passing year, they learn how to love themselves from the outside in. I call it resiliency training—the basis for power aging that allows for an active life of joy and contribution.

There have been thousands of scientific, peer-reviewed research studies on the green medicine of prevention. If you start traveling down the information highway, you'll quickly learn that quoting studies is in many ways like quoting the Bible. You can find a citation that substantiates your point of view if you look hard enough. My method was to find reputable research that talked about the green medicine of prevention. I've been careful to distinguish between published data and the clinical evidence that I have observed in my own patients and to be aware of how my clinical experience has influenced my point of view. One approach is to present the facts and nothing but the facts. However, even the driest of scientific literature can have a point of view and I think that it is more honest for me to state my prejudices and opinions right now and alongside the text. I invite you to question the material and ultimately form your own conclusions about what seems most reasonable to you.

WHAT'S OLD BECOMES NEW . . .

Today's fact may be tomorrow's quaint historical anecdote. The fantastic antiquity of *trepanation*, the cutting of the human skull to relieve headaches and mental illness, is still performed today in some remote societies around the world. Less than a hundred years ago, bloodletting was a common practice thought to cure a number of illnesses, and so blood-sucking leeches were applied to various parts of the body to do their work. In the late 1980s some doctors proposed a return to bloodletting for conditions such as high blood pressure, which is actually relieved by the ancient process. Whether or not these modern doctors proposed the use of leeches is unknown to me—although I can safely say that even the thought of a leech on my body would certainly raise my blood pressure, not lower it!

The work of scientists around the world continues as we strive to find a theoretical marriage between ancient common sense and modern scientific data. Perhaps another union between East and West will also help us to understand the human body. Dr. Ronald Melzack and Patrick Wall won the Nobel Prize twenty years ago for their explanation of the "gate theory" of pain. The theory states that while pain is transmitted through our central nervous systems and to the brain by specific nerve fibers, other nerve fibers could work to inhibit the pain message. In 1977, Dr. Melzack found that the "trigger points" reported in Western medical literature corresponded to acupuncture points documented by the Chinese more than 2,000 years ago. Chinese tradition ascribes the body of information regarding acupuncture, which is almost 4,500 years old, to Huang Ti, the Yellow Emperor.

AGING IS NOT A DISEASE

You can stay vital, strong, healthy, and sexy. Aging is not a disease. None of us are going to live forever, but we don't have to fear what time is doing to us. We can feel joyful about what we are doing to our time.

This is a thought that Daphne Rose Kingma writes about in her book *A Garland of Love*:

> The beautiful things you want to say to the person you love, say them now; the walks you want to take on the beach but don't think you have time for, take them now; the conversations that come from your heart, the sorrows you need to share, the shoulder you want to offer your sweetheart to cry on, offer them now.
>
> We need to say the words, have the fun, do the things, give the gifts, open our hearts, console one another. Time isn't forever. Whatever it is, do it *now*.

Do it Now.

Kingma's book was a recent find, but it was a passage from Ayn Rand's *Atlas Shrugged* that shaped my growing over the last several decades:

In the name of the best within you, do not sacrifice this world to those who are at its worst. . . . Do not let your fires go out, spark by irreplaceable spark, in the hopeless swamps of the approximate, the not-quite, the not-yet, the not-at-all. Do not let the hero in your soul perish in lonely frustration for the life you deserved, but have never been able to reach. Check your road and the nature of your battle. The world you desire can be won, it exists, it is real, it is possible, it is yours.

If you would like to explore these ideas further, then congratulations on wanting more out of life. It's earlier than you think. Now let's get to it!

WHAT IS AGING?

What is aging? I like the dictionary definition that says. "To mature, or ripen." that has a lovely ring to it, doesn't it? We're not *aging*, we're *ripening*, we're *maturing*!

Yet, regardless of the definition you choose, aging begins the moment we are born and it never stops. The only way to stop aging is to stop living. But what's going on inside of us that slows us down, or outside of us that makes us get wrinkled?

We now know that most of the processes we associate with aging are a result of free radical damage to cells and genetic codes on our DNA that actively limit our life span. Free radicals are actually different forms of the one molecular compound that we all know and need to live on this planet: oxygen. There are several forms of active oxygen and they are continually formed from the dissolved molecular oxygen in our tissues. However, our tissues also contain multiple 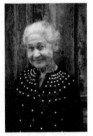 enzymes that rapidly remove these free radicals. But when we are exposed to chemical reactions that cause massive amounts of free radicals to occur on a continual basis and there are no nutrients available with which our bodies can manufacture these enzymes, the free radicals go wild and destroy cells. That's why it's important to consume *antioxidants*, like vitamins A, C, and E, so that free radical damage can be kept to a minimum. The exciting research on antiaging substances called *phytochemicals* is revealing miracle nutrients in the most humble plants that have the power to heal and protect us against cell destruction. Things like smoking, alcohol consumption, eating smoked meats and cheeses, exposure to pollution and ultraviolet light, even deep-sea diving, where the body is under great pressure of both carbon dioxide and forced oxygen, all of these activities and a host of others cause chemical reactions that can cause free radicals to occur.

In addition to the physical changes we experience over the decades, of course, there are many intellectual and emotional changes that occur as we mature. Famed psychoanalyst Erik Erikson, who was born in 1902 and lived ninety-two years, divided life into eight stages of crisis, the eighth being that of *ego integrity versus despair*. As they age, people strive to reach the ultimate goal: wisdom, spiritual tranquility, an acceptance of life and one's role in the world. Just as the healthy child will not fear life, said Erikson, the healthy adult will not fear death.

There has been much promising research. In Dallas, a scientific team found a way to make human cells live 100 percent longer. In a *Life* magazine story on aging, Dr. William Regelson, a professor of medicine at the Medical College of Virginia stated: "With the knowledge that is accumulating now about the nutritional and neuroendocrine aspects of aging, and if we develop ways to repair aging tissues with the help of embryonic cells, we could add thirty healthy years to human life in the next decade. And beyond that, as we learn to control genes involved in aging, the possibilities of lengthening life appear practically unlimited."

"Possibly in thirty years we will have in hand the major genes that determine longevity, and will be in a position to double, triple, even quadruple our maximum life span of 120 years. It's possible that some people alive now may still be alive 400 years from now," said Dr. Michael Jazwinski of the Louisiana State University Medical Center, the world's foremost authority on the aging of yeast. Want to live until your age is in the triple digits? Then spend more time getting into shape, less time at the doctor's office, and more money investing in your "savings" for the future.

What a lot of that research comes down to is that Mom was right when she told you to eat your vegetables, go to bed early, and get some exercise—a good beginning for constructing the foundation of health. Add a big dollop of the latest high-tech age-fighting weaponry and you've got a fortress on your hands. Who knew, for instance, that yams were high in DHEA and that this obscure-sounding hormone with the long name could be such a big gun, so powerful that it's being used on AIDS patients to prolong life? During the sixties, the average American was just starting to hear the word *cholesterol*. A few days ago, I had someone corner me at a party and pump me for the latest information on melatonin and pycnogenol. People are getting more

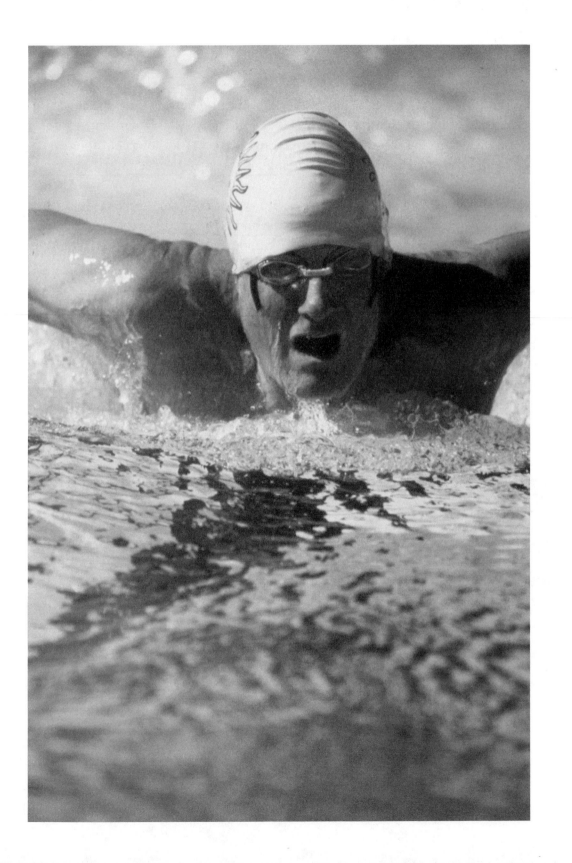

savvy. Yet our worst enemy may not be Mother Nature, but our own misconceptions about growing old. It doesn't have to be a shaky downward slide with one foot in the grave and the other on a bar of soap. How long? we ask. Not long, but long enough. There are no limits to our growing and being and doing. We are limited only by our imaginations.

To some, this may sound like a burden. But we should view it as an opportunity: There is always room to create a more wonderful vision and plan for your life. However, you have to sit yourself down and think about what that vision and plan might be. What are you holding on to? What myths or fears are you willing or needing to let go?

You don't have to decide right now. Albert Einstein once commented on the mysteries of life: "To know that what is impenetrable to us really exists, manifests itself as the highest wisdom and the most radiant beauty."

We can change our vision of what our lives can be whenever it feels right, but we do have to decide. As long as we're here, we can learn what we need to make us stronger, happier, more relaxed about what the future holds. Remember, a new century is on its way and science is on our side now.

2

Flying Lessons for Your Mind

> Only the heart knows
> how to find what is precious.
>
> Fyodor Dostoyevsky (1821–1861)

"Something strange and wonderful has happened, and it challenges much of what we thought we knew about living to be old. All over the country, the number of people who last beyond the age of 100 has been soaring." *Parade* magazine recently published this statement and went on to say that centenarians have become the fastest growing age group not only in this country (doubling every decade since 1970), but also throughout the industrialized world. Many researchers have calculated the genetic potential of humankind to be around 145 years of age. As we reach our potential, "middle age" will be from eighty to a hundred years and seniors will be those one hundred years and up!

Willard Scott, the NBC weatherman who's been sending birthday messages since 1981 to the newest triple-digit celebrators, now gets over four hundred a week. Not only are Americans living longer, they are staying active longer. For the most part, the hundred-year olds haven't been saved by high-tech bypass surgeries or miracle drugs. They simply haven't gotten sick.

"They're able to handle dietary problems and environmental insults that would devastate the rest of us," stated Dr. Thomas T. Perls, who heads the New England Centenarian Study at Harvard Medical School. And forget the myth of growing old and sick. Recent researchers are also finding that people in their nineties are in better general health than those ten or twenty years younger. The baby-boomer generation has the opportunity to rewrite the rules on aging. There's plenty we can do to stave off and even reverse the signs of time.

My friend Joanne had a ten-pound malignant tumor removed from her abdomen. She jokes, "The main thing is to get out of bed in the morning, even if the only reason you get out of bed sometimes is because you know your back is going to hurt if you stay in there. Some people just seem to procrastinate death twenty years longer. That's me—I've got too much stuff to do!"

You are what you think. That could sum up this whole book. The other pages can inform you about every super nutrient there is, but it's all worthless if your belief system is a negative work of art gone haywire. What follows are some flying lessons for your mind. They come from some very special people.

Your magnificent obsession. What is it you really love to do? Entertainer George Burns, scientist Linus Pauling, dancer Martha Graham—all had a passion for what they loved and pursued their excellence into a long and vibrant old age.

Volunteers at California Hospital Medical Center in Los Angeles started a "Cuddlers" program for premature incubator babies who must stay in the hospital after the mother has checked out. Gladys Yifter in Texas, age seventy-one, is organizing a statewide walking program to get Texans in shape by the millennium. Selma, an eighty-five-year-old woman on my street, walks two miles a day to get the bus to go to her day job—helping out at the information desk at a local hospital. Do what makes you happy and you'll stick around for the long run.

Don't wait for a catastrophe. Maybe this is what it takes sometimes to gain perspective on what's important. Ten years from now, when your kids are grown up, are you going to be glad you did the vacuuming or that you all went whale-watching or to the movies? Remember the anti–substance abuse campaign "Just say no"? That's what I

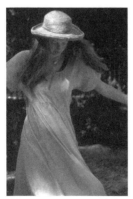

say when I find myself giving up a future memory for a trivial task of the present like doing the dishes right after dinner when I could be watching the sunset with my fiancé. The dishes will be there for you later. True, you will not be eligible for the Superwoman Sweepstakes this year if you put off some of your housework, but you may have a lot more fun and create some wonderful memories instead.

Spend some time with Mother Nature. You will never be lonely if Nature is with you. A Navaho medicine woman told me that once. For the shy creatures of the earth, the purpose of life is life itself. So they make every day their best day. Good advice on any level. It's been said—and it is true—that we are all made of the dust and molecules of ancient stars. Chief Seattle wrote the most beautiful and profound statement about the environment in 1854, titled *Our Earth*: "Every part of the earth is sacred to my people. Every shining pine needle, every sandy shore, every mist in the dark woods, every clearing and humming insect is holy in the memory and experience of my people. . . . All things are connected like the blood which unites one family. All things are connected. Whatever befalls the earth befalls the sons of the earth. Man did not weave the web of life; he is merely a strand in it."

Honor the ordinary things of right now. The small things in life are the most important. Be receptive to the moment. Be open to hear the joyfulness of the small sounds around you. When your husband snores tonight, think of how glad you are that he is by your side. When you drive by a school yard, open your car window and listen to the happy sound of the children playing at recess. Watch the smile of your friend or colleague today and imprint that vision in your mind's eye. Notice the dappled sunlight filtering through the leaves. Appreciate the closeness of a neighbor as you do common tasks at the same time. Frank Lloyd Wright once wrote that "everyday life is the important thing, not tomorrow or yesterday, but today. You won't reach anything better than right now, if you take it as you ought."

Keep a gratitude journal. A walking friend shared with me that she always wanted to keep a journal, but that with four young children and a full-time job, it was simply too time-consuming. Instead, she writes five things each day that she has to be grateful for. "You read in-between the lines here and it really does end up telling about what kind of day you had anyway—and it keeps you going on with things carrying an attitude of gratitude." Oprah Winfrey has recently included a moment of gratitude in her weekday TV show, and it is bound to reorient many lives toward the positive. What made you smile today? What blessings kept you going this afternoon? "I give myself a homework assignment every day to try and use the word *grateful* at least four times when I'm talking to the kids or my husband," says another friend, whom I can only describe as being full of the abundant joy of life. "That way I know that I'll remember to focus on those good things that happen every day and not get bogged down with all the frustrating stuff."

Give thanks today for the people and experiences and moments of joy and beauty that have been yours. Today, remember the truly magical things in your life that living and loving have given you.

Don't live for "when." Have you ever heard somebody say, "I'll take it easy this weekend—then I'm going to have some fun." Do you know anybody that's always living for the weekend, or for when they go on vacation, or when they retire?

Happiness is not a destination. That old saw has been around for a long time, and for good reason. You don't have to save up for a vacation before you can relax and be happy. How many "shoulds" are keeping you from enjoying life now? Are you putting off really living until you have more time? I met a man striding around a high school track early one morning. He was seventy-six years old and was telling me all about his new puppy and the typing class in which he had just enrolled. He laughed as he related to me the curiosity of his eighteen-year-old class mates who wondered out loud "why this old guy is taking up typing." He was getting ready to write his autobiography and wanted to be able to do it on computer. "I guess they thought that at my age, I shouldn't even be buying green bananas—go figure!" he laughed.

Here's a riddle I heard translated from an ancient Chinese proverb: " 'There' is no better than 'here', and when your 'there' has become 'here' you will simply obtain another 'there' that will, again, look better than 'here.' "

There's no prize at the end for sacrificing the present for the sake of the future.

From writer Robert Eliot: "Make three lists. The things you *have* to do, *want* to do, and neither *have* to do nor *want* to do. Then, for the rest of your life, forget everything on the third list."

HAPPINESS COMES FROM WITHIN, BUT WHO HAS IT AND WHY?

Optimism, strength of spiritual commitment, self-esteem, a sense of personal control, a tendency to be outgoing, a feeling of being empowered rather than helpless, an abundance of close relationships—these are the main trails that study after study identifies with people who rate their lives at the top of the satisfaction scale. How do you rate yourself?

Have you ever heard the expression that laughter is the shortest distance between two people? Are your spiritual beliefs and practices something from your childhood that got lost along your road to success? Have you gone through some hard times or been pained by a great loss and consequently not on speaking terms with God lately? Do you need to reappoint yourself as captain of your own ship?

"Your friend is your needs answered," wrote poet Kahlil Gibran. "He is your field which you sow with love and reap with thanksgiving."

For as long as I can remember, I have been interested to hear others' views on the meaning of life. It's almost like a hobby. And it beats talking about the weather when you meet somebody new at a social gathering.

Mostly I get nonanswers: "Give me a call when you figure it out," or "Is this a pop quiz?" But there have been some great answers. Some have been hilarious, but even while I was laughing out loud, they have vanished like a really funny joke that you wish you could remember.

The very best answer I received to the question "What is the meaning of life?" was "Love—to love well. That's all that really gives value and meaning to life. At the very end, to be able to say 'I loved well.' Without that, we're nothing."

THE FOUNTAIN OF YOUTH

Positive energy is like a magic spring. When you allow it to fill you up, it will just keep on overflowing out of you. No matter how stagnant and polluted the water around you, the fresh, clear water of your positive spring just gushes up and washes away all impurities, renewing and refreshing you continually. It is simply impossible to be filled and depressed at the same time. There isn't room in your brain for it.

Making better choices for your inner and outer self can make you feel better about things right away: Choose a better diet; commit yourself to an exercise program;

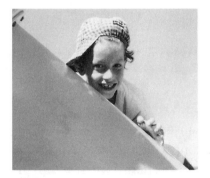

reestablish your value systems; put down that bag of chips and turn off the TV. Go for it. The more you do it, the easier it becomes. In this way you can begin to feel control over yourself—less passive and more the captain of your own ship. That's what power aging is all about.

When your body and mind are unified, you feel serene and tranquil, yet energized by that serenity.

Adversity, disease, aging—these are not disabilities. They are opportunities for us to learn to love ourselves and become the people we need to be.

One of my greatest privileges was working with Hollywood actress and stunt-

> While the forces blowing a leaf are easy enough to measure, the path and destination of the leaf are far from certain. All of us must be vigilant about where we are headed. Although we cannot stop progress, we can all lean together to steer its course.
>
> —William Knoke, *Bold New World*

woman Heidi Von Beltz, who was paralyzed from the neck down after a car crash. Bit by bit, I watched her work and sweat to recover minute improvements, building up day by day, until she was able to recover the use of her upper body and then actually sit up without assistance and even lift weights. She writes in her lighthearted and inspirational book *My Soul Purpose*: "The house is wired for electricity, but everybody's got to plug in their own lamp."

She found the spiritual and metaphysical lessons of healing and applied them to every aspect of her life. "I never realized what I was capable of until I had no choice," she says.

AS WE GROW OLDER . . .

It is unrealistic to think that our globe is going to become less complex. There is undoubtedly more and more going on all the time—scientifically, politically, emotionally. Life does not get simpler, it gets more involved: We meet more people, our financial status takes dips and curves, perhaps our children have children. Presidents win or lose elections and, regardless of who's in the White House, we fill up our garages with more useless junk from yard sales.

In the midst of this chaos and with the increasing mechanization of our society, we must construct our own calmness. All the designer nutrients, all the well-meaning trips to the gym and huffing and puffing are meaningless if we have not achieved self-mastery.

Everything changes based on how we perceive it. If you want to believe that aging is terrible and that you are doomed to live your life in misery and depression, then you will not be disappointed. You have to *want* to live longer; youth is not simply a matter of supple knees and smooth skin. We only lose our life energy when we abandon the dreams of our heart—when, as Ayn Rand described, we let the fire in our souls perish, "spark by irreplaceable spark."

The excitement that grows more intoxicating with time is that of being positive and thankful in our living, with respect for all forms of life. The respect that shows that we don't have to fight people or nations or ourselves in order to win or lose; the respect to love and nurture one another.

Giving and taking become one in this state of joyfulness. Not only as far as we interact with others, but also in each and every life situation we face. Nothing will become ugly and depressing then. In sickness, we can learn to heal our spirits. In our aloneness, we can learn the lessons that will cause us to appreciate loving and sharing with others even more when we have that opportunity again.

3

ENERGY: IT MAKES YOU FEEL SO YOUNG

If one lives a hundred years idle, without energy, better to live one day of steadfast energy.

—Suttapitaka (circa 500 to 250 B.C.), *Dhammapada* 1.5

*B*eing tired makes you feel old. Have you ever sat on the edge of the bed on a Monday morning and felt like you were trying to wake up from a coma? Have you ever fantasized at three o'clock in the afternoon about pulling the covers over your head and packing it in for the rest of the day? Do you ever find yourself having trouble keeping your eyes open after lunch, or relying on an extra cup of coffee here and there just to get through the day?

Chances are, you may be suffering from a syndrome I like to call The Irrepressible Recurring Energy Deficit. The cunning acronym for this insidious array of symptoms spells out, as you may have guessed, TIRED!

TIRED happens for a number of reasons. I like to think of it as the red idiot light on the dashboard of my car, telling me that the engine is overheated. Of course, you can choose to ignore it, but then the engine wears down. Unfortunately, mechanics and new cars are expensive.

Probably the easiest solution cure for TIRED is to get more sleep. Most of the cultures of the world have a siesta at lunch. Try going to bed half an hour earlier each night, until you wake up refreshed. Too wired to go to bed early? Check out Chapter 6 for some strategies on what to do while you're waiting for the Sandman to come.

HOW CAN YOU HAVE MORE ENERGY?

As a world-class marathon runner, I did plenty of research over the years on how to have and hold on to more energy. After all, 26.2 miles is a long way to run before you have breakfast in the morning. Not only that, but the long, lonely months of training in solitude gave me plenty of time and thousands of miles to think about it.

For some reason, the human mind tends to seek one answer to a question. But there's more than one answer to the energy crises that we all encounter on a daily basis. As I look back on my years of marathon running, and then the sleepless years of marathon studying in graduate school, there are, according to my own personal research data of just one person, a number of different components to the attainment of energy.

If you're really tired of being sick and tired, lifestyle changes, including diet, exercise, and spiritual nutrition are all important in the daily management of your energy. Are you thinking, I want energy and I want it right *now*? Then you may want to think about adding stress management to that list.

THE CHAIR WITH FOUR LEGS

Energy is like a four-legged chair: when one of the legs is missing, the chair falls down. In the pages that follow, I'll explain what I consider to be the key elements of increasing your energy without the use of drugs or other stimulants. (Please note: If you suffer from low energy, it is important that you get a physical examination by a doctor, because chronic fatigue can be a harbinger for serious disease. The following suggestions are not intended as a substitute for any treatment that may have been prescribed by your doctor.)

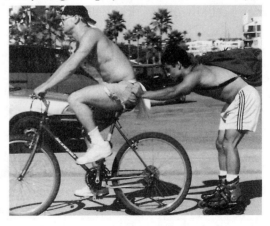

E is for exercise. The first letter of the word *energy* points to the first part of the equation. Exercise is one of the key secrets to having more energy. Yes, I know, you're too tired to exercise. So how do you break the cycle of fatigue?

Realize that aerobic exercise can actually give you energy. Here's why: First of all, it reduces stress and that alone can feel like a weight off your shoulders. Physiologically, aerobic exercise stimulates the body's production of new capillaries, the very smallest blood vessels, which are the final carriers of oxygen, blood, and nutrients to the cells. The end result is more oxygen and nutrients are delivered to the cells and more waste products, such as carbon dioxide and lactic acid, are carried away. So you feel more energy. Of course, the heart becomes stronger and more efficient, so you feel more capable of doing more on that count alone.

Power Energy Tip. When you feel your energy dropping, like at about 3 P.M., try going for a short walk around the block, or up and down a few flights of stairs. A ten-minute investment can stimulate your metabolism and your energy levels for up to a couple of hours.

N is for nutrition. Food is either your friend or your foe when it comes to energy. Jack LaLanne, the great fitness pioneer, once told me: "People ask me all the time about my energy. I ask them what they ate for breakfast and how they started their day. Would you wake up your dog, make him drink a cup of coffee and smoke a cigarette, and then give him a doughnut?"

Most folks reach for something sweet and sugary when they want a quick boost, but this is usually a big mistake, because it jerks around your insulin, gives you a surge of false energy for about thirty minutes, and then drops you down lower than where you were when you reached for the candy bar in the first place.

Also, fatty foods like fries, burgers, and desserts like cheesecake can really create some energy deficits. Within an hour of eating rich pastries or greasy junk food you can actually draw blood, centrifuge it, and see the fat globules swirling around like a blizzard. This fat causes blood cells to clump together, thereby reducing the individual surface area that absorbs oxygen. *Hemagglutination*, as it is called, robs the body of its ability to receive energy-giving oxygen.

As if that wasn't enough, too much alcohol and caffeine are well-known nutrient thieves that can deplete valuable minerals like calcium and magnesium. Calcium helps alleviate insomnia while caffeine causes it. Magnesium deficiencies are related to increased oxygen consumption and heart rate, which means the body may be working harder—up to 15 percent harder than necessary to meet energy demands. This results in physiological stress and fatigue, according to one study.

If you are a woman with heavy or painful menstruation, you could be iron-deficient. Ask your doctor for a blood test that checks for anemia.

POWER ENERGY GUIDELINES

1. **Read *The Zone*.** This book by Barry Sears, Ph.D., explains, once and for all, the energy/protein equation. I like the book because it prescribes the protein/carbohydrate/fat ratios (30:40:30) I ate for more than twenty years when I was a competitive athlete. I do, however, disagree with the negative assessment of the vegetarian diet, because I am celebrating my twenty-sixth year as a vegetarian and I know that it works for me. If you are a vegetarian, increase your veggie proteins like tofu and tempeh and cut your refined carbohydrate (white flour, refined breads, jams, etc.). Use flax products like flax seed oil and flour as vegetarian sources of omega-3 fatty acids, an option that Sears seems to have overlooked in his book.

2. **Lick the sugar habit.** Sugary snacks give you a quick boost, causing an insulin surge that gets you hyped up for about thirty minutes and then lets you down to a lower energy level than when you started. Go for a protein snack instead: pineapple and cottage cheese, plain yogurt, a one-inch cube of cheese, a small piece of baked tofu, or a hard-boiled egg.

3. **Try to eat "label free."** If you look at the label and can't pronounce any of the ingredients, chances are you may be better off not eating what's inside. As a matter of fact, maybe you should try to eat things that don't have a label.

    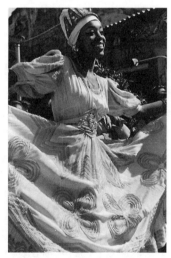

    There is tremendous energy in raw foods. The strongest mammals in the world are almost entirely vegetarian, and I have yet to see any photographs by Jane Goodall of a gorilla standing in front a bakery, eating a croissant before he swung from a tree. Try this challenge: For one week, include one raw food in each meal. (No, the parsley decoration on top of your steak doesn't count.) For instance, have an apple for a snack instead of a candy bar. Cut up a juicy pear for breakfast instead of jam on your toast. Eat a big salad as the main course of dinner instead of having it as a garnish on the side of the plate. Then evaluate your energy. Five servings of fruits and vegetables a day is the challenge.

4. **Don't get scammed by phony herbal "all natural" stimulants.** This includes ma huang, guarana, kola nut, and my personal favorite, coffee bean extract. Coffee

bean extract is caffeine! Sure, all these things are "natural," but so are cocaine, heroin, and poison hemlock—and they can kill you.

Ma huang is a Chinese herbal name for ephedra, which is the equivalent of herbal adrenaline. Guarana may be an all-natural plant from the Amazon jungles, but it is just another form of false energy that mimics amphetamines. I had a patient who mentioned she was suffering from heart palpitations. "Nothing serious, just every few minutes," she said. Turns out that she was on an herbal diet supplement that contained ma huang, guarana, kola nut, *and* a few hundred milligrams of caffeine. Her heart sounded like a syncopated jackhammer through the stethoscope.

The problem with the herbal and nonherbal stimulants is that they wind you up, only to let you down much lower than when you started. And they can be addictive.

5. **Use safer energy alternatives**. Ginseng, ginkgo biloba, cayenne, and aged garlic extract are herbs that may be energy-friendly without the heart-pounding side effects. Bee pollen is another, but as with any food substance, some people could be allergic. Foolishly, I once tried bee pollen for the first time right before a long-distance race, with the effect that I would have paid $1,000 to have been able to lie down on the starting line to a take a nap. Needless to say, the race was a disaster, so let the buyer beware. Bee pollen may be too concentrated for those prone to hypoglycemia.

A winning combination that works for many athletes is two or three amino acid complex capsules on an empty stomach, with water, before a workout. European athletes popularized carnitine, an unusual amino acid often called a B-vitamin. It has been used for everything from obesity and low sperm motility to improved endurance. It has the important function of increasing the rate of fat oxidation in the liver. The more carnitine that is available, the faster fat is transported across the membrane of the liver cell and then oxidized for energy. This energy is then stored as ATP, which is a body fuel for many functions, including muscle contractions. This is why both athletes and dieters became interested in carnitine.

Carnitine supplements are expensive, but the body makes carnitine from lysine. Foods high in lysine are: ricotta cheese (3.30g per cup), cottage cheese (2.50g per cup), wheat germ (2.10g per cup), yogurt (.7g per cup). For those who love pigs, pork comes in at the top of the lysine list with 7 grams per pound.

Speaking of fatigue, vitamin B-12 and folic acid are typically low in some vegetarian diets and many meat eaters may lack the ability to absorb it. Deficiencies here can cause low energy because blood cells need these nutrients in order to divide. Anemia deficiency syndromes can take years to develop, so if you think you might be anemic, get a blood test and find out for sure.

6. **Eat less and more often.** It's not the paradox it seems. Eating three big square meals a day leaves most people with several energy slumps throughout the day. Big meals take a long time and a lot of energy to digest. And, in between feeding times, most folks experience wide fluctuations of blood sugar levels.

 Consider that most people skip breakfast and their first intake of food is all too often coffee and a doughnut. So, after some sugary snacks and lots of morning coffee, many people typically eat a big lunch, then get really sleepy around three o'clock in the afternoon. Another candy bar and caffeine snack results. Then a big, late dinner feeding that often continues with several encores of snacky junk foods that are high in fat and sugar. Then a midnight snack to wash it all down and the digestive system is once again overtaxed all night long when the body is supposed to be resting. The alarm clock goes off and another tired employee trudges off to repeat the process.

 When Mom said <u>breakfast</u> was <u>the most important meal of the day,</u> she was right. However, the "don't eat in-between meals because it will spoil your appetite" advice was wrong. <u>Eat healthy food in between meals.</u> Then you won't be out of control by dinnertime. And you may find that you have a lot more energy with a lot less calories, which means you may be a lot less overweight, which means you may have a lot more energy . . .

7. **Load up on vitamins and minerals, naturally.** To load up on calcium, iron, magnesium, and other important energy minerals and nutrients, eat plenty of <u>greens,</u> <u>grains,</u> and <u>low-fat protein like tofu and nonfat cottage cheese.</u> Figs, prunes, leafy greens, millet, slow-cooking oatmeal, and barley are great ways to get in some power nutrients. <u>Blackstrap</u> molasses has more calcium in it measure for measure than milk, with only one tablespoon supplying 131 milligrams of calcium, 3 milligrams of iron, 585 milligrams of potassium, as well as other minerals. As a <u>hot</u> <u>energy drink,</u> try <u>one tablespoon dissolved in hot water, soy, or cow's milk.</u> It can be a real energy boost and is only 43 calories per tablespoon.

 B vitamins help give the body energy by helping convert carbohydrates to glucose (blood sugar, the body's fuel). They also play a key role in protein and fat metabolism. The nervous system is also heavily dependent on B vitamins. Try getting some hefty doses of B vitamins by eating whole grains like brown rice, oats, millet, and barley. Brewer's yeast is one of the richest sources of the B vitamins and one tablespoon daily is the recommended nutritional dose. If you are supplementing, it's best to take the Bs as a complex because they are so interdependent. However, a wonderful side effect of eating the fiber-rich food sources is that the fiber will help alleviate constipation, a well-known contributor to a feeling of sluggishness.

Chromium picolinate is a trace nutrient that is important for carbohydrate metabolism, but do be cautious with this one, because trace nutrients are meant to be ingested in tiny amounts. Chromium is a metal and can be toxic in megadoses. Clinically, I see a great deal of the "if one is good, then twenty must be twenty times better" type of thinking, which is often in error and can be dangerous. Chromium is found in brewer's yeast, honey, grapes, whole grain cereals, corn oil, and clams.

8. **Drink up, but make it Adam's ale and hold the coffee.** Don't forget the cheap and noncaloric energy booster known as pure water. You'd be surprised at how keeping your body properly hydrated can help ease energy swings. Eight to ten large glasses of pure water every day is considered a minimum requirement.

Alcohol and coffee mimic the effect of real food energy, but there's always a letdown, leading many into a cycle of addiction. It's best to avoid them. Additionally, they both have a diuretic effect on the body, washing away valuable vitamins and minerals that boost energy, like vitamin B12, calcium, and magnesium, to name only a few.

9. **Don't smoke and avoid the smoke of others.** Again, key nutrients are used up and smoking a cigarette is like lighting a torch for the Cancer Olympics.

E is for enthusiasm.

Contrary to the burgeoning phenomenon of caffeine emporiums on what seems to be every corner, enthusiasm does not come from a coffee pot. Something happened yesterday that really highlighted how we can build enthusiasm in our lives through very simple means. It's spring now, as I write this, and yesterday I was about to open my office door when I noticed a crowd of people outside. My office door opens to a natural courtyard with a path leading to a small lake. Everyone was frozen still and watching a small herd of fuzzy yellow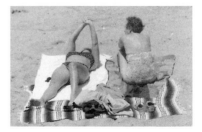

ducklings wandering around the shrubberies. I looked up and saw the stairwells lined with business people in suits pointing and laughing at the antics of this wandering little tribe of duck visitors. I slowly cracked open the door and listened to the growing crowd of passersby, some making silly quacking sounds and staring at the fifteen or twenty rambling ducklings. Nobody wanted to be the one who moved and scared them away. So we all stood there for about ten minutes and enjoyed the show. It felt really great. I looked around at all the smiling faces and took a deep breath and let it out slowly, memorizing how happy I was at that moment. I was so glad we all took the time to appreciate nature.

"Well, I guess we all got our free Prozac for the day," quipped a doctor on the stairwell. Everybody laughed. It *was* a free boost of natural enthusiasm.

"You'll never be alone if you are one with Nature," I was once told by a Cherokee medicine woman. I love the kind of quiet enthusiasm you can get from noticing spring, from inhaling an ocean breeze that has traveled four thousand miles to greet you, from feeling the fog brush up against your eyelashes.

What fills your cup with energy and enthusiasm? My friend Maura puts on classical music while she's preparing dinner for her family. "It just gives me a boost, and it's a jolt of enthusiasm that's better than two cups of coffee."

Another woman attests to affection as an enthusiasm booster. "When my husband walks in the door, regardless of the kids running around, their music blasting, or the dog chasing the cat across the room, we have an evening ritual of at least a thirty-second kiss."

Power Energy Tip. Nature, affection, music, the laughter and sharing of friends and family—these are important ingredients of our lives that help us bridge our temporary energy lulls. What will make you see the cup as half full instead of half empty? When you're overstressed, overloaded, and overwhelmed, force yourself to take a deep breath and recharge your batteries with what you know to be your own brand of inspiration. It's hard to stop and smell the roses when you're dying for enough time to smell a good cup of coffee. Are you old enough to remember that song "Accentuate the Positive"? It may sound corny, but it works.

R is for body rhythms.

Kahlil Gibran, the poet, philosopher, and artist, once wrote of marriage: "Let it rather be a moving sea between the shores of your souls." Love, as our highest from of spiritual energy, is a powerful metaphor that relates to even our daily tides of energy flow.

We all have natural biological body rhythms. Are you a night owl, someone who seems to get a second wind when the sun sets, someone who likes to go bed late and wake up late? When I asked my sister, an inveterate night owl, what the morning person would be called, you know, a catchy moniker for the person who cheerfully likes to rise and shine at the crack of dawn, her reply was, "Annoying?"

However, whether or not you are a night owl or an early bird, your individual patterns of energy ebb and flow may have certain trends. Sometimes these can be tracked to certain foods, or to consumption of coffee, alcohol, over the counter medications such as antihistamines, diet pills, or prescription medications.

Power Energy Tip. Keep a journal of your energy ebbs and flows throughout the day. I like to rate myself on a scale of one to five, with number five being peak energy and number one in the basement. This knowledge can be very powerful to you. Ask yourself if fluctuations could be substance-related. If you're hitting the basement at 4 P.M. then maybe you need a power nap. If you notice a low point first thing in the morning, ask yourself if you are getting enough sleep. Could alcohol or the caffeine in the hot chocolate before you go to bed be interrupting your sleep patterns? (More on this in Chapter 6, if you want to go there now.) Simply scheduling your toughest assignments during your peak hours could allow you to tackle the more routine or no-brainer tasks when your energy is lower.

G and Y: give of yourself.

Psychologist Abraham Maslow wrote: "When you select out for careful study very fine and healthy people, strong people, creative people, saintly people, sagacious people . . . then you get a very different view of mankind. You are asking, how tall can people grow, what can a human being become?"

Even on a very ordinary level, giving of yourself is a tremendous energy boost. It zaps depression and gives you a lift. Think of it: How easy is it to feel elated and enthusiastic and down in the dumps at the same time? Helping the world by using your own strengths helps build you at the same time.

Even physical fatigue seems to disappear when you give of yourself. There are times of stress and overwork when I drive to the office feeling tired. But during the day of teaching patients how to take care of themselves and ease their pain, I feel energized instead of exhausted. I feel happy that I have such a wonderful job, and that feeling takes away the tiredness.

Power Energy Tip. What rings your bell? Is there some way that you can have greater

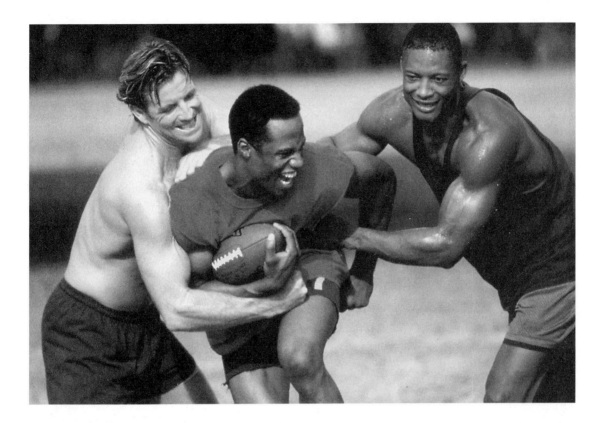

energy through doing something that you love? Is there a garden out there that needs to be beautified by you? Is there a special meal waiting for you to cook for a favorite person? My friend Edith Butler used play the pipe organ at a nearby shopping mall during the Christmas holidays. Another neighbor gets us organized throughout the year, one Saturday a month, to help out in a local soup kitchen sponsored by her church. A retired professional violinist I know helps out the harried music teacher at a local school one morning a week.

I read once that researchers actually analyzed the saliva of Mother Theresa and found that her saliva had higher concentrations of immune cells than a normal person's. The scientists speculated that the selfless dedication and committed spirituality in action in her clinic might have stimulated her body to a level of heightened immunity. What other scientific theory could explain her unrelenting and inexhaustible resistance to the most infectious and virulent diseases in the midst of the chaotic and unhygienic conditions in which she lived for so long?

THE ENERGY EQUATION

Energy is freedom, and acquiring it is the pinnacle of healthy living. It's the fountain of youth that allows us to quench our every thirst. With it, we feel alive in every sense of the word. Without it, life is depressing and can feel like it's not worth living.

Perhaps someday science will more fully understand the mysteries of energy. How does the ninety-eight pound housewife pick up the back of the family station wagon to save the life of her toddler? Where was that energy when she couldn't open the pickle jar on her own? How is it that Mother Theresa was surrounded by disease and never got sick, but your coworker comes down with the flu every time someone in the room sneezes? How is it that a skinny little ant can lift many times its own weight, and we often have trouble simply keeping up our spirits?

You could line up all the researchers clipboard to clipboard and it would still be a long time before we are able to understand the unique mix of science and magic that add up to energy. For now, it's up to us to build our own equation of personal energy truths. But then again, it always was.

4 SUPER SEX SECRETS

•

Sex and beauty are inseparable, like life and consciousness.
And the intelligence which goes with sex and beauty,
and arises out of sex and beauty, is intuition.

—D. H. Lawrence (1885–1930)

THE CULTURE OF DESIRE

Before you ever know a person's name, and long after you've forgotten it, you'll still remember what you first observed about that person: his or her gender. In fact, the first dictionary definition of *sex* I ever read, in a now much worn *Webster's* 1953 edition, lists four definitions of the word, the first two having to do with gender, and the next dealing strictly with "anything connected with sexual gratification or reproduction." The last definition acknowledged colloquial use of the word to mean sexual intercourse.

But sex is not just something a person does. It extends far beyond our cultural limitations of morality, machismo, and marriage. Our sexuality is expressed in so many other ways. Scientifically, our genetic inheritance of chromosomes is actually carried by every cell in our bodies. However, our sexual energy is a way of being, not only a way of doing. Human sexuality is the creative, explorative life force. We have often tried to define masculinity or femininity in words, or codes of behavior, but we are past the point where blue is just for little boys and pink is just for little girls. Music, dance, sweat, heartbeats: These are all an extension of our sexual energy, just as a song, a scent, a poem, or a sculpture can also awaken our senses and focus our life energy.

There is no physical reason related purely to age why we cannot enjoy our sexual energy as long as we live. But we'll have to get over some myths about aging and our sexuality in general in order to do this. Because, for most of us who are over forty, despite the "sexual revolution," we were raised with strict boundaries regarding our sexuality and with those boundaries came a set of myths and attitudes that may still make us feel embarrassed about discussing sex at all. I smile when I see the sexual mores and attitudes in reruns of old-time TV shows, like those with Lucy and Ricky retiring into separate beds: This type of reticence was part of culture of the 1950s. Turn on the TV now and, for better or worse, there is likely to be a talk show somewhere with a sexual theme, even if it's "Men who became women and the men who love them." One could say that we talk too much about sexual matters these days, but perhaps it is simply a reactionary swing of the pendulum away from the days when street wisdom dictated that if you masturbated, you'd go blind, or become addicted and spoil yourself for the real thing.

This chapter is intended to open a discussion about our sexuality in the second half of our lives, to explore some of the more common myths of aging and sex, and to help provide a basis for more openness and understanding. I hope that it will serve as a starting point for discussion for couples and singles, so that, through informed choices, we can enjoy our sexuality throughout our lives. A diet abundant in creativity and sensuality can fight depression, boost immunity, enhance imagination, shore up self-esteem, stimulate natural hormones and pain killers, burn calories, and help your cardiovascular system. It is the healing heartbeat of life itself that can lift our spirits, our souls, into the world of the creative. Are you getting the recommended daily allowance?

For the Forty- or Fifty-something Woman

Hormonal events help shape our physical and emotional selves from the moment of conception, and the complex interplay of these substances continues to be an important influence on our lives well into our later decades.

Women have the more dramatic changes, with significant declines in estrogen that can begin in the thirties and continue into the early fifties. Most women in North America, will stop menstruating by age 51, which is five years later than their mothers and ten years later than their grandmothers. As a woman over forty, you will likely be more self-assured and sexually secure than your foremothers because of the availability of information, support, and increasing commitment of other women over forty toward the goal of empowerment through understanding. The only hard and fast rule about the rate and extent of the changes that occur hormonally in a forty-something woman is that there are no hard and fast rules.

Menopause was thought to be an irreversible life event, but the research that comes to us now from the reproductive sciences has shown that women in their sixties can conceive and bear children. Fertility clinics currently have a cut-off for clients *at age fifty-five*! The italics and exclamation point are mine because I know that women get the "your clock is ticking" speech starting in their early thirties.

FOR MEN: A PAUSE

Men can not experience menopause, because the word itself literally defines the end of menstruation. However, the gradual decline of testosterone throughout a man's lifetime also brings its challenges to sexual libido, as do the life events that surround the decades of the forties and fifties for men. With children leaving the home—or *returning* home due to economic shifts—and with the added stress of a possible corporate downsizing, cessation or change of a job, there are also major psychosocial changes that men go through. Men have their own unique challenges as a result of this stage of life. Health changes that require medication, particularly those for hypertension, depression, high cholesterol, diabetes, ulcers, prostatitis, and arthritis can also begin the first wave of erection difficulties for men, causing emotions ranging from panic, to anger, depression, low self-esteem, and avoidance of sex altogether.

TESTOSTERONE AND DESIRE IN MEN AND WOMEN

But let's get back to sex. Most women don't report loss of sexual desire after menopause, even if they are not taking hormonal replacement therapy, which replaces the estrogen and progesterone that declines after the ovaries stop producing. That's because estrogen is not really the key player when it comes to stimulating sexual desire in a woman: It's testosterone that usually drives the libido for men *and* women. Freed from worries about pregnancy, some women report an *increase* of libido after menopause.

However, lower levels of estrogen and progesterone *do* affect vaginal, uterine, and other tissues. The health of a woman's genital and urinary systems, to name only two, are dependent on the highly complex and subtle interplay of hormones. We'll discuss a few of these concerns in the next section. For a more detailed discussion of hormone replacement therapy, you may want to review Chapter 22 and consider the options.

SEX AND AGING

Here are some of the more common effects of a slowing metabolic rate, declining hormones, and the associated physiological effects. You may experience none of these, or you may have a few to add. The bottom line is to realize that if there are changes, it's not all in your head and that in most cases the result will be only slight variations in your usual sexual script. If you need more information, then find a health-care professional, including a therapist or marriage and family counselor.

Your sexual health is as important as you would like it to be. In other words, understand that there is great variation from one person to the next, that one person might consider sex five times week a 200 percent improvement of activity while others might consider it a 200 percent decline.

CHANGES IN WOMEN

- The color of external genitalia may fade from a dark burgundy color to a lighter pink and pubic hair may become more sparse. Freed from waxing or shaving the bikini area, many women are okay with having less hair to worry about. The subtle shift in the color of the lips of the vagina is sometimes misinterpreted as a sign of bad health. But, this is a natural occurrence, just like gray hair.
- Vaginal walls may become thinner and less elastic, and the length of the vaginal canal may seem shorter because of decrease in elasticity, causing intercourse to be uncomfortable or painful. There may be less fatty tissues in the genital area. This is hormone related and may be helped by hormone replacement therapy, creams, and DHEA supplementation. Changing your love-making preparation to include a hot bath beforehand to stimulate circulation and promote relaxation, as well as use of lubricants or oral sex before penetration, may work well in addition to or instead of hormone replacement.
- It may take longer to lubricate vaginal tissues during arousal. Lubricants can be used in love-making, and even if they have never been used before, they may enhance the sensuality of sexual time together. Taking extra time to have your

partner massage them in, or even giving each other a gentle massage of the shoulders or back or thighs before proceeding to more direct sexual stimulation is something that many couples find erotic. Petroleum-based products are usually not recommended because they can clog sensitive pores, irritate delicate tissues, and promote infections. Astroglide, K-Y Jelly, and other sterile, water-based lubricants are available in drugstores. Replens, a moisturizer with the same acidity as the body, is formulated to last several days, so that it may be used ahead of time or before a weekend. And Kama Sutra oil, available through ads in magazines, has the advantage of tasting good and imparting a warm feeling when it is rubbed or blown on.

- Internal pelvic muscles may atrophy if they are not exercised. These muscles support the vagina and are both hormone- and activity-stimulated. Childbirth can also contribute to muscle laxity in this area. Urinary incontinence when sneezing, coughing, laughing, or lifting weights may occur as a result of the internal muscle weakness of the pubococcygeal muscle. The internal muscles of the pelvic floor can be strengthened with Kegel exercises. Incontinence has a high cure rate with these simple exercises and many women report improved responsiveness and better orgasms after practicing them. They are described in Chapter 19.

- There may be an increase in urinary or vaginal infection. Portions of the bladder walls and urinary tract may become thinner and more delicate, and therefore may become more prone to trauma during sex. Your doctor needs to be consulted, as frequent infections can be the first sign of diabetes and diabetes should be ruled out before self-treatment. Also, the changes in vaginal acidity may be due to hormonal fluctuation, so have your levels tested so that you know where you are in the process. Also, drinking a full glass of water immediately before intercourse and urinating immediately after may help. This flushes out the urethra and may help prevent bacteria from entering the bladder and causing infection. Additionally, unsweetened cranberry juice as a liquid or in capsule form is often an effective treatment.

CHANGES IN MEN

- Erections may become less spontaneous and less frequent than when you were eighteen years old, and may require more direct stimulation. Spontaneous erections aren't necessary for great sex. Having your sexual partner become more involved in foreplay is natural and normal, and something that most women like because it makes them feel needed. This may actually help both partners enjoy each other more.

- Erections may be less firm than they were in teenage years. While it's true that erections may not be as hard in a man of seventy as they are in a man of twenty, "So what!" says author Saul H. Rosenthal, M.D., in his book *Sex Over 40*. A long as the erection is hard enough for both partners to enjoy the experience, it doesn't matter. Skill as a lover has more to do with caressing, affection, fantasy, and caring than it does with the size or hardness of the erection. Unfortunately, the size myth is one that many men hold on to, avoiding sex and inviting heartache when they could be enjoying many hours of sensuality with their partners.

- Masters and Johnson, the sex researchers, have maintained that men over sixty need only one or two climaxes per week. This may actually add to love-making because it prolongs intercourse. If you are tired, stressed, or not feeling in need of a climax, it's not unhealthy. This is not an unhealthy or troublesome problem unless you think it is. By delaying or avoiding ejaculation, an older man can become erect again rapidly and enjoy more frequent sexual encounters with his partner.

- The *refractory* period may be longer, that is, it may take longer after a climax to renew the sexual energy necessary to achieving another erection. However, as noted above, there is a reduced need to climax in older men. By not climaxing, the refractory period may be shortened, enabling the man to become erect again rapidly. A mistake during the refractory period, which may be an hour or a day or several days, is not touching or caressing your partner in affectionate or sensual ways while your body is renewing its sexual energy. This type of sexual touching does not commit you to intercourse, and it usually heightens sexual tension to greater mutual satisfaction when love-making occurs next.

IMPOTENCE

Impotence is the inability to hold an erection long enough to achieve intercourse. All men have experienced impotence at some time in their lives and for various reasons. Years ago, impotence was thought to be psychologically based in most cases, but now it's widely acknowledged that there are many problems that can be contributing factors. The first thing to do is get a physical exam by a doctor. Ask to have your testosterone level checked. Your doctor will also want to rule out diabetes and other serious illnesses. Declining sexual function in men and women can result from: stress, financial worries, a change in career, illness, sleep deprivation, a heavy meal, alcohol, smoking, medications, and depression.

The accumulation of life fatigue is another factor. Masters and Johnson wrote: "This sensitivity to mental fatigue is the biggest difference between the aging population and younger men. There is no way to overemphasize that the role that 'fear of failure' plays in aging males' withdrawal from sexual performance."

Fifty percent of male impotence may be caused by arteriosclerosis, hardening of the arteries. That's a lot more than previously thought. And the list of medications that can cause difficulties with erections is quite long. Check with your doctor or pharmacist to see if your medication is on this list.

Heart drugs are the biggest foes, with the beta-blockers, anti-arrthymics, and anticholinergics most often causing erection problems. Antidepressants like Prozac and Elavil as well as muscle relaxants, ulcer medications, antiparasite drugs, antacids, and even over-the-counter antihistamines for allergies, colds, and sinus relief can all be responsible for impotence or reduced desire. Check with your doctor to find out if there are alternative medications. *Do not reduce or stop any medication without consulting your doctor first, as it can be dangerous.*

What can be done about impotence?

Cut down on the big thieves of libido: alcohol, marijuana, and nicotine. Make sure you take good care of your health. Long-term, poorly controlled diabetes, as well as chronic alcohol abuse, may result in nerve damage in the body that causes impotence. The preventive diet for diabetes, exercise, and a healthy body weight are all preventives. Atherosclerosis (hardening of the arteries) results in inadequate blood supply to the body's extremities, including the penis. Review Chapters 10 and 11 and and learn how a heart healthy diet and exercise program can help you to be healthier and protect your sex life.

The prescription drugs bromocriptine, isoxusprine, pentoxifylline, papaverine, and phentolamine are used for erection problems. Additionally, there are now penile suppositories that can be inserted into the tip of the penis via the urethra. They have been clinically proven to be quite effective in prompting a full-size erection.

If you have a hormone deficiency, testosterone and now human growth hormone have been approved by the FDA for human use. Your doctor can order a blood test to check your levels.

External devices, condomlike mechanisms that work via vacuum pressure to draw blood into the penis, are successful. A ring around the base of the penis helps the erection last. When removed, the penis returns to normal. The devices can be either hand-pumped or electronic. Unfortunately, after the urologist hands the device over to the patient, he often goes home and stashes it somewhere out of sight—in the sock drawer or under the bed, too embarrassed to even look at it, let alone bring it out at the first opportunity of a sexual encounter. It takes a certain self-acceptance to use it, because the idea can be overwhelming at first. But many couples use the devices as part of foreplay, just as would be done with applying condoms, much to their mutual enjoyment. It's in the same category as asking your mate to supply direct stimulation for getting an erection. It makes women feel needed and necessary and more involved in the process, and can enhance erotic play and a feeling of closeness.

Surgical implants have been around for almost thirty years, and three types are in common usage: semirigid, intermediate rigid, and completely inflatable devices. Some of the implants can be inserted using only a local anesthetic. Ask your urologist to discuss the advantages of each.

What if you are simply too stressed out to get hard? Impotence in itself is very stressful, even when it is only an occasional event. Fatigue, depression, anxiety, and stress—how easy is it to even seek intimacy in the first place when you're carrying the weight of the whole world on your shoulders? Men and women suffer equally from the increasing complexity of killer daily schedules. When it all gets too heavy, you *can* opt to stop carrying all the baggage and give yourself a break. Solving the stress/depression equation with professional therapy and medical intervention can help open up whole new worlds to enjoying life and sharing intimacy. It's up to you.

ROMANCE AND BREATHTAKING SEX IS A CHOICE

As far as I can tell from reviewing all the research, celibacy or lack of sexual activity is not associated with any fatal disease. But is there anything more life-affirming than the sexual passion of true love?

Couples who have been married for many years often forget to share fun times together and take time to express themselves sexually, as they did when they were newlyweds. The mutuality of years of problems and losses, child-raising, commuting, and struggling to simply keep their heads above water in the headlong rush of life may result in wonderful teamwork and companionship, but it can be the death of a passionate love life.

Romance in a relationship is a choice. The intensity *can* be recaptured, but it takes a renewal of your imaginations. Are you willing to put some thought into it or are you happy with being "married with children" instead of being lovers?

Now, please don't misunderstand me. I'm not saying that the solid qualities of a long-term relationship, the security and loyalty that you have built together, is not valuable. But we often have the capacity to slip into bad habits of complacency and taking the other person for granted as we stay glued to the television or socialize only with other couples instead of fuelling the fires of passion with each other.

When was the last time the two of you went away together someplace, alone? Can't remember? When was the last time you wrote each other an "I love you" message when it was not on a birthday or anniversary card? If you called him up at work today, just to give encouragement, would he think there was an emergency? If you brought her home an inexpensive romantic gift this week, would she wonder what was wrong?

Notes, small gifts, flowers, back rubs, weekend getaways, "date nights," and caresses, hugs, and kisses are all important, just like they were at the beginning. The problem is that couples allow themselves to be lulled into complacency, and stop putting effort into planning and being together as they did when they were dating and courting.

Love-making has to rank above doing the vacuuming, getting the car washed, watching television, and bumbling around in our overstressed world. Frequently, holding on to the irritations of the day, worrying about problems, and simply prioritizing other activities puts sensuality between couples on the back burner. Some couples might feel lucky if it even gets on one of the burners at all.

But breathtaking sex is a choice. Would you like to have an intimate and passionate relationship again? Think about it. Start dating each other again. Find a friend and promise to exchange baby-sitting for each other. Find a drive-in and make out. Go slow dancing someplace. Go hiking together. Meet for lunch at an X-rated motel. What would it take to light candles and take a sexy bath or shower together? Or go together to a lingerie store and pick out lacy lingerie and silk boxer shorts. What about staying in bed some morning and feeding each other fresh berries and cheese? Unplug the phone and the TV sometime. Go to a flower market and buy some day-old roses and heap the petals up all over the bed. Make love to each other in the bed of rose petals. Caress each other with feathers or massage each other with heated oil.

Sound too out of character for you? Think that it's too much work and you're too tired? Chances are, if you *stay* too tired, your mate *will* eventually experience the fun of sexual adventure again—but with somebody else.

The following passage is from sex therapist Dr. Ruth Westheimer's book *Dr. Ruth's Guide to Good Sex:* "Long sexual relationships offer pleasures you can't get any other way. Making love with the partner you've had for twenty years, who knows you better than anyone else, who has shared life's ups and downs with you, can be a royal pleasure."

What About Sexual Stimulants?

What's the most important part of the body to stimulate before sex? The mind. Much has been written on the psychology of desire, from spiritual transcendence to the most outlandish fantasy and the mindset of power as the ultimate aphrodisiac. And throughout the ages, there have been a variety of substances that were believed to cause arousal. Ibn Battuta, the great Arab geographer (fourteenth century A.D.), maintained that the fish and coconut diet eaten by the inhabitants of the Maldive Islands of the Indian Ocean had a "striking and unequaled power in the practice of sexual intercourse."

In our Western world, oysters appear on the list of modern aphrodisiacs. But they're not a new one. The Roman novelist Apuleius was sued in the second century A.D. for allegedly inducing a rich widow into marriage by giving her spice oysters, sea urchins, and lobsters.

The stimulant Spanish fly still makes the rounds in tabloid print every once in a while. It is the crushed remains of the blister beetle *cantharides*. It was written that the scheming Roman empress Livia (circa 20 A.D.) slipped Spanish fly into the food of members of the court in the hopes that they would commit sexual indiscretions that she could blackmail them with later. She was obviously a person with too much time on her hands. Spanish fly is not some magical sexual stimulant. All it does is irritate sensitive tissue, and because it's produced under highly suspect conditions, the actual ingredients and dosage could be harmful. So beware of ads in cheap magazines.

Cleopatra reportedly laced the meals of her intended lovers with garlic in order to increase their staying power. Along similar lines Martial, a first century poet, wrote, "If your wife is old and your member is exhausted, eat onions in plenty."

If you're not in the mood to eat oysters, onions, and garlic, here are some other substances that are being used today to enhance sexual health.

Fava beans. They have high levels of levodopa, a neurotransmitter (brain chemical) that seems to stimulate brain activity by increasing levels of dopamine. This may result in a temporary feeling of emotional well-being, which can boost libido. L-dopa is a prescriptive drug used for Parkinson's patients, but a sixteen ounce serving of fava beans contains a hefty amount, near prescription level. And if it doesn't stimulate sexual desire, at least you'll have had a high fiber meal and won't be constipated.

Yohimbe. This substance is from the bark of an African tree. Sailors returning from that continent centuries ago bragged about the effects of yohimbe, but it's only recently that scientific research has supported the plant extract's claims to helping sexual stimulation. Researchers maintain that it helps the neurochemical pathways that lead to erection. Yohimbe extract is available only by prescription from a medical doctor. There are no studies on the effects of the herb on women. Side effects of dizziness, nervousness, headaches, and muscle cramps have been reported, but generally fade over time.

Constriction rings and penile injections. These are medically approved and effective ways that patients are treated for impotence, but a word of caution: Leaving the ring on more than thirty minutes can result in tissue death from the tourniquetlike action of the ring. Overuse of the prescription injections can also result in permanent tissue damage, so be cautious, and follow your doctor's instructions carefully.

Vitamins and minerals. A healthy diet with a balance of at least five servings of vegetables per day and low-fat protein is, of course, good for your whole body and overall physical health and stamina is important for sexual health too. Vitamins C, A, E, selenium, zinc, and the B vitamins are important for the health of mucous membranes in the body, including those in your genitalia.

The amour amino. L-Arginine, an essential amino acid, has been linked to increasing growth hormone, better wound healing, and a positive effect on viability of sperm and erections. Biochemically speaking, it has been associated with the increase of nitric oxide (not the same as nitrous oxide, which is laughing gas) in men's bodies, which helps cause erections. L-Arginine is found in meat, nuts, eggs, milk, and cheese. Pork and wild game have the highest amounts, with 2.62 and 2.35 grams per half pound, respectively. But since both these are high in saturated fat, and a fatty meal is known to decrease libido, you may want to try something else. Vegetarian sources are: wheat germ, at 2.70 grams per cup (still high in fat); ricotta cheese,

1.60 grams per cup; cottage cheese, 1.40 grams per cup; and granola, .90 grams per cup. If you have herpes, be sure to keep your lysine levels high, because a low arginine to lysine ratio is linked to increased herpes outbreaks. Lysine is also found in substantial amounts in the foods listed above, which is good to know, since one drawback of supplementation is creating imbalances by a "shotgun" approach. Very high doses of arginine may be toxic (in excess of 40 grams). *Oral overdosage of arginine may be life-threatening to people with kidney or liver disease.* Amino acids are like everything in nature—they can have the power to heal, but occasionally they can do harm as well.

Have a drink—of water. It's a truism that alcohol stimulates the desire, but removes the means. Chronic alcohol abuse can depress performance and arousal in both men and women.

No smoke equals more flames. Smoking constricts blood vessels, so it can put a big damper on arousal. Also, kissing a smoker really is like kissing an ash tray. And stained teeth and yellowed fingernails are not usually considered to enhance physical desirability.

Check out your birth control pills. Birth control pills that use only estrogen and progesterone may eventually dull libido. Talk to your doctor about the new tricyclic contraceptives which contain a touch of testosterone, the libido hormone for both women and men.

Try wearing sweats before putting on the sexy lingerie. Libido is stimulated in men and women through regular aerobic exercise. In one study, after only nine months of exercise, the active male participants reported a 10 percent increase in frequency and a 26 percent increase of orgasms and passionate sensual contact like kissing and caressing. Researchers at Chicago State University surveyed 500 women and almost 60 percent stated that their satisfaction with their "sexual self" increased once they started to exercise.

Look your best. In a long-term relationship, it's easy to slip into fewer and fewer grooming habits and self-maintenance. But as they say: When you look good, you feel good. Good self-image is an important part of enjoying our sexuality. Few people can relax when they're running through the worry list of "Do I smell bad? Do I look fat? Can you really notice that food stain on my T-shirt? Maybe I should have shaved this week? Is that a

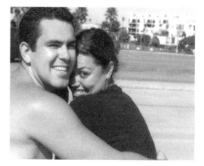

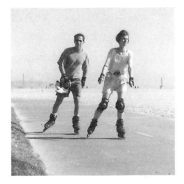

rip in my underwear? Will he notice that I'm a couple of weeks overdue on a pedicure? I think I have lint in my belly button. Will she notice that I ate onions for lunch? If he/she is not wearing his/her glasses, can he/she really notice the stains on my teeth/the dirt under my fingernails?" Etc. The details add up.

Reduce your fat intake. Testosterone, the desire hormone in both sexes, is decreased by fatty meals. So you'd be better off skipping that cheesecake for dessert and ordering the salad instead of the French fries and cheeseburgers if you want to keep your sexual thermostat out of the lukewarm zone.

Massage and caressing. Massage, touching, hugging, and caressing all stimulate the body's production of oxytocin, which is a "reward and pleasure" type of hormone. There are also hormone receptor sites for oxytocin in the uterus, and contractions of the uterus during orgasm are linked to oxytocin. Additionally, this hormone, stored in the pituitary gland, is also associated with feelings of nurturing and intimacy.

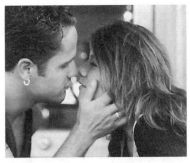

The power nap. How about trying to get some rest? Millions of people are sleep deprived and they wonder why their sex lives are lagging. They are simply too tired for sex. Schedule a nap somehow: Can you put your feet up and doze for a few minutes in your lunch hour instead of going out to eat? Would a portable tape player and a set of earphones help you relax for twelve minutes? Better yet, cuddle up and take a nap together.

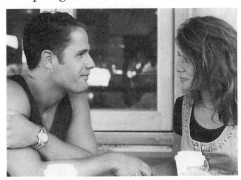

Prelude to a kiss. Remember all the private, intimate things you once did together? Walking under the stars—that's the kind of thing you did when you were dating, remember? The privacy of sharing a spectacular starlit sky together can create a quiet intimacy that's important for building desire. Remember slow-dancing together, enjoying each other's touch? Or the small, inexpensive, but romantic gifts you gave each other? Holding hands in the movies? Staring into each other's eyes over a candlelight dinner? These are all simple, but important preludes to a kiss.

Create the opportunity. This is probably the biggest stimulant of all. A momentary caress with a whispered promise of "later." Try calling your mate at work today and shock him or her with a partial list of all the sensual things that you would like to do tonight. Just make sure you're not on the speaker phone.

WHERE DO YOU GO FOR INFORMATION?

As our life expectancy continues to increase, we will have more people in their seventies, eighties and nineties. And as the generation that knew the wildness of Flower Power and the sexual revolution examine their lives, we will undoubtedly see this generation rewrite the book on human sexuality and aging. That's great news, because this generation reached sexual maturity amid debates aimed at keeping sex education out of the schools. Nowadays, it's not a matter of *should* it be taught, but *how early can we start?*

Dr. C. Everett Koop, the former surgeon general of the United States, was a pioneer when he tried to send out information about safe sex and HIV infection to every American. It's wonderful that schoolchildren have the opportunity to learn about their sexuality alongside their education in algebra and zoology. Long after they have forgotten the equation for an isosceles triangle, they may remember the rules for sexual good health.

Do your remember *your* schooling in sex education? I remember the extent of my high school education in human sexuality. On the last day of gym class, my gym teacher, very serious and frowning, told us, "Remember girls, there are always *those* types of men out there and be ever so vigilant to stay away from them." A belated speech, as it was never clear exactly what "those types of men" would do, and two girls from my class has already dropped out of school due to a failure of the rhythm method.

There aren't enough doctors trained in gerontology, and the training in aging and human sexuality is even more limited. There is new research constantly, but keeping up with it is a time-consuming job that few doctors have time for. But before you get angry, consider that those in the specialty fields spent at least ten years of their life completing the educational requirements to have the job. When we ask "Why isn't there more training?" it raises the question of how long a man or woman should study in order to become a doctor. Fifteen years? Twenty?

Even that wouldn't work. Think about it: Ten years ago, when the current set of hotshot specialists were sitting in a premed classroom for the first time, there wasn't any research on the fact that lifting weights could prevent compression fractures in elderly women. There was limited information on the fact that eating well and exercising could prevent heart attacks. It's only recently that vitamin E has been recognized to prevent heart disease. Even five years ago, it was far from mainstream, and considered quackery except by the "health nuts" who espoused it. A hundred years ago, we were happy if we lived to be fifty or even lived past retirement. Now, more than one-third of a woman's life will be lived after menopause.

Become your own advocate and expert by reading and seeking the information you need. Try approaching your general doctor for information. Don't be embarrassed to ask questions, because he or she has most likely heard it all before. If your doctor seems uncomfortable or unwilling to talk about your sexual health, find someone else. The Internet is absolutely loaded with resources on health, biotechnology, and just about everything else. The information is out there, just go for it. And of course, *practice safe sex*.

WHAT'S AGE GOT TO DO WITH IT?

Do you think young—or old? Perhaps one of the most misleading beliefs we have is that the beginning fires of hot emotion and sexual passion in a new relationship should be enough to keep us going forever. Yet many couples claim they're too busy for sex, and their love-making is a priority somewhere behind at least an hour of television watching a night, a night or two of meetings per week, and weekends scheduled hour by hour with taxi-driving the kids all over the place. Then, when passion fades, it's blamed on aging.

The best bonfire in the world needs more than a few twigs tossed on it every once in a while. Some may be "glad *that's* over with," while others may find ecstasy they never dreamed was possible, simply because they were open to communicating with their partner and committed to keeping their passion alive.

Everyone's sexual needs are different and the need for sexual release is both healthy and natural. If you are having sexual problems, don't avoid sex as a way of solving the problem. Find the answers you need. What's good for you may vary from day to day. If you are newly widowed, or without a partner, there are now plenty of manuals to describe different methods of self-stimulation.

Too stressed out for sex? The good news for any age, according to Dr. Ruth Westheimer: "Anything that's caused by stress—even a headache—will benefit from a good, satisfying sexual experience."

Feeling the aches and pains of sports injuries from years ago? "One orgasm can give some people six pain-free hours, whether they have arthritis or whiplash," says author Judith Sachs, who wrote *The Healing Power of Sex.*

Sometimes we may lose ourselves in a pit of disappointments, unwittingly letting the judgment of the world crash in on us, bruising our spirits. It's beyond "having a headache" or being too tired for sex. How about being just worn out by the world? Author Daphne Rose Kingma zeroes in on this familiar territory: "When you find yourself lost in the pit of unlovingness—blowing up, being sarcastic, slamming the door—you need to recognize that these are signs you have also stopped loving yourself. You have stopped seeing yourself with the compassion, which, if you could only reconstruct it, you could also offer to others."

She offers this wisdom in her book *A Garland of Love:* "Therefore make it your personal obligation, today, to treat it as a moral responsibility always, to give some very gentle attention to yourself."

What will it take to fill your own cup full of love again? My friend Maura creates inner peace with a quiet cup of tea in her best china teacup. Gazing out the window at the clouds while listening to classical music may work for another, while going for a walk in the park with your dog might create tranquility for you. What about buying flowers for yourself, or getting a therapeutic massage? Meditating, lifting weights, taking a bracing swim in the ocean, or hiking up a mountain trail may rekindle your inner fires. Being gentle and nurturing to yourself is a daily habit that can renew you for a lifetime. It sounds like a foreign, even selfish, idea to some, but self-care sends a strong message to your inner being that you matter, that your needs are important, and the result is that, reconnected to your own tranquility and sensuality base, you can offer it to others so that you can give and receive your sexuality as the powerful gift that it is. This is a strength that can grow in the safety of your affection, something that time can never take away.

When it comes to sex, what's age got to do with it? Only as much as you let it.

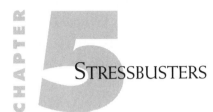

CHAPTER 5

STRESSBUSTERS

The old believe everything;
the middle-aged suspect everything;
the young know everything.

—Oscar Wilde (1854–1900)

*E*veryone has experienced stress, but few people can come up with a meaningful definition of it. Most of us think of stress as something bad—like sitting in freeway traffic when you're late for a meeting, or finding out you're going to be featured on *60 Minutes* and that Mike Wallace is in your office right now with a TV crew and he's *not* smiling. Most of us would agree that an IRS audit would be stressful, but so is falling in love, winning the lottery, or fulfilling a lifelong dream of being in the Olympics. The difference is that the wonderful stresses like falling in love activate positive biochemical events in the body and the negative stresses do the opposite.

Stress puts your life in the fast lane: When you can't sleep, your stomach is all tied up in knots, and you wake up more tired than when you went to bed, you can bet that your aging clock is speeding up. Chronic stress taxes your immune system, raises your blood pressure, and gives you frown lines, to name only a few hazards. I've had overstressed patients in their twenties with ulcers, high blood pressure, and other stress-related ailments that are common in people two or three times their age.

Almost twenty years ago Dr. Paul Rosch, the president of the American Institute of Stress, was interviewed in *Esquire* magazine and came up with an intriguing observation: "People today don't get sick for the reasons they think they do. They aren't killed by germs, risk factors, or cancer-causing agents. What's really killing people is the fact

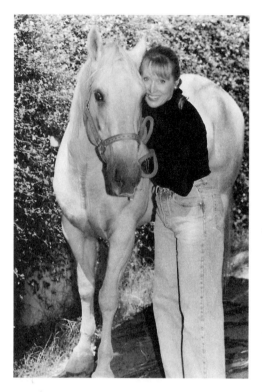

that we have been hit with about three hundred years of civilization in a few decades."

Dr. Hans Selye (1907–1982), the Canadian physician who dedicated his life to studying stress, noted that many things can cause stress. Heat and cold, pain and pleasure—all are stressors that can affect us at the most basic cellular level.

Dr. Selye noted that stressors force the body to respond by activating the body to either stay and fight or turn tail and flee. These reactions were real lifesavers in our more primitive times when clubbing down a wooly mammoth or fleeing from a saber-toothed tiger, but in modern civilization, our physiological alarm mechanisms are killing us. When you are stuck in traffic, you don't really need to pump more blood to your muscles so that you can run away from danger. When the IRS is auditing your taxes, you don't really need to sweat to dispose of excess body heat as if you were fighting for your life—even if it feels that way at the time.

However, Dr. Selye did not propose that we design a stress-free life. I remember hearing him answer a question on the topic in a live interview. He said, "A stress-free life is an impossible goal—we need some stress to be alive. . . . After all, we call it blood *pressure*. Without some pressure, we are dead."

Stress *avoidance* is not a goal. It's stress *management* that's most important to power aging. We would absolutely hate a life without stress. Think of it: What is the ultimate punishment for inmates in maximum security prisons? Solitary confinement, a situation where you're totally isolated from any elements of a normal day or any stimulation at all. Yet it is so stressful it can produce insanity.

We need the daily stress of challenges so that

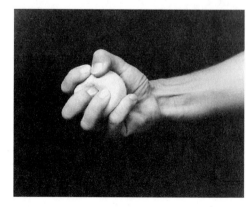

we can grow and become complete human beings in a healthy way. Problem-solving skills, coping mechanisms, learning to deal with each situation, and feeling the sense of accomplishment when we reach a goal—these are a part of the stress package too. Learning how to manage stress effectively so that we don't feel overwhelmed prevents the wear and tear on our minds and bodies that can cause illness and premature aging.

Dr. Selye pointed out that psychological or emotional stresses are as significant as physical stresses like pollution or excessive heat. A counterbalance of positive factors, like an excellent diet, can attenuate the effects of toxic chemicals. Of course, the opposite is also true: poor nutrition plus exposure to pollution can certainly make the whole equation worse. Taking control of our daily health needs, maximizing our potential physically, helps establish a baseline message of strength and respect that can only add to the positive outcome for us mentally.

PERSONALITY AND PERCEPTION

After Selye's pioneering research, scientists found that stress is not a purely biological condition that results in illness. The personality of the person being stressed and his or her perception of that stress is also key to understanding how stress affects us. It's the old "one man's meat is another man's poison" scenario. Your neighbor may love life in the fast lane working in a hospital emergency room. You might get overly hyped up simply watching "ER" on television.

Additionally, *how* we react to stress when it occurs is essential to understanding how the stress will affect us. Do you drive too fast, smoke too much, drink too much, and kick the dog after a hard day at work? All of these things can increase your health risks. For one thing, you could get a speeding ticket, which will add to your financial stress, get lung cancer, or suffer a nasty dog bite from those poor habits. Some people feel alive on four hours of sleep or with a big deadline looming. If you're not one of them, don't get stressed out over it.

Finally, a stress definition: Psychological stress occurs when a person believes a situation is overwhelming and threatens his or her ability to cope. It is a function of the relationship between a person and an environment.

You see, it's *not* the stress itself that matters most: It's whether or not you feel that you are in control of it. It's not the stress of the job that causes the executive to drop dead of a heart attack, it's his *reaction* to the stress of the job that did him in. Hostility in itself does not lead to heart disease. Researchers have found that *neurotic hostility*, the type that is felt by irritable complainers, is not related to increased cardiac risk. It's the *antagonistic hostility* of the rude, aggressive, confrontational cynics that puts them at greater risk.

Rule 1: Don't sweat the small stuff.
Rule 2: It's all small stuff.

> "There'd be nothing wrong with us fast-moving Type As if it weren't for all those slow-moving Type Bs."
> —Bumper sticker

TOP TWENTY STRESSBUSTERS

To effectively manage stress, you need more than an ambulance at the bottom of a cliff. The stressbusters that follow will help you build a guard rail at the top to keep you from falling over. A general word on managing stress: Use common sense. Eat nutritious food, go to bed early, and get some exercise. Don't smoke and go easy on the alcohol. A ten-year-long study of 7,000 people in California found that these habits all related to good health and a lack of stress symptoms. No big surprises here!

1. **Catch a few zzzzzzzs.** Depression loves to ride in on the heels of fatigue, and we all know that stress can make you feel depressed.

2. **Sweat it out.** Exercise is a time-proven stress reliever. A half-hour of vigorous aerobic exercise relaxes tense muscles and helps burn off unhealthy stress-related chemicals in the body.

3. **Eat your fruits and veggies.** A lot of stress seems to turn our digestive system into cement. Ever had that "punched in the stomach feeling" when you've been hit with a big stress load all of a sudden? The extra fiber in fruits and veggies will not only keep you regular, but will help keep you away from junk food binging, which adds fat to your body, which adds work for your heart, which adds to your body stress and risk of heart disease.

4. **Have a drink of water.** I've noticed that when I offer my most hard-driving, stressed-out patients a drink of cool water they immediately begin to relax. Often, they will have several cups of water in a row—evidence that they've been going too fast to realize that they're down a quart. Chronic dehydration leads to chronic constipation. The water also helps the body wash out the stress-related chemicals.

5. **Relax.** This is the simplest way to reduce your stress. You can lower your heart

rate, blood pressure, and breathing within seconds. Practice tensing and then relaxing your muscles starting with your neck and shoulder muscles and work through all the muscles in your body. Studies show that relaxation techniques can improve your immune system activity. Try taking a deep breath in and then letting it out slowly. Cheap and easy.

Eastern cultures have meditation built in to religious philosophies. Yoga, t'ai chi, and similar exercises as well as various forms of transcendental meditation are all excellent stressbusters. The ultimate goal of these practices is not simply relaxation, but the attainment of spiritual harmony and wisdom. That has to be the ultimate stressbuster if there ever was one.

6. **Make a list—a short list.** Efficient people who don't let stress build up have a secret: They make a list of things to do and then do them, starting with the most important one. I find that prioritizing the list is a stressbuster in action. Making the list too long, though, can *add* to your stress, so stick with a few major items. Is it *really* that important? I have never heard anybody on their deathbed say "I wish I would have done more housework!" Have you? I found a list of New Year's resolutions I made eight years ago and there's the same stuff on that list that I put down this year: Organize the garage this year, lose eight pounds, do your taxes early. You have to laugh about it, which brings me to my next point . . .

7. **Get in a few laughs.** My fiancé is wonderful on this one. He reminds me to laugh when I get too serious. Watch a funny sitcom, read a humorous book, rent *The Three Stooges* on video if it will make you chuckle. Remember that laughing is also very good for your abdominal muscles in addition to being a great stressbuster.

8. **Learn how to say no without feeling guilty.** Stressed-out people are often ones who try to do everything themselves, get in over their heads, and then feel overwhelmed by it all—which, of course, leads to more stress. I often tell working mothers that they don't have to enter the Superwoman Sweepstakes this year. People who can't say no without feeling guilty need to learn how to assert themselves and delegate tasks. Start small. Join a car pool. Ask your spouse to help you with the bills. Get help from your family in preparing dinner. If saying yes to a social situation is going to stress you out, then say no. It's unfair to expect others to be mind readers and it's ineffective to rely on that type of intervention as a communication skill. There is support out there if you can be clear about what it is you want and set limits.

9. <u>Solve the problem.</u> Once you're in a stressful situation, you'll be more effective if you spend 95 percent of your time and energy on problem-solving actions and only 5 percent of the time venting your spleen or wallowing in your worry, anger, and pessimism. The opportunity to develop coping skills comes with the stress. It forces us to grow and learn techniques that can last a lifetime. Financial problems yield well to this approach. One friend traded in her Lexus and bought a secondhand four-by-four truck. That reduction in monthly expense was enough to take the pressure off.

10. <u>Seek excellence, not perfection.</u> It's been said that demanding perfection is simply another way of beating yourself up. If you were perfect, you'd be the only one! This stressbuster is particularly important for people living with a health ailment or a chronic stress situation. Sometimes folks have too strong a sense of control. The most harmonious approach is to take responsibility for getting well without blaming oneself for getting sick.

11. **Cultivate your garden of friendship.** <u>Closeness and sharing with others</u> is a basic human need. Friendship lessens our suffering and increases our joy.

12. **Keep a personal journal.** This type of reflection and confession is good for your soul and it can do wonders for your body as well. Researchers have found that <u>keeping a journal can speed up the normal coping process associated with</u> major <u>life changes.</u> College freshmen who chronicled their feelings had fewer bouts of flu and visits to the infirmary than the control group who wrote only about less intimate topics.

13. **Kick the coffee habit.** This is a tough one, so ease off slowly. I love coffee and the <u>effects of caffeine,</u> so I tried really hard to come up with some positive research saying that coffee was good for you. It didn't happen. In addition to frazzling your nerves, it temporarily raises your blood pressure and heart rate and causes insomnia.

14. **Reach for your mate instead of your plate.** <u>Sex is a wonderful stress reliever.</u> As an added benefit, it burns calories and <u>releases pain relieving endorphins,</u> which give a mild sense of euphoria, into the bloodstream—as if you needed another reason.

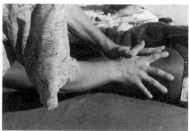

15. **Watch out for the land mines.** <u>Chronic high-stress lifestyles</u> can lead to poor choices when it comes to coping. Dentists have one of the highest suicide

rates, my dentist told me. Abuse of drugs, alcohol, and long-standing depression or feeling out of control are danger signals that stress has gone haywire. You don't have to be a perfect person or have all the answers yourself. Seek professional help if you feel you are stepping on land mines.

16. **Take a bath.** It's a cheap mini-vacation that can soothe achy muscles and give your body a well-deserved reward for keeping you on your feet. Light a few candles, lock the bathroom door to keep the kids and the dog out, and turn to Chapter 8 to learn about some time-tested herbal baths.

17 through 20. The Big Four Stressbuster Exercises.

17. **Door stretch.** This is probably the number-one stretch that I teach my stressed-out patients. Starting position: Stand in line with the door frame, as shown. Then, slowly take a baby step into the room, keeping your arms against the door frame. Hold for a count of 20 and then repeat on the other foot. Remember to keep your chin tucked in as pictured.

18. **Shoulder shrugs.** Your body understands full contraction of muscle fiber. The killer is the half-contracted spasm of stressed-out tension states. This exercise teaches the muscles the fully contracted

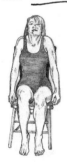

state once again, bringing total relaxation when the tension is released. Circulation to the flexed areas is a welcome side effect. Starting position: Hold for a slow count of eight, then relax. The door stretch and these shoulder shrugs are great traveling de-stressors on long plane flights.

19. **Scalp massage.** The circulation and relaxation stimulated by this simple act are positively heavenly. If you can trade a scalp massage with a friend, do it. The old-time strong men like Vic Boff (see his profile on page 326) are great believers in scalp massage as a source of vitality for the body. They are famous for their full heads of vigorously vital hair, so try this exercise on for size and perhaps even the hairs on your head will show their appreciation by sticking around in the years to come. Start at your temples. Apply firm pressure with your fingertips and move the scalp in small circles. Most people are surprised to see how much tension they have outside their head when they have a lot of tension on the inside!

20. **Sight for sore eyes.** Other exercises for strengthening and relieving tension in the eyes are described on page 156. This one is very relaxing and restful, especially if you read a lot, work on a computer, or do long-distance driving. Starting position: Simply cup your hands over the eyes. This blocks the light and gives tired pupils a chance to rest. Resting your elbows on your desk and breathing slow, deep breaths of air into your abdomen will relax you further. Think lovely thoughts. Five minutes of this and you can feel as refreshed as if you had a nap.

SNACKING FOR LESS STRESS

What food do you reach for in times of stress? Chocolate bars? Potato chips? Ice cream? Eating to relieve tension by reaching for these "binge classics" can backfire. Sugar hypes you up and then saps your energy as you crash, making you even more stressed. Excessive sweets and fats can also take their toll on your immune system, leaving you more vulnerable to illness.

Instead call on "low glycemic" carbohydrates (see Chapter 11) to boost levels of serotonin, a brain chemical that relaxes you. Try crunching on raw veggies or unbuttered popcorn. They have carbs, and the mechanical action of the chewing eases tension in your jaw. Some other good comfort foods are hot oatmeal or a baked potato. A bowl of split pea or minestrone soup is also a good choice. Stir-fried rice with veggies, toast, a bagel, or a banana—take your pick. Sorbet is a better choice than ice cream because the of the fat in ice cream, as any fat-phobe will tell you. The best choice would be frozen orange juice or fruit juice popsicles you make in your own freezer. I fill the ice cube trays with fruit juice and stick in a tongue depressor when it starts turning to slush. And, to wash it all down, a glass of water is always healthy and better than coffee or soda.

6

SLEEP ON IT

Sleep that knits up the ravel'd sleave of care . . .

—William Shakespeare (1564–1616), *Macbeth*

What if there really *was* a Fountain of Youth? What if:

- you knew of something that would make you look and feel younger?
- it might add years of good health to your life?
- it would make you feel more energized throughout the day?
- it might increase your sex drive?
- it could make you feel more motivated and less depressed?
- it wasn't going to cost you anything?

If you knew of something like that, wouldn't you want it? Well you can have it. It's called *getting enough sleep at night*.

As kids, how we railed against our bedtimes! "*Please*, can I stay up just a little bit longer?" beg children from the Atlantic to the Pacific. However, as adults, many of us have had days when we would gladly give up our entire kingdom if we could just sleep in some morning.

Do you wake up in the morning more tired than when you went to bed? Are you feeling really overwhelmed with stress on the job lately? Are you the parent of a newborn? Are you a student? Do you work nights on shift work? Are you going through menopause right now? Are you getting up several times a night to go the bathroom? Have you ever wished that you could just put your head down on your desk in the afternoon and take a nap?

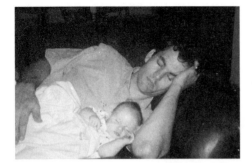

If you have answered yes to any of those questions, chances are you are sleep deprived. One in three Americans doesn't get enough sleep, according to the National Commission on Sleep Disorders. Some experts estimate the number of chronically sleep-deprived people in this country to be closer to one in two. That's 100 million people who are shuffling through life, too tired to cope. Sleep deprivation can have serious consequences: It can make headlines. Remember the Exxon *Valdez* oil spill? The grounding of the tanker was ultimately blamed on the sleep-deprived third mate.

Last year, a young man sped through a red light at an intersection and totalled another car. He also narrowly missed hitting the police car stopped at the intersection. "I'm so sorry!" he told the waiting officers. "I fell asleep at the wheel and I didn't see the red light." I was sorry too—it was my car he totalled. He had just finished his shift as a nightwatch security guard. I was pretty badly injured, but knew it could have been much worse, and I sincerely hope that he is seeking another line of work at this time. If only he had gotten more sleep! According to the *Journal of the American Medical Association*, 13 percent of all automobile deaths are caused by people who fall asleep at the wheel.

WHO HAS TIME FOR SLEEP?

We expect twenty-four-hour-a-day service and accessibility for everything from supermarkets, banking, and photocopying to catalogue shopping, stock market advice, and television programming. Police protection, hospital and emergency care, and other public services like fire departments provide services that we *demand* on a continual basis.

We want to be able to take an airplane ride, call a plumber, or order a pizza any time of the day or night. And with the advent of cellular phones, fax machines, and the Internet, even the office can follow us home and go with us on vacation. Who has time for sleep? I once attended a lecture on stress and the speaker started the speech by saying, "The American Dream leaves little time for dreaming."

HOW MUCH SLEEP DO YOU NEED?

There is no magic number. We've all heard of at least one person who can function perfectly well on a couple of hours a night and accomplish superhuman, wonderful things on a daily basis. "Plenty of time to sleep when I'm dead" was the mantra of one person I knew. The rest of us need about eight hours. We're all familiar with the sluggish, "syrupy" feeling that occurs toward the end of a long period of staying awake, and scientists have noted that a person can become irritable or even psychotic following prolonged periods of forced wakefulness.

Sleep restores balance to our bodies. One researcher likened it to the "rezeroing" of electric analog computers after prolonged use, for all computers of this type will gradually lose their "baseline" of operation unless they are rezeroed, just as we will gradually lose our functioning after prolonged sleep deprivation.

Here's the straight scoop: You need as much sleep as you need to feel rested in the morning. If you feel like you have jet lag and you haven't been anywhere, chances are that you are sleep deprived.

WHY IS SLEEP SO IMPORTANT?

Sleep has two major physiological effects on the body. The first one is on the nervous system, and the second is on the different structures and organs of the body.

Over the past few years, there has been growing evidence suggesting that _mental depression psychosis_, which affects about 8 million people in the United States at any one time, is associated with severe insomnia. These patients suffer from symptoms of grief, unhappiness, despair, and misery in addition to losing their appetite and sex drive. There are measurable and significant decreases in important brain chemicals

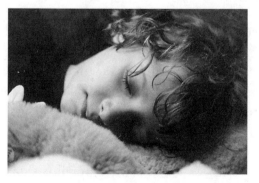

such as serotonin and norepinephrine.

In addition to its effect on the nervous system, sleep has a major impact on every cell in the body. Sleep allows the body to rest and repair itself. Arterial blood pressure falls as the tension of the day melts away, heart rate decreases (allowing the heart to catch a rest), and the blood vessels of the skin dilate (allowing nourishment to be brought to the skin). Muscles fall into a relaxed state and the overall metabolic rate of the body decreases by 10 to 30 percent

Paradoxically, during sleep some parts of the brain may have an *increase* in metabolism of up to 20 percent while the muscle tone of the body severely declines. In fact, this stage of sleep is actually called paradoxical sleep, because the muscles of the body are extremely inhibited, but the brain waves show the same type of marked activity characteristic of wakefulness.

And if you still need another reason to catch come *zzzzzzs*, take note of this: During the first two hours of sleep, the body produces its highest amounts of human growth hormone, which repairs cell damage and is now being marketed as an anti-aging substance. Getting enough sleep is one way you can save money—and you won't have to go to the doctor and get a prescription. Additionally, immune system soldiers like natural killer cells, which help fight infection, are highest in animals who get enough sleep. We've all had the experience of burning the candle at both ends and getting that "run down" feeling that often precedes a cold or the flu. Now you know why. It's pretty simple: When you sleep better, you feel better.

THE WIDE-AWAKE FACTS ON INSOMNIA

Having trouble getting to sleep at night? You're not alone. An estimated 2 to 3 billion doses of sleeping pills are taken each year in the United States. Ralph Nader's Public Citizen organization called them "dangerously overprescribed." The *Berkeley Wellness Letter* stated that sleeping pills are "one of the biggest rip-offs in the drugstore." As many insomniacs learn, most sleeping pills don't work the same after a couple of weeks of use. And, of course, sleeping pills combined with alcohol and tranquilizers can cause illness and even death.

Avoid sleeping pills because they are addictive. While they are often a necessary evil when, for instance, a patient is postoperatively in intense pain, they actually interfere with the body's normal sleeping rhythms because they temporarily alter the activity of your brain cells. Then some of the most important dreaming and other cycles of sleep are not possible. The result: a dreamless, unsatisfying sleep that frustrates insomniacs even more.

Sleep apnea is the main symptom of a group of sleep disorders characterized by the cessation of breathing during sleep. The person with apnea actually stops breathing for about ten seconds at a time. The apnea sufferer then wakes up with a start, and the breathing starts again. This could happen thirty to a few hundred times a night. In the morning, the person wakes up exhausted, often without even knowing why. Most commonly, the spouse of the apnea sufferer reports the condition because there are often loud snorts, snoring, and gasping sounds that wake the partner during the night as well. Obesity can be a cause, most likely because the extra fat around the neck actually presses down on the esophagus when the person is horizontal, resulting in a kind of choking. Chronic obstruction of the nasal passages because of allergies or sinusitis is another cause of apnea. The American Sleep Apnea Association, 202-293-3650 or www.sleepnet.com, can offer more information.

The *New England Journal of Medicine* reported that sleep apnea affects 9 percent of women and 24 percent of men in the general population. It has been suggested that melatonin supplementation may be a way to manage this condition.

Nightmares occur in both children and adults during a kind of mentally active sleep known as REM, or rapid eye movement, sleep. Most of the time, the bad dreams are of no clinical importance, and children in particular seem to outgrow them. But nightmares could be an indication of stress, chronic drug or alcohol abuse, or withdrawal from drugs such as barbiturates. One simple precaution is to avoid watching horror movies at bedtime—the main themes of most bad dreams are falling, death, and fear of attack.

THIEVES IN THE NIGHT

Are any of these robbing you of a good night's sleep?
- **Caffeine:** it (or its close relatives) is in in chocolate, hot cocoa, tea, coffee, and some painkillers like Exedrin and prescriptive drugs including antihistamines
- **Nicotine:** from cigarettes, snuff, chewing tobacco, and secondhand smoke
- **Appetite suppressants:** they suppress sleep as well
- **Cold remedies:** including decongestants
- **Alcohol:** it can be a hidden ingredient in cough syrups and decongestants
- **Prescription Drugs:** for asthma, hypertension, heart rhythm, and thyroid problems, to name only a few. Read the insert sheet that is included with the medication or ask your doctor or pharmacist about possible side effects associated with your prescription.

- **<u>Shift work:</u>** The *New England Journal of Medicine* reported that eight out ten shift workers have sleep problems, and they are <u>more likely to have heart and digestive problems</u> than people who work regular day jobs.

MELATONIN MANIA

There has been a recent wave of publicity about the wonders of melatonin supplementation in books, magazines, newspapers, and television specials. People have been flocking to health food stores to snap up this latest miracle pill. The research on melatonin has been intense and extensive. There are enough facts in the scientific literature to put you asleep just reading about melatonin, never mind actually taking the supplements.

What is it? Melatonin is a hormone produced by the pineal gland, a pea-sized little structure buried in the center of the brain. The hormone's chemical name is N-Acetyl-5-Methoxytryptamine. The pineal gland is influenced by the amount of light seen by our eyes each day, and production of the hormone is cyclical. Our daily and seasonal cycles of waking and sleeping, sexual cycles, and the function of the hypothalamus, thyroid, thymus, pancreas, and adrenal glands are all related to the tiny pineal gland.

The pineal gland also plays a role in *narcolepsy*, which is the opposite of insomnia. People who suffer from this disorder could fall asleep in mid-sentence during a conversation or even while driving. It is a serious problem named from the Greek word *narke*, which means numbness, and *lepsis,* which means seizure. It occurs in families and is thought to be controlled by a specific gene. Changes in sleep patterns similar to those of narcoleptics have been shown when the pineal gland is removed.

How does it affect sleep? Melatonin helps produce a substance called *arginine vasotocin*, and this secretion inhibits an adrenal gland stress hormone called *cortisol*. Cortisol is a normally occurring hormone that has multiple functions, including protein, carbohydrate, and fat metabolism. During periods of prolonged stress, cortisol production is increased, causing the body to remain in an agitated state. Insomniacs tend to have high nighttime levels of cortisol. So <u>melatonin helps induce sleepfulness by providing arginine vasotocin to inhibit cortisol production. Immune functioning is also improved when cortisol production is curbed.</u> Earlier, we discussed how sleep promotes production of human growth hormone, which helps regenerate cells, so in this way you can see how different hormones work together in complex ways and with far-reaching effects.

Melatonin is linked to prevention of osteoporosis and is thought to be a free radical scavenger, possibly preventing cancer and promoting longevity. In France, melatonin is marketed with progestin as a birth control pill.

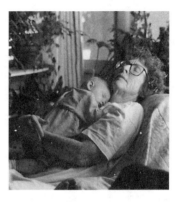

Is melatonin toxic? Melatonin has been researched for more than thirty years and given in doses over 200 milligrams without any adverse side effects. Drug researchers determine the LD 50, which stands for the median *lethal dose* of a substance, or the dosage that will kill 50 percent of the animals receiving it. The LD 50 tests on animals have yielded no toxic levels for melatonin. In fact, scientists were unable to find a concentrate strong enough to kill a mouse, and Italian researchers have found melatonin to boost the performance of immune systems compromised by drugs, stress, or aging.

How much do you need to fall into a good sleep? Controlled studies have shown that as little as one-tenth of a milligram will induce sleep. British Columbia's Children's Hospital in Vancouver uses 2.5 to 10 milligrams at bedtime to help kids with problems like autism to get a sound sleep. The typical dose is three to five milligrams per night. Up to 6,000 milligrams were fed to human volunteers for thirty days. Volunteers reported some stomach discomfort and were also very sleepy, but those were the only reported side effects. Vivid dreams are fairly common the first few nights, but usually subside after that.

SOMNOLENCE MADE SIMPLE

Perhaps some of the following ideas will help you snooze. Sleep well, and may all your dreams be in technicolor.

Count your blessings. As Peter Pan said, Think lovely thoughts. When you are tired, you are often prey to negative thoughts and worries that would otherwise be kept in perspective.

Realizing this can prevent the negativities of the day from taking over and keeping you awake at night. Thinking about the really important things, like the people you love and the good things in your life, is a way to go to sleep with an attitude of gratitude.

Avoid caffeine. Caffeine can stay in your body up to six hours after you drink that cup of tea or coffee or eat that chocolate bar. Caffeine keeps you awake, so cut it out.

Have a cup of herbal tea. Chamomile has a long tradition as a sleep inducer. It contains calcium and tryptophan just like milk, but without the calories or fat.

Consistency is the key. Philosopher Friedrich Nietzsche said that we prepare for our sleep all day long. The body loves routine. World-class athletes in training maximize their potential by establishing a regular daily rhythm of meals, exercise, and waking and sleeping. You can do the same by eating at regular intervals, going to bed at the same time each night, and waking up refreshed and on schedule. By doing this, you are preparing yourself for quality sleep at night.

Create a sleepy environment. A comfortable bed, quiet, and cool temperatures can all contribute to restful sleep. Try turning down the thermostat at night, wearing earplugs if your neighbor's dog seems to wake you up all the time, and allow fresh and circulating cool air in your bedroom.

Eat better. Try to eat a more natural diet. Fresh, raw foods keep you free of the toxic buildup that occurs when your body is constipated. This could make you feel sluggish regardless of how much you have been sleeping. Also, avoid late-night, heavy, fatty, or spicy snacks. Assuming that you're not allergic to milk or that you are not a fat-phobe, maybe Mom was right after all about that warm glass of milk.

Don't drink and sleep. Alcohol can make you very sleepy. But it is also known to disrupt the pattern of rapid eye movement (REM) sleep that is important for quality rest. So even if you spend more time in the sack, it won't be quality time and you'll wake up feeling crummy.

Don't pull the covers over your head. This could cause a lack of free-flowing oxygen and give you a "turtle headache" in the morning.

Exercise. Do work out during the day; it relieves stress and makes you more relaxed. Remember how great it felt when you were a kid, outside playing hard all day?

Don't work out vigorously any less than two hours before your bedtime. Your metabolism will still be too revved up for sleep.

Wind down. Just because your eyes are closed doesn't mean your brain is going to shut down automatically. Spend some time in the evening doing relaxing things like taking the dog for a walk, having a warm bath, or listening to music before you go to bed. (See other stressbuster strategies in Chapter 5.) Paying bills, worrying about your work, and calculating your taxes are *not* ideal ways to unwind. How about reading a good book? What about listening to a bedtime story from a books on tape library or

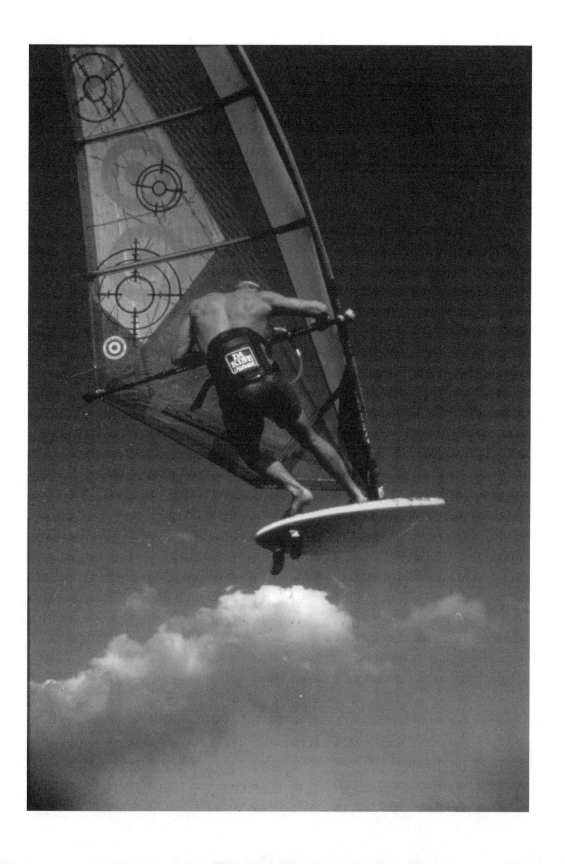

to soft music? I have a lecture on tape from a old pathology class that is an absolute cure for insomnia. Whatever works for you.

Don't drink a lot of liquids late at night. For obvious reasons. Although, during my student years I found drinking a few glasses of water before bed to be more reliable than an alarm clock for waking me up, especially if I only had a few hours to sleep.

Have sex. Isn't it better than counting sheep?

7 FORGET ABOUT LOSING YOUR MEMORY

It is the fight itself that keeps you young.

—Colette (1873–1954)

After spending an entire day with me, two older friends of mine, ages eighty-two and ninety-seven, dissolved into a fit of giggles. "You've made us feel so great!" said the younger of the two. I smiled and was glad that they had enjoyed going out to lunch in Beverly Hills and all the fun of window shopping on Rodeo Drive in the afternoon.

"First, you locked your keys in the car. Then you forgot where you put your appointment book, and then you left your sunglasses at the restaurant. We're always afraid we're getting old and feeble and it's so great to see someone your age even more forgetful than us! Wait'll we tell our friends!" I guess you just never know what kind of entertainment your guests will like the most.

Forgetfulness _can_ make you feel that your brain is going soft. Stress in itself is usually the culprit, as it was that particular afternoon when I had a million things on my mind. It's simple common sense to realize that the less attention you pay to details, the more absent-minded you'll be. But many of us worry that such forgetfulness is a harbinger of things to come. Get over it!

According to some recent research, our mental muscles may actually flourish with age, a fact that is punching holes in the widespread myth that intellectual faculties diminish as we grow older.

This is certainly good news. Because these days, "The fear of dementia is stronger than the fear of death itself," writes Mark Williams, M.D., in *The American Geriatrics Society's Complete Guide to Aging and Health.*

FOREVER SMART

Get out your paper and pencils and listen up. A group of professors at the University of California, Berkeley, recently taught the rest of the world a lesson about minding our memories. If you skipped class that day, here's the scoop, as reported in *Science News*: "Intelligent people who stay mentally active into their sixties and beyond can give their memories more staying power."

A battery of memory and cognitive tests were given to professors from a wide range of disciplines on the Berkeley campus who were divided into three age groups: young professors, from age thirty to forty-four; middle-aged, forty-five to fifty-nine years old; and senior professors, ages sixty to seventy-one. While the older professors had comparatively lower scores on pairing names and faces and on pushing a computer button quickly in response to commands, the senior professors held their own on two memory tests that required mental planning, organization, and problem solving. In a recent issue of *Psychological Science* (September 1995), the investigators of the study proposed that because professors must frequently integrate new information into an existing knowledge base, they may devise memory strategies that overcome some of the biological glitches of the aging brain.

However, before contemporary researchers devoted years to cognitive analysis of the qualities of learning, knowledge, and erudition, this application of gray matter was simply called *wisdom!*

In another study reported in the *New England Journal of Medicine*, early verbal ability also seems to help our brains later on. Ninety-three nuns in their eighties and nineties were examined and compared to versions of themselves as depicted in autobiographies they had written sixty years earlier. The nuns who remained the sharpest were the ones who had made the most articulate, complex, and dense recordings of their lives when they first joined the convent more than a half century earlier.

THE BIG FOUR THAT GET YOU MORE

The studies above relied upon a relatively small number of subjects. Clearly, we need more information, and on bigger groups. However, 1,192 healthy and mentally fit people between the ages of seventy and eighty were tested and measured by scientists from Harvard and Mt. Sinai medical schools and from Yale, Duke, and Brandeis universities. Twenty-two different variables were studied, including blood pressure, blood fats, nicotine habits, psychiatric symptoms, lung function, and level of education. The testing began in 1988 and the seniors were tested again in 1991.

The factors found by the study to be most related to mental fitness were:

1. **Physical activity.** Regular exercise may stimulate blood flow to the brain and also nerve growth. Both of these create a greater number of densely branched neurons, which apparently make the nerve cells stronger and more resilient to disease. At least 25 percent of people age eighty-five and older suffer from some degree of dementia. In reading these statistics, I compared that rate to the number of seniors who suffer from hypertension resulting from plaque-hardened arteries; nearly two-thirds of the population will eventually develop high blood pressure at some point. How much of dementia is due to arterial plaquing? The smaller diameter of the clogged up arteries prevents blood flow to the brain. Just as in any part of the body deprived of blood and the oxygen it contains, the nerve cells of the brain may be functioning less from simple oxygen deprivation.

One study of one hundred adults revealed that people with higher blood pressure scored lower in short-term memory-retrieval tests. Another reason to keep your blood pressure under control.

Wonder what kind of shape your arteries are in? Get your blood pressure checked. Turn to the cardiovascular health section in Chapter 16 and plan your heart-healthy strategies. You have to exercise, eat right, and control your toxic emotions if you want to stick around, have fun, and keep your brain intact so that you'll be able to enjoy it all. You can make a difference in your future by making better choices for yourself today.

2 and 3. **Level of education and early linguistic ability.** This would seem to parallel the findings of the nun study mentioned earlier. Perhaps people who have challenged themselves with at least a college education or those who developed early linguistic ability are actually stimulating neurons in their brains to develop more

synapses. The hypothesis is that this may provide them with a bigger reserve to fall back on in later years.

So, as much as may have hated algebra or English composition and even if you have forgotten all your geography and can't name the capital of Togo anymore, that <u>early flexing of your mental muscles really *was* good for you.</u> Keep your neurons busy and you'll be set for the long run.

4. <u>**Personality.**</u> According to Marilyn Albert, Ph.D., of Harvard Medical School, who was involved in the landmark study of 1,192 seniors mentioned above, research indicates that <u>elevated levels of stress hormones may harm your brain cells and help to destroy the brain's hippocampus, a part of the brain critical to memory.</u> "It's not a matter of whether you experience stress or not," Albert concluded in an recent article in *Psychology Today*. "It's your attitude toward it."

If you would like to learn how to deal with your stress effectively and mind your memory, turn to Chapter 5 and develop some stressbuster strategies.

BUILDING MENTAL MUSCLE

Feeling absent-minded lately? Here are some things that might help you hold on to your thoughts.

1. **Get some regular aerobic exercise.** It boosts circulation to the brain and has the added benefit of reducing your risk for heart attacks and stroke. Brisk walking would do it.

2. **Can the brew.** Alcohol slows your reaction time and kills brain cells. Moderate use of red wine (one glass per day) can protect against heart disease and promote longevity, according to French studies. In another twenty-year study of 4,000 male twins, men who drank one alcoholic beverage per day had better learning and reasoning abilities in their sixties and seventies than their teetotaling siblings. Others say that even one drink of alcohol can reduce your reaction time and make it difficult to store information. If you can limit yourself to one glass, most experts say go ahead and drink up. But more than that one glass per day can lead to a host of other problems, especially if you drive. For women, who are affected by alcohol to a greater degree than men, there is more liver damage. Some experts say that more than four drinks a week increases the risk of breast cancer, though it reduces your heart disease and osteoporosis risk.

As usual, the door swings both ways. There are well-documented health risks for heavy drinking, including increased risk of cancer, liver disease, and heart attacks as well as increased spousal abuse.

3. **Kick the caffeine.** It causes insomnia and raises cholesterol and therefore may lead to arterial plaque, which of course is related to hypertension, stroke, and circulatory problems to the brain cells.

4. **Feed your brain.** There are many vitamins, minerals, and amino acids that help feed your brain. See Chapter 11 for a full description. Your brain isn't stupid. It wants protein, fruits, and veggies and all the B vitamins and minerals and amino acids so it can handle running your body. You think it's easy being a brain?

   Your brain can't work for you at top speed all your life if you load up on sugar, refined carbohydrates, and junk food. Author Barry Sears, Ph.D., who wrote *The Zone*, says, "Genetically, there's virtually no difference between you and your ancestors who walked the earth 100,000 years ago. In fact, mankind's genes have not changed substantially for the past one million years." And there were no doughnut shops back then either!

   Important minerals for your brain include zinc (eat your pumpkin seeds) and boron (high in dried fruits like dates, prunes, and raisins).

5. **Ginkgo who?** Ginkgo biloba. It's an extract made from the leaves of the ancient Ginkgo biloba tree. Living fossil records date these trees back 200 million years, so I really do mean ancient!

   In the 1950s German researchers began studying the medicinal properties of the ginkgo leaves. There are currently more than four hundred published studies on the effect of ginkgo leaves in treating memory problems, circulatory problems, depression, and Alzheimer's and on its nerve protecting properties. For patients recovering from stroke and minor head injury, it has also been a boon. It is devoid of any serious side effects. One clinical study showed an improvement in memory, mood, and even ringing in the ears after only eight weeks of taking 120 to 240 milligrams a day of the ginkgo leaf extract.

   At the Sixth Congress of the International Psychogeriatric Association held in Berlin in 1993, investigators reported on a six-month study of 212 Alzheimer's patients who showed significant improvement in memory, attention, and mood after taking 240 milligrams of the standardized extract per day.

   How does it work? Ginkgo's seemingly magical benefits come about because of the powerful bioflavonoid antioxidant action of quercitin, kaempferol, and isorhamnetin and by the action of terpene lactones, which <u>increase circulation to the brain and protect brain and nerve cells in the body.</u> Ginkgo biloba extract is available at health stores.

6. **Dust off your notebooks.** Take a course in something, read up on the classics, but pay attention and use your mind daily. It pays off in the long run. You've heard that old saw "Use it or lose it." Perhaps the reason that saying has hung around so long is because it is so true. I've also noticed that people who are learning new things are interested in and interesting to others. One of the greatest complaints I hear in families is that their parents are living in the past, or that they sit around and have competitions with other family members about who's the sickest. Older people often complain about being lonely, but to be honest, who wants to hear only negative, depressing stories about the past or the daily monologue and each health complaint? Meet new people, take a class, read a book, keep yourself interested in life and interesting to those around you.

7. **Call on some stressbusters.** It's not about whether or not you experience stress—because a life without stress is impossible and undesirable—it's about how you perceive it and deal with it. If you feel that you are the captain of your own ship, you'll do better than if you feel out of control and overwhelmed by the events of your daily life. Your brain function is the beneficiary when you keep the stress hormones at low levels, because scientists think that the hippocampus, a small area of the brain that's critical to memory storage and retrieval, may atrophy under a constant load of stress biochemicals. If you're not too stressed out already check out some of the stressbuster strategies in Chapter 5.

8. **Melatonin.** In addition to helping the body toward more restful sleep, melatonin may be a free radical scavenger capable of protecting the brain against aging. Melatonin is a hormone of the brain's pineal gland that decreases in abundance over the years. In *Neuroscience and Biobehavioral Reviews*, researchers state that: "Melatonin promises to become a powerful pharmacological agent with its unique properties as a nontoxic, highly effective free radical scavenger which provides protection eventually from neuro-degeneration as well as from mutagenic and carcinogenic actions of hydroxy radicals."

9. **Get some sleep.** Who can think when you're too tired to stay awake? Most populations on the planet take a siesta at lunchtime. Sounds good, doesn't it? Have lunch, get cozy for a little nap, and then take on the world.

10. **Meditate on this.** People who meditate regularly have higher levels of DHEA. In

addition, *Psychology Today* recently quoted research that people who meditated daily had higher levels of melatonin than those who took 5 milligram supplements.

11. **Estrogen.** Estrogen replacement therapy has had a very controversial history and while doctors know that this drug can shield women from osteoporosis and cut the risk of heart disease, it is still unclear whether it can magnify the risk of breast and endometrial cancer. While that debate rages, a plethora of studies indicate that hormone replacement treatments may prove an antidote to forgetfulness, boosting memory and improving reaction time, verbal ability, mental alertness, and complex cognitive functioning in post-menopausal women.

In one interesting project, researchers recruited thirty-four postmenopausal women who were not taking estrogen. These women were subjected to a battery of tests, including a simulated driving test in which the subjects had to make fast decisions about road hazards. Compared to the control group of twenty-four women of childbearing age, the older women were not as quick in their responses. Then estrogen replacement therapy was given to the older women for sixty days and the tests were repeated. The women did significantly better and some of the older subjects scored results which were indistinguishable from those of the younger subjects. The results of this paper were presented in July 1995 at the International College of Neuropsychopharmacology meeting in Washington, D.C.

Almost 8,900 female residents of a Southern California retirement village called Leisure World were studied by researchers from UCLA Medical School. Among women who used estrogen replacement therapy Alzheimer's was 30 percent less likely than among the non-user control subjects. Another study of more than 1,000 women age seventy and up conducted by Columbia University's School of Public Health concluded that women who had taken estrogen for just a year were significantly less likely to develop Alzheimer's. Researchers estimated that taking estrogen for ten years may reduce Alzheimer's risk by approximately 40 percent.

Is estrogen the antidote for depression, Alzheimer's, and forgetfulness—or another double-edged sword with a controversial risk-benefit ratio? The research is very promising, but *caveat emptor*—let the buyer beware.

Forgetfulness, confusion, anxiety and depression are all symptoms that can overlap. In his book *Hypericum (St. John's Wort) & Depression* (Prelude Press), Harold Bloomfield, M.D., writes: " . . . depression often goes untreated because of the standard justifications 'It's just a phase' (for young people) and 'That's just part of getting older' (for older people)."

He recommends that depression should be considered if the "phase" continues for more than two weeks. St. John's Wort, a medically proven herbal supplement available in supermarkets and health food stores, is gaining rapid acceptance because it does not have the negative side effects of the prescriptive antidepressants like Prozac. He advocates a dose of one 300 mg. capsule of the herb, three times a day. Those taking antidepressant or MAO inhibitor medications should consult their doctor first.

MEMORIES FOR THE FUTURE: WHAT'S HOT

Phosphatidylserine. It's a natural phospholipid—the stuff brain cells are made of. It seems to enhance brain glucose metabolism and increase neurotransmitter receptor sites. In one small study, subjects aged fifty to seventy-nine who were suffering from memory impairment associated with aging were able to "roll back the clock" to a level twelve years younger than they were at the beginning of the study by taking the substance.

Ampakine. This is a prescription drug being developed by Gary Lynch, a psychobiologist at the University of California at Irvine, to increase memory in mild cases of dementia, stroke, and Alzheimer's disease.

Piracetam. Another prescription drug that may enhance cognitive function, this does not have FDA approval yet.

An antibody that might make you smarter. Jan Leetsma, M.D., of the Chicago Institute of Neurosurgery and Neuroresearch, put an antibody into rabbit brains and they learned more quickly. No word on how it works on pet owners yet.

Nicotine. Yep, it's the same thing you get from tobacco. It has some of the effects of a major brain neurotransmitter called acetylcholine, and it may improve brain functioning and memory tasks. Low concentrations may slow or prevent formation of plaque that is found in the brains of patients with Alzheimer's disease. Of course, tobacco use in the form of cigarettes or chewing tobacco is a known factor in developing cancer, so this cure for forgetfulness may kill you.

Deprenyl. It does not have FDA approval, but is used now for Parkinson's disease in some countries and may be tested as a new "smart drug" in the future.

DMAE. It stands for dimethylaminoethanol bitartrate, an ingredient that is found naturally in fish like anchovies. It's hot in Europe right now, and early clinical trials show promise in using DMAE to boost cognitive functioning of the brain.

Novel antioxidants. Nitrones, novel antioxidants designed to trap free radicals, have been shown to prevent the damage to brain proteins that leads to brain impairment. A nitrone named PBN is now being tested on humans by a research team in Kentucky to see if it can prevent the plaque formation of Alzheimer's disease.

Fetal nerve growth factor and Parkinson's disease. In Parkinson's disease, for no clear or determined reason, brain cells that produce dopamine deteriorate. Dopamine is a chemical messenger in the brain that controls muscle activity. When it is destroyed, tremors, balance problems, senility, and depression result. Eventually rigidity of the body occurs when 60 to 70 percent of the dopamine producing neurons are gone.

Neurosurgeons at Good Samaritan Hospital in Los Angeles are seeing success with clinical and surgical procedures using fetal cells that are seeded into the disease-destroyed parts of the brain.

JUST REMEMBER THIS . . .

More research is being done on memory all the time, but you *do* have to use your mind or you will lose it, because our minds can become couch potatoes too. Try turning off the TV tonight; watching TV is a passive experience for your gray matter and does little toward developing the incredible power of your brain. How about reading or doing a crossword puzzle or learning to play chess? Have you always yearned to play the piano? Sign up for some lessons. Studying a foreign language can be very stimulating. Or try your hand at pottery or perhaps an art or creative writing course at your local community college. Ever watch an old-time movie and sigh when you see Fred and Ginger cutting up the dance floor? Learn to tango this year. Clear your head by joining a choir. Save money on expensive Christmas gifts and learn woodworking or take a guilt-free dessert-making class.

Even listening to classical music can help stimulate your hidden brain power. A December 1993 study at the University of California at Irvine demonstrated that listening to *Piano Concerto for Two Pianos in D Major* by Mozart actually raised the listener's IQ by nine points. Even meditation and relaxation techniques didn't compare to classical music for the temporary swell it provoked in the intelligence quotient.

Goethe summed it up the best when he wrote: "Whatever you can do, or dream you can, begin it. Boldness has genius, power, and magic in it."

8 SKIN DEEP

To a newspaperman, a human being is an item with the skin wrapped around it.

—Fred Allen

$\mathcal{A}$s usual, there was a lot of commotion on the street. Commuter trains roared and screeched on the rusting steel structures overhead. Street vendors shouted back and forth as customers negotiated the price of fruits and vegetables at Brooklyn's famous 86th Street open-air market. Today, however, red flashing police lights and patrol cars blocked the street and all the delivery trucks, cars, and yellow checker cabs behind them honked their horns. Frustrated drivers leaned out of their car windows to yell obscenities at the cops, the crowd and anybody else within earshot.

Finally, officers strong-armed a young man out of a building and shoved him into the patrol car. "He's the guy up for murder one," said one of the bystanders. "But he has the face of an angel," countered another.

I've never forgotten that scene and the comment, "But he has the face of an angel." As if only an ugly person would be able to commit a crime.

We have many expressions in our language about appearance: "A face that would stop a clock." "Let's face it." "Let's not take this at face value." We talk about the "face" of a mountain, "putting on your game face," "a real poker face." Or we discuss a business "interface."

As we grow older, we are "faced' with our changing appearance. We get wrinkles. Hair retreats, and, if it sticks around, it turns gray. Makeup manufacturers and plastic surgeons harvest our fantasies about cosmetic perfection.

Looking older is hard on some of us, joy-producing for others. I remember finding my first gray hair and feeling a rush of excitement. I called up my big sister long distance in Canada and reported the news with a feeling of accomplishment. I was finally grown up. It felt great. Later that week, she sent me a card scrawled with the word, "Congratulations!"

But when a department store clerk urged me to try the latest skin cream "for your crow's feet" I was slightly less than pleased. Go figure. The key here is that, no matter what, there *is* probably some adjusting and acceptance to be done.

Most people assume that they are prisoners of time and that there is nothing that can be done to help their skin except plastic surgery. This is simply not true, but it is precisely that feeling of not having any control that drives people into depressions and anxieties over their skin. There are many new weapons in the arsenal to help keep your skin fresh and healthy.

HOW YOUR SKIN AGES

Most skin seems to show squint lines and other faint signs of aging around the age of thirty. By age seventy, wrinkles have usually formed just about everywhere. Liver spots, the large freckles of deeper pigmentation, can usually be seen on the face and neck, arms, and hands. These are primarily caused by exposure to ultraviolet light.

One of my oldest patients, at age one hundred, had been a construction worker most of his life, working outside in a short-sleeved shirt. When he took off his shirt, he looked like he still had it on: his head and neck and forearms were dark and leathery, and looked, well, a hundred years old. But the skin on his upper arms and chest and back looked brand new, like a ten-year-old's! It was amazing to see how young and soft the unexposed skin looked: not a wrinkle or spot. It was smooth, tight, and firm.

Exposure to sunlight causes various reactions that lead to thick and tangled fibers in the skin. The leathery look is due to the buildup of these fibers. The good news is that using sunscreen faithfully and avoiding tanning for a decade can help to heal the damage and, in some cases, reverse it. Some of the chemical peels can also reverse *photoaging*, the damage done to the skin by the sun.

Experts agree that sunlight produces more than 90 percent of the signs of aging skin and that it is the number-one cause of skin cancer. "Prevention and protection are going to be the biggest trends of the future," states Dr. William Fisher, M.D., a teacher of plastic surgery at UCLA and a board certified plastic surgeon in Southern California, who has his share of celebrity clients. Your children will probably look younger than you at the same age.

"As teenagers, they will be able to prevent the severe scarring of acne. By decreasing smoking and increasing ultraviolet protection early on, the skin will stay young and healthy-looking for a very long time," says Dr. Fisher.

WRINKLES

Dark, oily skins are the least wrinkle-prone, while fair-skinned people who sunburn easily usually notice wrinkling soonest. Wrinkles are caused primarily by damage to the dermis, the supportive tissue that underlies the skin we see. The dermal layers contain the firming collagen and stretchy elastin fibers that give our skin resiliency and strength. As the years go by, oil production, fibroblast cell renewal, and blood supply to the dermal layers, which are related to hormone and other metabolic changes, tend to slow down.

SAGGING

Our fat cells have a tendency to shrink with age. With the skin becoming less elastic due to decrease of elastin and collagen production, the skin doesn't reshape to the newer dimensions of the body and sagging occurs.

Some sagging on the body can be prevented. If the muscles atrophy from disuse, then regular weight training can keep the muscles "pumped up," causing the skin to appear tighter.

STRETCH MARKS

Most pregnant women worry about and suffer from stretch marks. But they're not the only ones. Weight lifters and body builders, children undergoing growth spurts, yo-yo dieters, and anyone who suddenly gains weight may develop stretch marks. They are caused when the skin is stretched beyond what the collagen and elastin fibers can handle. The result are striae, the silvery scar-like stripes that remain for life. Some nutritionists have used therapeutic doses of vitamin E (up to 600 milligrams per day), the B-complex, zinc, and vitamin C to prevent and help reduce the visible signs of stretch marks. The time-honored topical application of vitamin E during pregnancy to prevent stretch marks may be helpful, but it seems that one out of two women get the striations, so it is difficult to evaluate the success of this. Surgical tucks and some laser treatments have been successful in reducing the appearance of some of the larger striae.

UV INDEX: WHAT THE NUMBERS REALLY MEAN

Have you every wondered what the talk about a UV index is all about when you hear it on your local weather report? The ultraviolet index was developed by the National Weather Service. It's meant as a guide to predict how much sun exposure you're likely to encounter on any given day. The scale ranges from zero to fifteen.

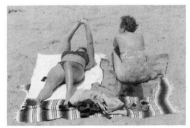

0–2 Minimal UV: It could take up to thirty minutes for unprotected skin to develop a sunburn.

3–4 Low UV: Unprotected skin could sunburn in fifteen to twenty minutes.

5–6 Moderate UV: There's a good risk of sunburn on exposed skin within ten to twelve minutes.

7–9 High UV: In about eight minutes, unprotected skin will probably burn.

10+ Very high UV: This is the most dangerous time for unprotected skin to be exposed to sunlight. At this rating, in less than six minutes, you'll be toasting.

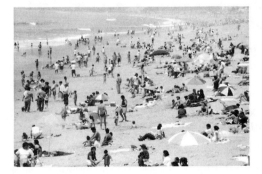

While it's true that your body converts certain elements of sunlight into vitamin D, which is essential for strong bones and teeth, given the increasing skin cancer rates in this country, you're probably better off taking a multivitamin. You only need 400 International Units (IU) per day.

Actually, there is no such thing as a safe tan. Like the sun, tanning parlors and sunlamps are very damaging to your skin. The ultraviolet light beamed on your skin at a tanning salon is five times the rate you'd get on a tropical beach. It is not somehow safer because you are getting the radiation out of a lamp. Given that over 90 percent of all the visible signs of aging of the skin are due to ultraviolet light exposure, perhaps tanning salons should be renamed *aging salons*.

Halogen light has also been linked to skin cancer. Keep all 20 watt halogen lamps at least twenty inches way from skin and all 35 to 50 watt lamps thirty-nine to fifty-nine inches away. On another safety note, be sure to keep halogen lamps from tipping, as a number of recent fires in college dorms were caused when the high-heat bulbs came in contact with flammable materials.

SKIN QUIZ

Most factors that age our skin are within our control. The first step toward improving your skin is learning something about it. Then you'll be ready to face the world with a smile, because regardless of whether you are seventeen or seventy, skin care begins with you. Test your skin savvy by answering true or false to the following questions:

1. A man's skin ages slower than a woman's.
2. A good soap is essential to hygienic cleanliness of the face.
3. Isometric exercises will prevent sags and wrinkles on your face.
4. Cold or ice water firms your skin.
5. Oily skins need to be washed more frequently.
6. A bracing aftershave is a must after a man shaves in order to close the pores and prevent skin irritation.
7. The best time to get a tan is between 11 A.M. and 3 P.M.
8. It is better to use hot water on the skin, especially in winter.
9. Collagen creams help replace lost collagen and prevent wrinkles.
10. Deodorant soaps are more hygienic and superior to regular soap because they help reduce skin bacteria.
11. Blepharoplasty is genetic.
12. If you rub garlic on your skin, the scent can be detected later on your breath.
13. Skin cells are regenerated every twenty-eight days.
14. Skin odor can be an indication of mineral deficiency.

15. Vegetarians' skin smells different than that of meat eaters.
16. Regular sunblock should never be used on your face.
17. Fair-skinned redheads and blondes are more wrinkle-prone than everyone else.
18. The nicotine from smoking enlarges the tiny capillaries that nourish the skin.
19. Smoking causes wrinkles around your lips.
20. If you live in a hard water area, you should use synthetic soap.

And here are the answers.

1. **True.** A man's skin is generally oilier and thicker than a woman's and does not age as quickly.

2. **False.** You don't have to use soap at all. Cleansing creams are gentler and, with them, you avoid drying the skin. Dry skin doesn't make wrinkles, per se, but it can accentuate your fine lines, making your skin appear older.

3. **False.** This is a tricky question though, so give yourself some freebie points on this one, regardless of how you answered. Isometric exercises firm the muscles under the skin, but not the skin itself. However, cardiovascular huff and puff exercise improves your circulation, bringing blood to the skin and flushing impurities out of the body. The glow of skin that sweats daily looks healthy.

   Consistent exercise retards skin aging because the skin's temperature can rise up to 15 degrees, which is thought to stimulate production of collagen cells.

4. **True.** Some scientists say nay, but I'm with the physical culturists who say yea. If you've ever taken a cold shower, you'll have to agree that the stimulating effects seem to affect not only your skin, but your psyche.

5. **False.** Repeated daily washings of oily skin doesn't get rid of the problem. It can actually stimulate the skin to produce even more oil to counteract the excess washing. Excessively oily skin could be caused by hormone imbalances, stress, a junk food diet, caffeine intake, or a combination of all these factors.

6. **False.** If your skin is dry, then a moisturizer will do the most toward helping to minimize the wear and tear of shaving. Aftershaves are typically alcohol-based, which is drying to the skin and useful only if skin infections are a problem.

7. **False.** This is when the sun's burning, destructive radiation is at its worst. There *is* no good time to tan, because sunlight is the number-one cause of premature aging of the skin and skin cancer.

8. **False.** In a cold-winter climate, your skin is so beat-up by the extremes of indoor/outdoor temperature differentials and drying indoor heat that using extremely hot water is adding insult to injury.

9. **False.** Collagen is a big protein molecule. If our skin pores were big enough allow the collagen *in*, they'd also be big enough to allow the collagen flow *out*. It doesn't happen. If you apply collagen cream to your skin, the collagen basically just sits there on top of the skin.

10. **False.** Deodorant soaps are harsh and they can create an imbalance in your skin's pH (acidity) levels. These soaps can also increase the skin's sensitivity to sunlight.

11. **False.** Trick question. Blepharoplasty is the medical term for an "eye lift."

12. **True.** An old folk remedy for colds and fever is to rub raw, cut garlic on the soles of the feet. A few minutes later, the garlic scent can be detected on the patient's breath.

13. **True.** In fact, in an average lifetime, we shed approximately forty pounds of dead skin.

14. **True.** A deficiency of the mineral zinc has been linked with strong body odor. Who could ever forget the mnemonic: "Take zinc, don't stink"? White flecks on the fingernails may also indicate a zinc deficiency. Zinc helps speed healing of wounds and increases resistance to infection, among other things.

15. **True.** Hunters and trappers of wild game often go on a strict vegetarian diet for several months before a big hunt so that the animals they are stalking do not smell danger from a meat-eating predator.

16. **False.** Get that sunblock out and use it. Sunlight is the number one cause of skin cancer.

17. **True.** Heavily pigmented skin and dark, oily skin is protected more from sun damage.

18. **False.** The opposite is true—yet another reason to quit.

19. **True.** The wrinkles occur from the way smokers inhale on the cigarette by pursing their lips and drawing in the smoke.

20. **True.** They rinse off your skin more completely, leaving less of a filmy soap residue to irritate your skin.

Give yourself 5 points for every correct answer. Check your score against the list below for your skin care IQ.

80–100 You're loaded with skin savvy. Keep up the good work. If you are putting into practice what you already know, your skin will be grateful to you for years to come.

60–80 You could stand a little refresher course on the facts of your body's largest eliminative organ—your skin. Arm yourself with some more facts and be nicer to your skin.

0–60 Your skin is crying out for help. Start a skin-deep fact-finding mission for yourself and launch a preventive program today. Your skin will thank you in the future.

SIX USEFUL TIPS

1. **Sunblock.** Use it early and use if often. You can get tan even from driving around in your car on a sunny day, because there is a lot of reflection from the hood of your car and your windshield does not block ultraviolet rays. Use a 15 SPF rated formula in the winter and a 30 SPF in the summer. Formulas containing titanium and zinc oxide are the most effective in blocking rays.

2. **Water.** Not the kind you wash with—the kind you drink. Eight to ten glasses a day of pure water will help flush out toxins and moisturize your skin from the inside out.

3. **Sleep.** If you're waking up more tired than when you went to bed, chances are you're not getting enough of this essential skin ingredient. During the first two hours of uninterrupted sleep, human growth hormone (HGH) levels are at their highest. HGH is the key factor in initiating cell repair. If counting sheep is not working for you, check out Chapter 6. Lack of sleep can make your skin puffy, blotchy, or sallow. Think of a cat nap as a mini-facial.

4. **Stop smoking.** It ages your skin. "Not only does regular intake of nicotine often give skin an unhealthy-looking grayish cast and less attractive texture and feel, but it literally diminishes skin's ability to heal itself," said Thomas D. Rees, M.D., clinical professor of plastic surgery at the N.Y.U. School of Medicine, in a study published in the *Journal of Plastic and Reconstructive Surgery*. In an examination of more than 1,100 face-lift patients, Dr. Rees and his colleagues found that heavy smokers were twelve times more likely to experience skin healing problems soon after surgery than were nonsmokers. Secondhand smoke is also identified by surgeons as an increased risk factor in healing after surgery.

5. **Sleep on a neck pillow.** This is a time-honored tradition for many Hollywood stars. It helps prevent creasing and wrinkling of the neck on the outside, and helps reinforce the natural curve of your cervical vertebrae on the inside. While we're on this

topic, avoid sleeping on your stomach; it's very hard on your cervical vertebrae from a wear and tear point of view, not to mention encouraging permanent press creases on your face.

6. **Feed your skin.** Eat your five servings of fruits and veggies per day and consider antioxidant supplements. Getting enough antioxidants is the key here. (See more details on antioxidants in Chapter 11.) The reason: As cells age, they accumulate lipid breakdown products called *lipofuscin* (ceroid pigments), which appear on the skin as brown spots, commonly called liver spots. Antioxidants are the main saviors as they help to minimize this lipid destruction. There are many antioxidant-rich foods that you can eat to enrich your daily intake. Additionally, flax seed oil has shown great promise as a skin healer in a number of preliminary studies because it supplies essential fatty acids that are often lacking in our modern diets. (Vitamins A, C, and E and Beta carotene are antioxidants that are abundant in fresh fruits and vegetables and whole grains. Examples: fresh carrots, oranges, green peppers, yellow squash.)

HERBAL SKIN CARE

Cosmetic companies make big money from our fantasies about youth and beauty. When you look at the labels on the various products, it's quite amazing to read those tongue-twisting lists of ingredients. Who knew that you could get that many chemicals for your money? Did you know that one hundred of the ingredients in cosmetics are suspected of being toxic? So says the National Institute of Occupational Safety and Health. Lipsticks, for instance, may contain dyes that cause cancer in laboratory animals.

After the outrageous price, one of the biggest surprises in antiwrinkle creams, especially eye creams, are that they contain petroleum distillates or hydrocarbon derivatives. Take mineral oil, for instance. It is manufactured from crude oil, a mix of liquid hydrocarbons separated from petroleum. Here's another good one: Have you ever read one of the cosmetic cream labels and seen "propylene glycol"? It's a popular moisturizing ingredient, and also an ingredient in industrial antifreeze. It is also well known for causing allergic reactions and sensitivities in skin. Other chemicals can act as deep irritants, causing increased blood flow to the area and modest swelling. Put into a crow's feet formula that increased blood flow and swelling causes the wrinkle tissue to puff out a bit, "reducing the appearance of fine lines and wrinkles," to borrow from an oft-repeated claim of the cosmetics industry.

One last wrinkle on this information: Hydrocarbons in skin tissue, when exposed to ultraviolet light (that is, sunlight), set off a cascade of biochemical free radical reactions—the very reactions that cause wrinkles in the first place. The petroleum distillates in the eye cream formulas may actually accelerate these reactions. The cream may have "seemed to be doing so much good" at the beginning, but, as time goes by, more free radical damage adds up to more wrinkles, so more cream is used and bought. And another consumer gets hooked in the cosmetics merry-go-round.

Our skin is our largest eliminative organ. And as we just discussed, it can be equally *absorptive* as well. A wise person once told me that you shouldn't put anything on your skin that your wouldn't put in your mouth. If you are tired of paying big money for a lot of chemicals, here are some time-honored recipes for a more natural approach to skin care. Herbs are nature's gifts to us, to be used with prudence and understanding.

SKIN CARE "RECIPES"

Herbal Bath

Luxuriating in a bathtub and inhaling the steamy fragrance of sweet herbs is surely one of life's sweetest natural pleasures, and it is a wonderful tonic for your skin and muscles. You need a muslin bag or a large square of soft mesh material for the herbs. Mix all the herbs listed below (or a mix of your own choosing) together loosely in the bag, tie the top securely, and then place in the tub. Pour on the hottest water that comes out of the tap, enough to cover the bag, and let it soak for ten minutes. Then fill the tub the usual way and climb in. You deserve it! Think virtuous thoughts.

FOR RELAXING NERVES AND SORE MUSCLES

1 handful of dried lavender flowers
1 handful of rosemary leaves
1 handful of chamomile flowers
1 handful of mint leaves

Any single one of the above or any combination of the above could be tried. Triple the amount when using only one herb.

Massage Oil

Touching the skin has healing powers. Swedish physiologist Kerstin Uvnas-Moberg found that gentle stroking can stimulate the body to release the hormone oxytocin, which blunts pain and blocks the release of other stress hormones.

    1 cup of sweet almond oil

    4 to 5 drops of an aromatic oil of your choice (even vanilla extract is very nice)

Apply the oil with caring hands to the tired body of a deserving person. A small amount of eucalyptus, cajuput, or arnica oil could be added for a deep penetrating action for relief of sore muscles. *Caution*: Keep oils away from eyes and mucous membranes.

Oatmeal Facial

This is good for blemishes and combination oily/dry skin.

    ¼ cup ground oatmeal (you can use quick oats)

    2 teaspoon honey

    1 teaspoon milk

Blend the honey and oatmeal well. If it seems too thick and unwieldy, add the milk. Apply to clean face and neck, avoiding the eye area. Leave it on thirty to forty minutes, and lay down with your feet up if you can. I've made this facial with just milk and oatmeal, heating the whole thing in a small enamel pot or double boiler first. After half an hour, use a washcloth with warm water to remove the facial. Finish with a mild astringent. *Caution*: If you do the milk and oatmeal recipe, do *not* laugh while it's drying. You will feel like your face is cracking.

Astringent

Astringent helps close the pores after a facial and is useful in helping to reduce blackheads and blemishes by removing excess oils. For an easy one, add two parts witch hazel with six parts rose water. Shake well in a glass bottle and apply with cotton balls. Refrigerate between uses.

Another old-time favorite that is exceptionally mild is to simply boil barley in water, then strain the water. After it has cooled, it can be applied liberally to the skin, stored in a glass bottle, and refrigerated.

Age Spot Remover

Freckles or age spots may be reduced by rubbing with castor oil. My great-grand-mother swore by the following recipe. She was Ukrainian, so I am surprised there is no garlic in this treatment. She grew her own horseradish, but you can buy it fresh at most better supermarkets these days. I am unaware if she did any double-blind studies with this recipe, so I offer it with a "proceed at your own risk" motto.

2 teaspoons of grated horseradish

4 tablespoons of old fashioned buttermilk

2 teaspoons dry oatmeal

Gently simmer the horseradish and the buttermilk in an enamel pot, covered, for about ten minutes on a medium heat. Add the oatmeal and make it all into a paste. Apply to freckles. It takes a week or two of daily applications to see the age spots fade. I usually leave the paste on for about ten minutes. In the meantime, stay out of the sun, as that will only increase the amount of age spot freckling. *Caution*: Avoid the sensitive eye area and mucous membranes of the body.

Note: If the above preparation is too much trouble for you, lemon juice or over-the-counter skin lighteners with hydroquinone will also fade unwanted age spots. Of course, you must use sunblock to keep the spots from reappearing.

Moisturizer

You can buy vegetable glycerin suitable for cosmetic purposes at most drugstores. The following glycerin and rose water formula has been around for a very long time. It's easy to make and smells wonderful.

3 parts glycerine

4 parts rose water

Keep in a glass container and shake well before using.

Also try rice bran oil. Added to bath water, it is so light that it's barely noticeable, but it helps counter dryness. I use one tablespoonful per tub.

Brittle Nails

I appreciated this one because I use an alcohol-based bactericide on my hands all day between patients and it is very drying to the hands and nails. You can buy the oil at a health-food store.

Place one drop of squalene oil (derived from fish liver) on each nail. Buff only about four or five times in one direction. It adds luster to the nails without nail polish.

Skin Care 101

Skin care does not have to be expensive or complex. The rules of the road are actually quite simple:

1. Cleanse your skin daily with a gentle soap or nonsoap formula lotion. Be sure that whatever you use does not leave a film. Wash a wine glass with it and you'll see whether or not a film has been left.
2. Use a moisturizer daily on the face, neck, and forearms.
3. Use sunblock daily. Make it part of your morning grooming habits: brush, floss, apply sunblock.
4. Drink plenty of water daily, eight to ten glasses per day.
5. Don't smoke or inhale the secondhand smoke of others.
6. Consider using an alphahydroxy, Retin-A, or the newer ascorbic acid (vitamin C) exfoliative products at night.

Anyone for a Peel?

If you still think a peel is something that grows around an orange, then we need to welcome you to the nineties. We're talking *chemical* peel here: a procedure performed most commonly for cosmetic reasons to enhance appearance and decrease fine lines and wrinkles. Chemical peels may also remove precancerous skin growths, soften acne facial scars, and even control acne.

Peels are not a substitute for plastic surgery if you feel the need to reach for cosmetic perfection, but they are becoming increasingly popular as the average person's affordable answer to the quest for "skin harmony," as we say in California.

Peels use chemical solutions, typically alphahydroxy acids, such as glycolic lactic or fruit acids, trichloracetic acid (TCA), or phenol. The principle at work is to improve and smooth the texture of the skin by removing its damaged outer layers. Sun-damage, superficial blemishes, and pigmentation changes may be corrected. TCA, for instance, is one of the few chemical procedures that works well on skin of color, because it does not depigment. The precise formula used may be adjusted to meet each patient's needs, but the results can be very good.

Are They Completely Safe?

Normally, a chemical peel is safe and gives good results when performed by a qualified plastic surgeon. While peels can improve the texture of your skin, they can also

PLASTIC SURGERY STATISTICS

According to the American Academy of Cosmetic Surgery, these are the number of surgeries performed in 1994.

Type	Women	Men	Total
Vein removal	327,467	12,233	339,700
Plumping (with collagen or fat)	243,769	31,711	275,480
Chemical peel	217,742	36,290	254,032
Liposuction	189,001	37,743	226,744
Hair transplant/restoration	13,234	197,276	210,510
Eyelid lift	72,139	18,350	90,489

cause stinging, redness, irritation, and uneven pigmentation changes and crusting of the skin. This certainly adds a wallop to the phrase "Suffer for beauty."

For one thing, in some states, it seems amazing that you must have a license to catch a fish, but you can drop acid on somebody's face with a minimum certificate of training. Leave it to the professionals and be sure to locate a board certified plastic surgeon. You can telephone first to check on this.

The strong phenol peels could have serious consequences like uneven color changes to the skin. Although infrequent, infection and scarring are still possible risks and phenol may pose a risk for patients with a history of heart disease. Normally, a chemical peel is a safe procedure if its performed by a qualified certified plastic surgeon with lots of experience.

"We have thirty-years of experience in our field with chemical peels," states Dr. Fisher. "In the hands of a skilled physician, the results can be quite wonderful."

Regardless of the peel formula or strength, sunscreen must be used diligently afterward.

PLASTIC SURGERY GLOSSARY

I've seen some really good plastic surgery results on patients and acquaintances, and I've seen some shiny, tight faces that look as if the skin is being traumatized when the person blinks. Going under the knife is certainly a personal choice. The following glossary of some of the most popular procedures is provided whether you are "window shopping" right now or simply trying to understand what you're reading and hearing about these days on the news and perhaps from your friends.

Having plastic surgery doesn't stop the clock. Your face will continue to age with time, but the effects can last for years.

Blepharoplasty (eyelid lift). For droopy upper lids and puffy bags below the eyes: removal of fat along with excess skin and muscle. Recovery time: Back to work in a week to ten days, and back to normal activities in three weeks. Risks: double or blurry vision, asymmetrical healing or scarring, infection, swelling, a rare condition called *ectropion*, in which the lower lids get pulled down, requiring a second surgery.

Botox. Botulism—yes, the same deadly toxin you worry about from eating poorly canned food—is injected in minuscule amounts between the eyebrows to paralyze the frowning muscles. Then you can't frown and the vertical frowning crease is attenuated. This procedure is not for those with overactive imaginations! Results last a few months and then the procedure is repeated. Risks: allergic reaction, infection, scarring.

Browlift (forehead lift). Drooping eyebrows, "hooding" over the eyes, forehead furrows, and frown lines are attenuated when the muscles and skin are removed or altered. Either an ear to ear behind the hairline incision or a newer endoscopic technique with a few smaller incisions is made. Recovery time: Back to work in seven to ten days. Risks: infection, scarring, nerve injury, asymmetrical lift, numbness.

Chemical peel. Alphahydroxy (AHA), phenol, or tri-chloracetic acid (TCA) and even Vitamin C derivatives are used to peel off the skin's outer layers, removing fine lines, wrinkles, and sun-damaged skin. Recovery time: If it's a mild AHA peel, same day. With the other peels it can take a week to ten days before you go back to work or up to six months until the pinkness disappears. Risks: infection, scarring, allergic reactions, uneven pigmentation, and heart arrhythmias (with TCA and heart patients).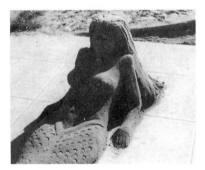

Collagen injections. For crow's feet and feathery wrinkles around the lips, the skin is plumped with injections of collagen. Risks: allergic reactions, infection, scarring.

Dermabrasion. Not as popular a procedure these days as it once was. Outer layers of skin are scraped with a motorized wheel to remove acne scars and fine wrinkles. Risks: scarring, infection, allergic reactions, herpes symptoms.

Face-lift (rhytidectomy). Jowls, sags, wrinkles, deep creases, and folds—this procedure is the granddaddy of them all for "setting back the clock." We're talking redraping the skin, removing the fat, tightening the muscles, getting rid of the excess skin. Recovery time: Back to work in two to three weeks, back to a normal routine in about a month. Risks: scarring, infection, poor healing of the skin in smokers, and temporary injury to the underlying nerves.

Laser. High-tech lasers are used in general surgery, in treating rosacea (an inherited skin condition) and in removal of tattoos and scars and wrinkle reduction. Laser resurfacing of the face involves perhaps the longest recovery time, with skin reddened for up to six months and a return to work only after a month or more. Basically, the process is similar to dermabrasion, but the skin is being burned instead of scraped. Some plastic surgeons are cautious about using lasers over large areas of skin at one time and may combine a variety of techniques, such as a traditional eye lift, laser around the mouth, and botox for the frown line between the eyes, to name only a few. Risks: scarring, infection, poor healing in smokers, and rare occurrences of a rash while the new skin is forming.

Nonsurgical scar removal. For recent or scars up to sixteen years old, there is a new method for removal that does not use drugs or surgery. Soft, pliable polymer sheets are applied over the scar for a few hours a day. An electrostatic ionic bonding process helps the skin actually rebuild from the inside out. It's effective on scars from surgical incisions, burns, cystic acne scars, and scrapes and cuts. This new product is available over the counter without a prescription under the brand name Rejuveness.

Tummy tuck. Excess fat is liposuctioned, excess skin is removed, and the abdominal muscles are tightened. The endoscopic technique with a few small incisions leaves less of a scar than the side to side incision. Recovery: Back to work in two weeks to one month. The scars can take up to two years to fade.

Vein Removal. More than 300,000 people had this done in 1994, according to the American Academy of Cosmetic Surgery. A saline solution is injected into the varicose or spider veins, which then collapse and disappear in a few weeks. Recovery time: Back to work in one day, while avoiding strenuous activities and prolonged sitting or standing for about two weeks.

WHAT YOU SHOULD BE ASKING IF YOU'RE THINKING ABOUT PLASTIC SURGERY

1. Is your doctor board certified in plastic surgery? This is an important question because anybody with a medical license can do cosmetic procedures. Call the

American Society of Plastic and Reconstructive Surgeons at (800) 635-0635 to find one.

2. Who is giving the anesthesia? Be sure it's a qualified anesthesiologist.

3. Does your doctor have hospital privileges anywhere? Hospital privileges mean that your doctor has been reviewed by his or her peers.

4. Has the office surgery center been accredited? The American Association for Accreditation of Ambulatory Surgical Facilities at (847) 949-6058 will tell you.

5. Who will be doing the surgery? Make sure you meet with the doctor who will be doing the actual surgery to raise any concerns you may have and to make sure *that* doctor is the board certified plastic surgeon who will be doing the entire surgery.

6. Also find out how much experience in your surgical procedure the doctor has; will there be a charge if you need a touch-up or "re do"; what are the risks of the procedure and what is the recovery time?

A QUICK WORD ON SKIN CANCER

The two most common types of skin cancer are *squamous cell carcinoma* and *basal cell carcinoma*. Squamous cell is seen in men more than often than women, except in the lower leg. The cancer appears as red, scaly plaques on the surface of the skin. Basal cell is a slow-growing cancer that is usually pigmented with melanin. These are both highly treatable and curable by surgery and exfoliating prescription creams. *Melanoma* is the deadly skin cancer that is highly malignant and is more common in lightly pigmented skin. It is usually diagnosed when a patient reports an existing mole that changes shape or color or bleeds. As always, your best bet is prevention, so schedule a skin examination with a dermatologist annually to have your skin inspected.

LOVE ME, LOVE MY WRINKLES

They say that beauty is only skin deep. As if anyone really wants to look all the way inside to your pancreas! Certainly, there is a lot more to us than how we look. You'll never get wrinkles if you never laugh or cry or frown or squint or pucker up your lips for a kiss. But if you never do all those things, then you're not alive.

Prevention is really the key. Don't smoke and avoid the smoke of others is the first rule toward protecting your skin and body. Prevention does *not* mean going around with a poker face all your life, but prevention in the form of an enthusiastic attitude toward life, sunscreen, a smoke-free environment, healthy eating, lots of water to drink, enough sleep, and plenty of exercise.

THE ABCS OF SKIN CARE

Here are warning signals of skin cancer you need to watch for:

A. If you have a freckle or mole that is asymmetrical in shape, see your doctor.

B. If the borders of a mole or freckle are uneven or changing, or if it bleeds, see your doctor.

C. If there is a change in color of a mole or freckle, see your doctor.

D. If the mole or freckle gets larger in diameter, see your doctor.

9 THE BARE FACTS ON HAIR

What he hath scanted men in hair, he hath given them in wit.

—William Shakespeare (1564–1616),
The Comedy of Errors

*Y*ou know how it goes . . . somehow you avoid combing your hair, because it's upsetting to see so many hairs left in the comb afterward. You try not to think about the alarming number of hairs you notice clustered around the drain every time you take a shower. You start examining old family photographs to compare your hairline then and now. You get that sinking feeling in your stomach when you look in the mirror, because it's hard to deny: You're losing your hair, and feeling older by the minute.

It's probably not that comforting to know, but hair loss typically occurs between the ages of twenty-five and forty. That seems so unfair when forty is not even considered middle age anymore.

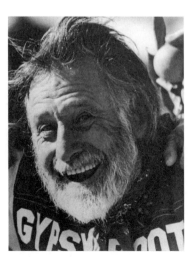

Most men worry about becoming bald as soon as they get their driver's license and resign themselves to it long before they receive social security.

"I have bad dreams at night about losing my hair," one man told me. "I wake up and keep trying to console myself with the fact that my father, at age eighty, still has most of his hair, but then I look at my brother, who is ten years younger starting to get a receding hairline, and I can feel crummy all morning."

Women worry about getting wrinkled, men worry about losing their hair. But women also experience hair loss as the years go by—an estimated 20 million of them, according to some experts. Women are protected somewhat from hair loss by higher estrogen levels, but if there is hair loss, it tends to be more uniformly over the entire head, while men lose their hair first at the crown or the hairline.

A man's hair tends to grow out of his head from follicles at a 90-degree angle on top. Women tend to have hair that is angled in the follicle. Some speculate that

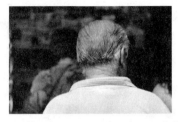

women's hair is therefore more capable of "running off" the oil or sebum which is produced, thereby preventing buildup which could eventually choke off the production of hair from the follicles on the crown of the head.

We have put rocketships on Mars and unravelled some of the deepest mysteries of the ocean, but to date, nobody really knows why hair falls out. What we do know is that baldness is most closely related with the following:

1. Age
2. Genetic inheritance of male pattern baldness
3. Testosterone, the hormone found in both genders, but in greater abundance in men
4. Nutrition
5. Prescription medications with a possible side effect of hair loss

THE HAIR-RAISING FACTS

Even children lose hair everyday. This is part of the normal cycle of hair growth and renewal. It takes nearly two to three months for a single hair to grow about an inch. And that same hair will continue growing for two to six years until it "rests" and falls out. This is the stuff you see in your hair brush, the resting hairs. It is normal to lose between fifty and one hundred hairs a day. In view of the fact that most adults have more than 100,000 hairs on their heads, that's not a lot.

The hair we brush and style and shampoo all the time is actually dead tissue composed of about 98 percent protein. There are two different kinds of hairs on our bodies. The fine *vellum* hairs that have very little pigmentation, are soft in texture, and almost invisible. Then there are the terminal hairs, which are thicker, coarser, and pigmented.

When a person begins to bald, the thick, terminal hairs are converted over to fine vel-

lum hairs. The size of the follicles shrink due to
normal aging processes. It happens only in the follicles that are programmed to do so by genetic
information that was present from the moment of
your conception.

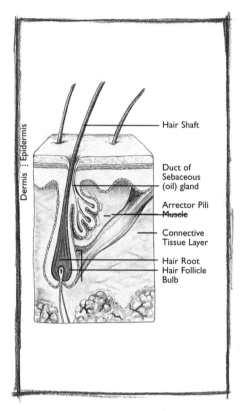

Therefore, if you are experiencing hereditary
balding, there is little that can be rubbed or eaten
or poured on the scalp that will alter the genetic
facts of your hair inheritance. At this point, we
could coin our own phrase and call it our
"inhairitance."

According to *The AMA Book of Skin and Hair
Care*, male pattern baldness becomes noticeable
in 12 percent of men aged twenty-five; 37 percent
of men aged thirty-five; 45 percent of men aged
forty-five; and 65 percent of men aged sixty-five.

IS ALL HAIR LOSS HEREDITARY?

There *are* some other conditions that could cause hair loss, and in these cases, hair
regrowth may occur in some individuals. Let's go through these one at a time and see
if anything here could be causing your hair loss.

1. **Major stress events.** Divorce, death of spouse or loved one, general anesthetic,
   stress, high fever, menopause, and childbirth are a few of the most common stressors. In the case of menopause and pregnancy, hormonal changes are the culprits.
   What seems to happen in the other cases is that the many of the resting hairs take
   a break—all at the same time, so the hair seems to fall out at a fast rate. These
   hairs usually comprise about 10 percent of all head hairs at any given time. A
   twenty-year old with a full head of hair has about 100,000 hairs—slightly fewer
   for redheads, slightly more for blondes. If you do the math, that amounts to a lot
   of hair, but the good news is that the hair usually grows back.

2. **Fad diets.** Fad diets are hard on the whole body, never mind your hair. If the diets
   are low in protein, scarce in carbohydrates, or supplemented by stimulants, then
   the body has to jump through hoops, as it were, to maintain its equilibrium. A

fad diet is a nutritional shock to the body. One unhealthy and dangerous practice I've seen is the use of cocaine to aid in weight loss. Data is scarce on this, but from my own experience in observing patients, I've noticed significant hair loss associated with the drug habit. As I took a friend to an eating disorders clinic at a prestigious hospital, I remember looking around the waiting room and noticing that many of the anoretic appearing patients were experiencing diffuse hair loss. The key is really simple common sense: You need to eat healthfully to maintain strong body tissues, which includes skin, hair, nails, and all the millions of other cells in the body that we cannot see, but which are just as important. Protein, complex carbohydrates, the B vitamins, vitamin C, minerals such as iron, zinc, magnesium, and sulfur as well the sulfur-bearing amino acids cysteine and methionine, are all major players. Between 4 to 6 percent of the body's total sulfur content is in hair.

3. **Anemia.** Women in their reproductive years may experience hair loss because of heavy menstruation combined with poor eating habits and resultant anemia. However, there are other causes for anemia: alcohol intake, hemorrhoids, thyroid dysfunction, aspirin intake, ulcers, fibroids, colon cancer, and chronic colitis and diverticulitis. All of these should be medically corrected. Iron absorption can be hindered by the phosphates in soft drinks, vitamin C deficiencies, copper deficiency, tea, antacids, and the oxalic acid in spinach. You need to eat iron-rich foods—like leafy green vegetables, whole grains, dried fruits, legumes, and molasses—to prevent anemia.

Symptoms of fatigue, tiredness, lack of stamina, and inability to concentrate may all be symptoms that the trace mineral iron is lacking, because iron is a constituent of hemoglobin, the red pigment of the blood which functions as an oxygen carrier. There are other forms of anemia due to folic acid and vitamin B12 deficiencies, and the symptoms are similar, so the exact cause of the anemia is important to diagnose. A simple blood test can give most answers.

Yet while a blood test can give a snapshot of what is occurring at the moment the blood is drawn, it does not show what is stored in tissues. Blood cells only live a few weeks, but hair grows slowly and mineral deficiencies or toxicities will be indicated by the hair and nails, for instance, over a long period of time. Hair is composed of 98 percent protein, but that remaining 2 percent will indicate much about minerals of the body. Even heavy metals will be detected if an analysis is performed on a hair sample.

Iron is an important mineral to the body because oxygen uptake by the hemoglobin in red blood cells fuels all the body's metabolic processes, including tissue regeneration and protein synthesis for products like hair and nails.

4. **Drugs.** Anabolic steroids, the illegal muscle-building drugs used by athletes, are a known cause for hair loss. Balding can be caused by blood pressure drugs (the betablockers), blood thinning agents (heparin), ulcer and arthritis medications, birth control pills, and a host of other prescription medications (cholesterol-lowering drugs, Parkinson's disease drugs, ulcer drugs, anticoagulants, gout drugs [Allopurinol], anti-arthritics, indomethacin [an anti-inflammatory], naproxen, tricyclic antidepressant drugs, and anabolic steroids [male hormones]). If you are on medication and have noticed hair loss recently, ask you doctor or pharmacist if it could be a side effect of your medication. Or, you could check out the *Physician's Desk Reference* at your local library and look up the prescription yourself. Always check your prescription drug insert sheet (that rolled up piece of paper stuck in the box of medication with all the small print).

5. **Physical conditions that affect hair growth:** Low thyroid output, arthritis, lupus, psoriasis, eczema, seborrheic dermatitis, low pituitary gland output, fungal infections, and polycystic ovarian syndrome, as well as the effects of chemotherapy and radiation can all lead to hair loss. Most of these conditions can be diagnosed by a blood test. The skin conditions of psoriasis, eczema, fungal infections, and seborrhea can be treated with topical solutions or creams. A low thyroid output is often noticed when the outer two-thirds of the eyebrows become sparse. Check it out with your doctor if you think your hair loss could be related to any of these conditions.

6. **Traction.** We're talking traction of the hair itself. Tight hairstyles such as chignons and ponytails, sleeping in or using rollers, tight braiding of the hair, or nervous habits of twisting or pulling on the hair all help to pull it out. It may or may not grow back after all the abuse. Even brushing the hair the old-fashioned one hundred strokes a night can cause excessive hair loss. Comb or brush your hair only enough to style it, say the experts. Avoid any hairstyle that creates tension on the scalp.

7. **Metal or other poisoning.** Aluminum, lead, and mercury are probably the most common.

    Cooking exclusively in uncoated cast aluminum pots could be a problem. Check your cookware for pitting of the inside surface. My mother was experiencing hair loss and after a very thorough workup we were still mystified until I noticed that she was cooking in the pots given to her as a wedding present almost fifty years before. The inside of the pots were quite pitted and rough. It was very hard wrestling those pots away from her because of the sentimental value, but, after a year or so, her hair started to grow back. I had another interesting find when a patient in her thirties complained of hair loss, and it turned out to be due to metal contamination from her well water.

The blood test that reveals the most information about heavy metal toxicity and amino acid deficiencies is called serum amino acid fractionation and it can be ordered by your doctor. An interesting auxiliary point is that the amino acid cysteine is often deficient in people with hair loss due to heavy metal poisoning as well as hair loss in general. Cysteine, like all other amino acids, has the important function of contributing to the structure of protein, in the form of cystine. Preliminary findings indicate that daily dietary supplementation of cystine does increase hair shaft diameter and hair growth density in certain cases of human baldness and hair loss. Note: Sometimes I am asked about the difference between *cystine* and *cysteine*. Cystine is created when two cysteines bond together; hydrogen is left and they become cystine. My research is that cysteine is a better supplement than the oxidized cystine. Cysteine levels have been found to be low in patients suffering from allergy, asthma, depression, rheumatoid arthritis, and hypertension (high blood pressure). Foods containing cysteine include: egg yolks, red peppers, cabbage, brussels sprouts, broccoli, cauliflower, mustard, and horse radish.

8. **Megadoses of vitamin A.** It's the "too much of a good thing" syndrome. The doses have to be very high and prolonged for this to happen in an adult. Yellowing of the skin, primarily the palms of the hands, can be a tip-off of vitamin A toxicity. The condition can be produced by "monster amounts of carrots (rabbits and carrot freaks take note) or by an inborn error of metabolism" states the classic textbook, *Robbins Pathological Basis for Disease*. If it sounds like your hair loss could be due to this overdose of vitamin A you need to stop eating pounds of carrots every day.

9. **Cosmetic trauma.** Bleach, perms, hair color, excessive blow drying, harsh shampoos, and back combing or "teasing" of hair can also lead to hair loss, especially in women.

GROWING IT BACK

Some men have made baldness a handsome look. The late Yul Brynner and Telly Savalas and the very much alive Montel Williams and Michael Jordan come to mind.

Given the general social acceptance of male balding and the general rejection of female balding, the shaved head look seems to work best with men, aside from the efforts of female entertainer Sinead O'Connor. Since baldness is not a disease, it seem ludicrous to talk about a "cure," however, there are a few options currently available.

Minoxidil. Minoxidil, sold under the brand name Rogaine, was originally developed to control high blood pressure. Not all people with thinning hair are candidates for it, but it is successful in 20 to 30 percent of those who try it. Rogaine is used by both men and women; it helps grow new hair as well as helping you keep the hair you have. For hereditary hair loss, it is approved by the FDA as a prescription drug and it takes about four months to see a difference. Unlike some more outlandish and unsuccessful preparations that have been used for centuries, Rogaine is colorless and odorless, but it is rather expensive. It must be applied twice a day for at least four months before you can tell if it's working. The only drawback is that if you stop using it, you will lose all the new hair plus any of the hair you would have normally lost as part of your hereditary cycle.

Tricomin solution. It works by preventing the existing follicles of the hair from going into the dormant cycle. New follicles were also stimulated in clinical trials. Expect FDA approval in a few years.

Diazoxide. This drug appears to dilate blood vessels in the scalp and thereby stimulate new growth and encourage existing growth to remain. Rogaine works via the same biomechanism. Diazoxide was initially developed as a pancreas drug, but seems to help hair growth when applied to the scalp.

Electrical stimulation. There are spas and beauty parlors that offer these treatments. Galvanic electric current is used and it feels slightly tingly, but not painful. Galvanic stimulation is used on the body for physical therapy treatments to relax muscles, and facialists also use the low volt current when relaxing the musculature of the face. I use galvanic stimulation for muscle relaxation in my office on patients, and it is very effective. I've also had it used on my face by a facialist and it was very relaxing (I fell asleep) and healing to the skin. It felt like I was getting a high-tech massage on my face. But does it work on your scalp to grow your hair back? Scientists in Canada are at work on this one, but in the meantime, it does feel very good and you might, as I did, at least get a good nap out of it.

Risks: Electrical stimulation is contraindicated in the presence of infection, cancer, diabetes, or active tuberculosis. It should not be used over the eyes, over recent scars, or over the carotid arteries.

Hair transplants. These have changed a lot over the years. The early transplants from about thirty-five years ago involved taking whole clumps of up to twenty follicles of hair at a time and transplanting them from the back of the head into bare parts of the crown. Unfortunately, the results were very easy to spot and often resembled an aerial view of the corn rows in Iowa.

Thankfully, both technology and the surgical techniques have improved with micrografting, which allows one hair at a time to be transplanted. A more natural look can be achieved. Risks: infection and scarring. This procedure is usually used on women, who do not generally lose hair in any one area, but experience a more diffuse hair loss over the entire head.

Scalp reduction. The bald scalp is cut away and then the scalp with hair on it is stretched from the sides and back of the head, up and over the crown. It's mostly done on men with typical male pattern balding. Risks: infection, large scars.

Hair weaves. This is a cosmetic procedure in which either real or synthetic hair "extensions" are spliced into existing hair. The weaves must be redone every six weeks or so as the hair grows in.

Also, it is important to keep the hair you do have healthy. The important hair nutrients are: the B complex of vitamins including B6 (in whole grains), vitamin C (in citrus fruits), as well as the minerals iodine (for proper thyroid function), sulfur (in cruciferous vegetables like broccoli and brussels sprouts), magnesium, manganese, and the "ZIP" hair factors: zinc, iron, and protein. If you eat green, leafy vegetables and whole grains, you'll be looking after the minerals. Magnesium is an essential element of chlorophyll. Concentrate on getting as much protein as possible from vegetarian sources like tofu and tempeh. It'll make your heart happy and healthy as well.

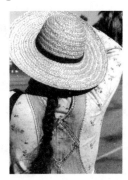

THE FUTURE OF OUR "INHAIRITANCE"

We talked earlier about how, from the moment of conception, we are either programmed for hair loss or we're not. But the story gets more interesting. Recent research has shown the way toward a spate of new products that will target only those follicles programmed to give up their hairy tenants.

Each follicle seems to be genetically programmed with a predetermined number of receptor cells for *DHT*, dihydrotestosterone, which is converted from the more well-known, plain old testosterone we're all familiar with. Those follicles that are programmed to go bald have been found to contain twice as many receptors for DHT as their hairier counterparts. DHT also appears to make the follicles go into their resting phase faster, which then causes the hairs produced by those follicles to become thinner and thinner with each growth cycle.

Recently a U.S. patent was granted to a product called Kevis that has been successful in clinical trials in Europe. It is a liquid which, when rubbed on the scalp, acts as a blocking agent on the DHT receptors sites at the follicle level. By binding the 5-a-dihyrdotestosterone receptors, the follicle remains intact and keeps producing hair. However, if a man or woman is already bald and shiny on top, there is little that DHT can do. Double-blind placebo studies on Kevis have already been initiated and, so far, there are promising results. Further testing is being planned as the product scrambles for an FDA approval process.

Regardless of our "inhairitance" though, hair does thin as we age. Hairs are generally thickest in diameter when we are in our twenties. At that point, strands measure in at about 101 microns wide. (For those of us who have not completely made the conversion to the metric system, a micron is one-millionth of a meter and a meter is just a little over a yard.) After our second decade, there's a fairly consistent rate and pattern of thinning, unlike balding or graying. Each decade sees a small decrease in strand size until we reach the half-century mark. From age fifty to age seventy, hair slims down to about 80 microns, the fine diameter we knew previously when we were babies.

THE GRAYING OF AMERICA

What color is gray hair? Not as dumb a question as it seems. You see, the odd thing about gray hair is that it really isn't gray. What's happening is that the pigment of the hair that is produced in the hair follicles is slowing down. Eventually, when most people reach their seventies or eighties, there is no pigment produced at all, and then the hair is colorless, or white.

The time schedule and pattern of the graying is mostly genetic, although a B12 vitamin or paraaminobenzoic acid (PABA) deficiency or even anemia may all lead to premature graying. In these cases, it is possible that graying may be reversed when the deficiency is corrected. However, if you are thinking of reversing the gray by using hair dyes and colorings, read on so that you can use the safest products.

DANGER IN A BOTTLE

A lot of people's gray hair stood on end when, in January 1997, the *Journal of the American Pharmaceutical Association* published a report stating that some popular dyes for darkening gray hair have so much lead in them they endanger children and adults and should be pulled from the market. Scientists at Xavier University in New Orleans, led by environmental toxicologist and professor Howard Mielke, singled out five leading cream, foam, and liquid formulas with lead acetate contents ranging from just under 6,000 parts per million to just over 2,000 parts per million.

The research team said that some shampoos contain up to ten times the lead concentration permitted in household paints. Paint may contain no more than 600 parts per million of lead. All of the products listed in the report as unsafe were of the "progressive" type—they worked gradually to change hair color over a period of several days to weeks.

Lead acetate works to accomplish the slow shift in hair color because it binds with the protein in hair and darkens it. The problem is that the lead acetate also leaves a residue on the hands. Users of the shampoos will retain between 17 to 20 micrograms of lead on each hand, even after hand washing. The federal limit for daily intake of lead is 6 micrograms for children and 30 for adults. The problem is that the lead can be transferred to other common household surfaces, such as a telephone receivers, hair dryers, or faucets, used by other members of a household, which is especially hazardous for children.

The tests done by the Xavier research team caused the scientists to state that "a user of such products becomes a living purveyor of lead contamination."

What can be done about all this? Check the ingredients of the hair coloring you use or are thinking of using. Does it contain lead acetate? Until federal regulators get tough on the manufacturers, consider switching products. Or, think about coming out of the bottle and "going gray" like the rest of America. The good thing about going gray is that at least you have the hair to go gray!

WHAT ABOUT DANDRUFF?

The skin of the scalp, like skin in general, seems to become drier with age. Normal dandruff from drying of the scalp is seen as dry, white scales. If the flakes are a yellowish-gray, gray-brown, or oily yellow scales, they could be due to a skin condition called seborrhea. If the skin is also inflamed and irritated, the nutrition of the hair follicle could be impaired, and baldness could result. So, if dandruff persists in spite of the usual over-the-counter shampoo remedies, consult a dermatologist. For a simple dry scalp and dry hair, I offer the following, which has been helpful to me.

Natural Hair Remedy for Dry Hair and Dry Scalp

Hot showers, saunas, sunshine, and jet air travel really give my hair a beating. A very kind elderly lady from Paris first mixed up this hair ointment for me. She recalled a time more than half a century before when, as a young girl, she had worn her hair down to her waist. Her mother had told her to care for her hair this way: apply the mixture, shampoo with castile soap, and then finish with a rinse of chamomile tea to assure highlights. My hair seems to thrive on this formula, which I use every six weeks.

> 1 cup of honey
> ¼ cup of olive oil
> ¼ cup of almond oil

Mix ingredients a few days before you intend to use the ointment and store it at room temperature. No need to refrigerate. Shake well before using.

I massage this gently, but very thoroughly into my hair and scalp and leave it on for at least thirty minutes. Be careful about going outside with this on your hair—bees, wasps, and all kinds of insect creatures will go wild over you. Wash out with your favorite shampoo.

FEED YOUR HEAD ON THIS

In gathering data for this chapter, I conducted an informal poll among friends and associates. Two important findings of this unofficial survey with no affiliation to any major university or medical center are as follows.

Of the things that upset women about men's appearance, baldness does not even

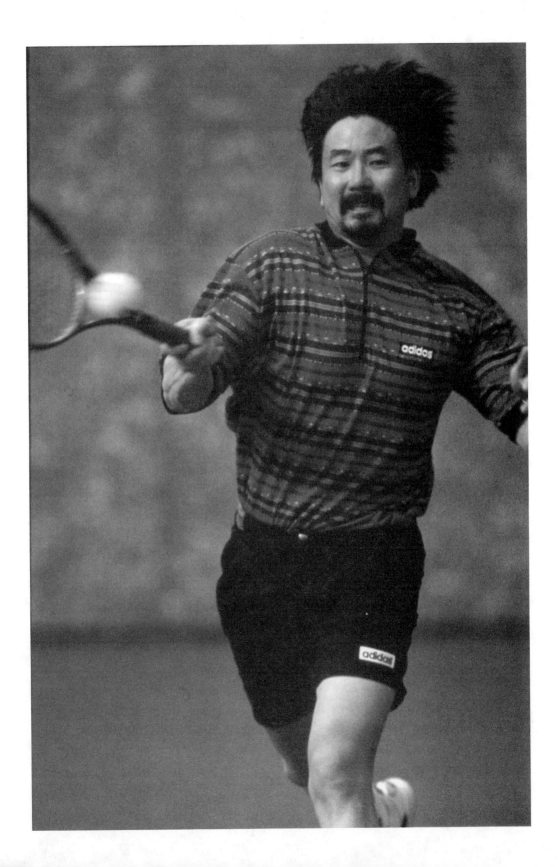

make the top ten. Unattenuated boorishness, a big, saggy buttocks, untrimmed nose or ear hair, and body odor are the most consistent top five turnoffs.

Of the things that upset men about a woman's appearance, hair loss is also *not* on the list. Lack of physical conditioning, poor grooming, body odor, bad teeth, and boorish behavior, including annoying speech habits ("like, ya' know" and cursing) are the most frequent on men's pet peeves lists about women.

Do you see a trend here? Perhaps what we need to focus on is the fact that a fit, vital person will always have personal power and magnetism far beyond what could be provided by mere pile of protein on your head.

10

WINNING THE WAR ON GRAVITY

Being entirely honest with oneself is a good exercise.

—Sigmund Freud (1856–1939),
Origins of Psychoanalysis

*I*f you could have all the riches in the world . . . or your health, which would you chose? Odds are you'd choose the latter. The good news is that staying healthy for a long, long time is amazingly simple to achieve. The first step? Get in shape.

Everyone can get stronger, and every time you do something for yourself in the fitness department, it is an investment in your future. The effects of a lifetime of fitness are cumulative, like money in the bank, like savings you work for in your thirties, forties, and fifties that accumulate so that you can enjoy your seventies, eighties, and nineties. Just as the money you've already saved is still in the bank even if you temporarily stop saving, should you happen to fall out of a fitness plan for a week, a month, or even a year, your body retains memory of the route to fitness, and you have only to guide it back. The return trip will be much quicker than the original journey.

It's a tragedy that so few people really learn to be as strong and alive as they can be. Why live a half-life, always feeling too tired to cope? Socrates said, "No person has the right to be an amateur in the matter of physical fitness. What a disgrace it is for a man to grow without ever seeing the beauty and strength of which his body is capable."

Getting stronger is not only important for athletes. Muscular strength and sculpting a new shape for your body is exciting and fulfilling, and it doesn't matter whether you are rich or poor, tall or short, female or male. It feels good to feel strong. And that can do wonders for your self-esteem. Thank goodness nobody has figured out how to tax it yet! At the times in my life when I've been poorest, I was living on a skateboard budget. Yet when I ran down the street, my body handled like a finely tuned Porsche. The state of the economy, pollution, and the actions of others are all things over which we have little or no control. We all have a need to feel good about ourselves, and having physical control over the strength and energy of your own body is something that no one can take away from you. Not even time. It belongs to no one but you. And as the world moves toward harder times, this precious self-mastering takes on increasing significance. In the chaos that is happening around us, we need at least to be in complete physical command of ourselves—to have the strength to cope, to remain rational and to retain positive values. This is to have achieved personal freedom.

Vic Boff, one of the world's pioneers in physical fitness, has said, "Always remember—the care of one's body is a sacred responsibility—the first you accept and the last you lay down."

WHY EXERCISE IS THE KEY TO POWER AGING

1. **You'll live longer.** Those who are physically fit and participate in regular exercise throughout their lives have substantially and dramatically lower risks of many diseases. Lower incidences of heart disease, high blood pressure, stroke, and diabetes. Exercise raises your immunity and protects you from illness ranging from cancer to the common cold. HIV-positive patients are advised to exercise to improve immune functioning. Exercise can cut your risk of heart attack by half. One ten-year study of 17,000 Harvard alumni, ages thirty-five to eighty-four, found that when the least active men were matched against those who exercised the most, the least active men had a 200 percent increase in death from cardiovascular disease.

   Another 7,000-person study of life expectancy in Alameda, California, demonstrated that a healthy regime of regular exercise, not smoking, moderate alcohol consumption, good eating habits, and regular, sound sleep, could add up to twelve years to a person's life.

2. **You'll live better, as well as longer.** Here's a list of some of the many functions and systems of the body that benefit from exercise.

- Arthritis. Weight lifting builds muscle and flexibility. Less stress is then put on the joint. A Finnish study found that when it comes to knee pain, exercise did more to relive the pain than antiinflammatory drugs or rest.
- Balance. It's a skill that you need to practice. It's important for preventing falls.
- Blood clotting. Your blood likes exercise too! Regular aerobic exercise seems to thin the blood by expanding plasma, the fluid part of blood. It also lowers the level of fibrinogen, a blood protein related to clotting, and makes platelets less sticky. Platelets are the tiny parts of blood that also work to help blood clot. Altogether, your risk of stroke and heart attack are lowered, because exercise dissolves or prevents blood clots.
- Blood pressure. Regular aerobic exercise helps to lower blood pressure.
- Blood vessels. Capillaries are the smallest blood vessels in the body and their job is to deliver food and oxygen to cells and help carry off waste products. Active people actually have more capillaries than sedentary people. The body grows more to meet the increased demands by the cells during exercise. The end result is more oxygen and nutrients delivered to the cells, and more waste products, such as carbon dioxide and lactic acid, carried away. End result—you feel more energy.
- Bones. Exercise strengthens bones and helps prevent osteoporosis.
- Breast Cancer. Exercise decreases the risk up to 60 percent.
- Cancer. Exercise helps reduce all cancers by enhancing immune system function.
- Cholesterol. Cholesterol levels are lowered by exercise.
- Constipation. Exercise promotes bowel contraction. That's why exercisers have up to 80 percent less colorectal cancer; the increased contractions speed irritants that could be cancer causers and reduces their contact time with the lining of the colon.
- Depression. After a workout, the body releases opiatelike substances called endorphins and enkaphlins that reduce pain and contribute to a sense of well being, even euphoria.
- Diabetes. One of the best ways to avoid getting it is to keep in shape, because obesity is a major risk factor for adult-onset diabetes. And those with Type II (adult-onset) are often able to reduce their insulin needs through a disciplined exercise program monitored by their doctor.
- Fatigue. Many folks shuffle through life, too tired to cope, simply because they lack the body strength to stand up straight and cop an attitude. Working out is like putting high-octane fuel in your system to fight stress and fatigue.

- Fertility. Women who are too skinny or overweight may have trouble conceiving. Keeping your weight in line with a moderate exercise program may help.
- Hearing loss. Some experts think that hearing loss may be due, in part, to hardening of the arteries that feed the ear and high blood pressure. Exercising aerobically on a regular basis will help keep blood pressure down and stimulate blood circulation.
- Heart. Exercise strengthens your heart, improving circulation and oxygenation to every cell in your body, and cutting your risk of heart attack.
- Incontinence. Urinary incontinence has a high cure rate when Kegel exercises are done. Turn to Chapter 19 to read all about it.
- Lung capacity. Exercise helps increase your lung capacity.
- Mental acuity. In a study done at Scripps College, in Claremont, California, highly active exercisers ages fifty-five to ninety-one were compared with a same-age sedentary group. The researchers found the exercisers had higher performances on all the reasoning tests and on two out of three memory tests.
- Metabolism. Exercise stimulates your metabolism, helping you feel more energetic.
- Muscles. A firm body is always in style, and toned, fit muscles also contribute toward stimulating body metabolism, sometimes up to 15 percent. This means that you can eat more and not gain weight, a bargain by any standards.
- Pulse. Exercise lowers your resting pulse rate. This means that your heart, by getting stronger and more efficient, can have more of a rest between each heart beat. This also helps you feel more relaxed.
- Sexuality. Research has shown that regular aerobic exercise, twenty to thirty minutes, at least three times a week, can improve sex drive and performance. One study at Bentley College in Waltham, Massachusetts, found that women in their forties who swam regularly were, when compared to sedentary counterparts, as sexually active as women ten to twenty years younger.
- Sleep. Active people with a healthy active lifestyle that de-stresses, tend to sleep better, which is common sense. One caveat though: Save intense workouts for earlier in the day, because the postexercise boost in metabolism can keep you wide awake.
- Snoring. Being overweight may cause you to snore more than a thin person, because of the pressure of fat tissue in the throat area. If you would like to snore less, then trimming body fat through regular exercise and good eating habits may help.

- Stress. Regular aerobic exercise is thought by some experts to be more effective as a de-stressor than drugs. Exercise stimulates the production of endorphins—natural, opiatelike substances that release the mind and body, causing relaxation and a sense of well-being. Of course, regular exercise strengthens the heart, helps you get a better body and can increase your self-image, and because it's free (except for the cost of sneakers), it's got to be the cheapest psychotherapy around.

- Stroke. Study after study supports the fact that exercising will reduce your risk of stroke. A study from Britain showed that the earlier in life you start exercising, the greater you cut your risk: Women who started between the ages of fifteen and twenty-five had a 63 percent less risk; those who started to huff and puff aerobically between the ages of twenty-five and forty cut their risk by 57 percent. Even the late bloomers who waited until the ages of forty to fifty-five were still able to cut their risk of stroke by 37 percent.

- Weight reduction. This one is really a no-brainer, because it's a simple equation of energy in versus energy out. Do you know that if you didn't change one thing about how you are eating right now, but walked briskly for just three miles a day, that you would lose approximately one pound every seven to ten days?

SIX REASONS WHY WORKOUTS WORK

I read this little piece in a newsletter, and the author was listed as unknown, so we won't know who to thank for this wonderful bit of inspiration that was entitled *Why Workouts Work*:

A workout is 25 percent perspiration and 75 percent determination.
Stated another way, it's one part physical exertion and three-parts self-discipline. Doing it is easy once you get started.

A workout makes you better today than you were yesterday.
It strengthens the body, relaxes the mind, and toughens the spirit. When you work out regularly, your problems diminish and your confidence soars.

A workout is a personal triumph over laziness and procrastination.
It's the badge of a winner, the mark of an organized, goal-oriented person who has taken charge of his or her destiny.

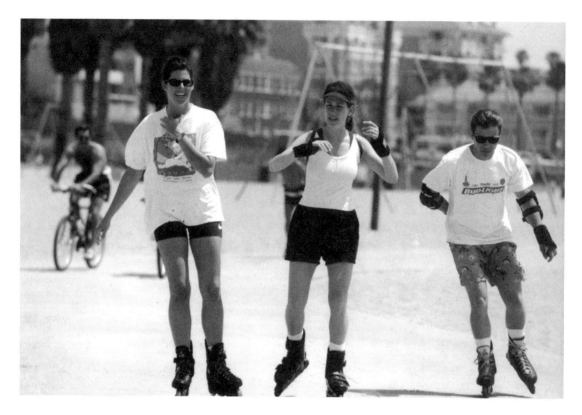

A workout is a wise use of time and an investment in excellence.
It's a way of preparing for life's challenges and proving to yourself that you've got what it takes to do what's necessary.

A workout is a key that helps to unlock the door to opportunity and success.
Hidden within each of us is an extraordinary force. Physical and mental fitness are the triggers that can release it.

A workout is a form of rebirth.
When you finish a good workout, you don't simply feel better—you feel better about yourself.

THE FOUNTAIN OF YOUTH: CARDIOVASCULAR FITNESS

A few years ago, the word *cardiovascular* was heard only in the hallowed halls of academic institutions. But now, this odd word that comes from two ancient cultures is a

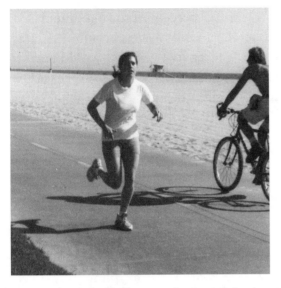

likely candidate for the evening news. *Cardio* comes from the Greek word *kardia*, for heart. *Vascular* comes from the Latin word *vasculum*, which means "small vessel." So when we use the expression "cardiovascular fitness," we mean the strength and condition of your heart and of all your arteries, right down to the smallest capillary, which is so tiny that the blood has to march through one blood cell at a time. The biggest blood vessel, the aorta, which stems directly from the heart, is about as big as a garden hose. Can you imagine the force of the blood as it ricochets around the curving aorta when the full muscularity of the heart is pumping out blood?

Exercise that makes you huff and puff—biking, running, walking, rowing, swimming, cross-country skiing—is considered *aerobic* exercise. Aerobic activities use your body's major muscle groups, stimulate your heart rate and breathing, and are something that you can keep up for at least twenty minutes to an hour. This combats aging and makes you feel younger, with more energy and a leaner body. Not only that, but aerobic exercise helps you to live longer by cutting your risk for heart attack, stroke, cancer, and a host of other health problems.

Most experts agree (and that's quite something in itself) that the minimum of aerobic activity needed to give you all the wonderful effects of cardiovascular fitness is thirty continuous minutes of exercise that raises your heart rate between 60 to 85 percent of its maximum.

HOW TO DETERMINE YOUR HEART RATE

Find your heart rate by lightly touching your fingers on the radial artery at your wrist (that's the thumb side of your wrist). Here is a matrix to help you find a safe range from the American College of Sports Medicine:

1. Subtract your age from the number 220. For instance, if you are forty-five years old, your maximum heart rate would be 175 beats per minute.
2. To get the best cardiovascular health from workouts, a forty-five-year-old should

aim to get his or her heart rate to between 60 and 85 percent of the maximum 175. That 60 to 85 percent, in this case, would be 105 to 149 beats per minute.

3. Now for the last part of this fitness equation: A forty-five-year-old would need to keep a heart rate of 105 to 149 beats per minute for thirty minutes at least three times a week to achieve the maximum cardiovascular benefit.

WORKOUTS TO MAKE YOU LOOK AND FEEL YOUNGER

How do you know which aerobic activity to chose? The most important thing is to pick one that you will enjoy. If you hate getting your face wet, then that certainly kicks swimming out of the picture. But you may enjoy a water aerobic class where you don't even have to get your hair wet. You stand in the pool at the shallow end, usually up to chest high in the water. Advantage: You don't have to spend the whole workout worrying about the physique you have versus the one you want because you're submerged.

A big advantage to walking as a form of exercise is that it takes no training—everyone over the age of two already does it well. With start-up costs limited to a good pair of walking shoes, you're off on the right track.

Remember how much fun you had as a kid, when you were finally old enough to ride your bicycle around to wherever you wanted? There's a lot of fun in a regular bicycle. And it's so much easier to cycle the time away riding around and seeing the sights versus riding indoors on a stationary bicycle. This is the whole idea—to have fun doing your exercise.

Cross-country skiing is a way to make winter fun—getting outdoors in some fresh air and building up an appetite with some fat-burning workouts. I used to love this sport when I lived in Canada. But with little snow in Southern California, I can still have all the nonjarring exercise I want in my living room on a cross-country ski

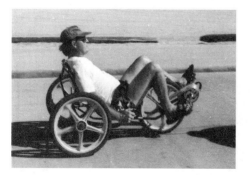

machine, listening to great music, or watching a video. It's a total body workout.

The whole idea is to pick something, anything, that will be fun. Running, walking, rowing, cycling, cross-country skiing, snowshoeing, aerobic dancing, handball, soccer, stair-climbing, walking on a treadmill—these are all aerobic activities. If you join a gym, you could try ten minutes on each piece of aerobic equipment and make it interesting that way, by going from the treadmill to the stair-climber to the bicycle to the rowing machine. Monitor your heart rate and try to keep it within the exercising zone for the required amount of time (see page 109). You will feel yourself getting stronger and more alive with the possibilities.

POWER AGING BY PUMPING IRON

Pumping iron, weight training, or resistance training: They're only different words to describe the ancient art of strength training. Call it what you will, it's very often something a lot of people neglect when they're planning their exercise programs. But I bet that if more folks knew that you could increase your metabolism up to 15 percent by weight training, thus enabling you to lose weight even while you sleep, there would be a line around the block to get into health clubs across the country.

But there's more to it than that. Strength training can improve your bone strength, muscle strength, and the shape of your body so that you can deter what used to be thought of as the inevitable signs of aging: muscle atrophy and weakness. We know now that muscle strength can be improved throughout life, and it's never too late to start.

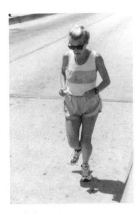

Only a decade ago, it was believed that muscle loss was simply an inevitable process of aging. Here is a fascinating study that was reported in *Science News* magazine. In a joint study by Tufts University and the Hebrew Rehabilitation Center for the Aged, nursing home residents between the ages of seventy-two and ninety-eight years old were put on a fitness program of high intensity physical resistance training. Now, it's important to note that the one hundred subjects were *not* retired professional athletes or superstar senior fitness champions, by any means. As a matter of fact, eighty-three out of the one hundred used either a cane, a walker, or a wheelchair. Two-thirds of them had fallen the year before, and 44 percent had such weak bones that they had sustained bone fractures.

In the research project, the elderly participants did two exercises only. In one, while they were seated on an exercise machine, they extended their legs in front of them against resistance. The other exercise was to push against resistance while they were lying on their backs. Both exercises were done three times a week.

At the end of ten weeks of this simple program, the participants doubled the strength of their trained muscles and increased their stair-climbing power by 28 percent. Other studies done by the Tufts team showed that with only twice-a-week workouts, women over fifty not only increased strength throughout the one-year-long study, but they also gained skeletal muscle. Meanwhile, women in the control group who remained in their sedentary lifestyle showed measurable declines in strength and muscle mass.

The crippling effects of wasting muscle robs people of their independence, subjecting sedentary people to the vulnerability of falls, fractures, and a life of restriction to canes, walkers, and wheelchairs. And of course, there is the loss of cardiovascular health: 50 percent of Americans die because of cardiovascular disease. Tufts researcher Irwin H. Rosenberg acknowledged how muscle loss is robbing the elderly of their freedom. "We want to give it back," he said in the *Science News* interview.

Think of strength training as a free body lift. It helps firm sagging breasts, flabby underarms, and middle age spread and will give your self-esteem a boost while you're at it.

Don't Wait to Lift Weights

You don't have to join a gym or health club to gain the benefits of strength training. There are plenty of videos you can watch to help with your technique and reinforce the proper warm up and breathing patterns that can guide you safely through your early workouts. You may consider a personal trainer. If this is the road you're traveling, be sure the instructor has some certification from a reputable organization. The American College of Sports Medicine and the National Strength and Conditioning Association are two good choices.

THE BASIC EIGHT

There are so many great strength exercises for every part of the body. When I was an athlete, discovering new workouts and feeling the strength growing in my body was part of the fun. If you haven't made up your mind about joining a gym yet, or if you're not sure about buying a set of dumbbells, there are many exercises that use

THE BASICS OF GETTING STRONGER

1. Get a physical exam from your doctor and he or she can clear you for liftoff.

2. Get smart before you use dumbbells. Professional instruction is always a plus and may help you keep motivated.

3. Breathe. This is really important. Many people hold their breath when they lift, and this can suddenly increase your blood pressure to dangerous levels. The best breathing technique is to blow the air *out* during the hard part of the exercise. For instance, if you're doing the chair dips (see page 115), you would *exhale* when you are straightening your arms.

4. Start easy. Use a weight that you can lift ten to fifteen times in a row before resting. This is called one *set*. When you can do three sets of ten to fifteen times, then you can gradually increase the amount of weight.

5. Take your time. Focus on what you're doing and think about *squeezing* the weight up rather than swinging it up. A slow count of three works for most exercises.

6. Lower it slower. It's the easy part of the exercise, so it's tempting to let gravity take the weight down for you, but you should keep roughly the same amount time to lower the weight as you did to raise it.

7. Work out with a friend. It's more fun, and safer too, because you can help each other keep good form and stay motivated.

8. Work out with weights at least two times a week. This will keep your muscles strong.

9. Enjoy the results. You'll see the changes in your body and improvements in your strength in about two weeks.

Exercise warning: Before starting on this, or any other exercise program, get checked out first by a doctor. He or she will be taking your family history, looking at your blood pressure, listening to your heart for murmurs or irregularities, and evaluating your blood tests to assess your cardiac risk factors, among other things. It's important to have a complete physical so that you know the basics of your own health: For instance, what your cholesterol and triglyceride levels are, what you need to look out for, and what kind of exercise and nutrition you may want to concentrate on, given your personal and family history. This way you can shorten the path to your maximum potential.

your own body weight to help you get stronger. Think of the great bodies that gymnasts have: Moving themselves against gravity is one of the main reasons that they have such great shapes.

The following are exercises that provide maximum results in minimal time.

Abdominal Muscles

I've included two exercises for the abdominal muscles, because, let's get real here—our bellies are the first thing to go, and usually need twice as much attention. If you've never done an abdominal exercise before, start with whatever time or number of repetitions you can do. If you find you have trouble doing one, keep trying until you can complete one. Then try two after a few days. You'll get stronger a lot faster then you think. Before you know it, you'll be doing fifty easily.

Cradle Crunches. This is a wonderful abdominal exercise because you're not always crunching your neck. Also, because you hold your position, there's no strain on your back. Lie on the floor, hands behind your head, the small of your back pressed flat against the floor. Bend your knees and with your knees bent bring your heels up off the floor *one inch only.* Now, raise your trunk off the floor and hold this position. When it feels like your stomach muscles are catching on fire, count to fifty. *Beginners:* Hold the position for thirty seconds, rest for one minute and then try it again for a total of three times. Increase the amount of time when it starts feeling too easy. *Tip:* The farther your heels are from the body, the more work your abdominal muscles have to do. When you get to holding the position for five minutes and it feels too easy, then add ankle weights.

Girondi's. An old-time strong man named Vince Girondi taught me this exercise. The key is to try to raise your trunk off the floor instead of crunching your neck and trying to rock your trunk up. Lie on your back, with your fingertips against your temples at the 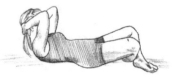 side of your head. (This is to prevent you from crunching your neck.) Cross your legs as shown. Raise your trunk off the floor as straight as possible, remembering to breathe out as you raise your trunk. I like to hold the top position for at least two seconds by counting "one steamboat, two steamboats." *Tip:* Keep your back pressed into the floor. If your neck feels crunched-up when you do this exercise, think of lifting up your trunk with your nose pointed up toward the ceiling. *Goal:* beginners twenty-five repetitions; advanced, fifty repetitions.

Lower Legs

Calf raise. This is a good one, because you can be stirring your pasta sauce on the stove or brushing your teeth and you can get these in without making a big deal out of it. Stand straight, with good posture. Don't stick your butt out and keep

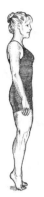

your chin in. Slowly raise yourself up on your toes and then slowly lower, counting two "steamboats" on the way up and two more on the way down. You do not rest your full weight back on your heels, merely touch the ground lightly with your heels and raise up again. *Tip:* Try ten with your toes pointed straight ahead, ten with your toes pointing inward, and ten with your toes pointed outward. *Goal:* Start with ten times and then rest.

Upper Legs

The Horse. This exercise uses not only your thigh muscles, but your willpower as well. Feet apart, back straight, and knees bent as shown. Now just stay there as long as you can. Time the effort, trying to increase time with each session. *Goal:* beginners, one minute; advanced, five minutes.

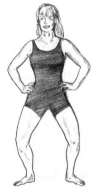

Triceps

Chair dips. This is a fun exercise because it works the major muscles of the arms all at once. Most folks feel it on the back of the arm, the tricep area, where many of our species seem to develop flabbiness as time marches on. Well, now you have the opportunity to defy time and turn back the clock on that dough that's been trying to pass itself off as your arm muscles. Your shoulder muscles also get a lot out of this exercise as well. Position yourself between two chairs or benches. You could also try simply resting your heels on the floor as shown. Extend your arms, but do not lock elbows at the top position. Lower yourself and repeat. **Goal:** beginners, ten repetitions; advanced, three sets of ten repetitions.

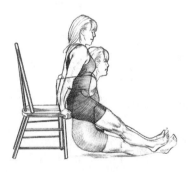

Biceps

Bicep Curls. Be sure that the door handle is in good condition and that no one is going to try to use that doorway from the

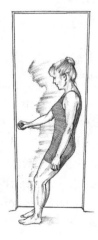

other side when you're doing the exercise. Grasp the door knob firmly with one hand. Stand right up to the door with toes right up to the door. Keeping your body straight and rigid, lean away from the door and then pull yourself back to it. Only lean as far back as you comfortably can. Do not lock your elbow when your arm is extended straight out. *Goal*: beginners, two repetitions; advanced, five repetitions.

Glutes and Hamstrings

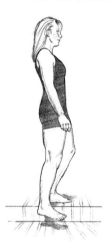

Find a stair or a block of wood. Start in the position shown. Raise and lower yourself by straightening your leg and then flexing it, as shown. If you are only feeling this in your thigh muscles, then bend at the waist a little and you will feel it in your glutes and hamstrings. The idea is to just touch your flexed foot to the stair below and then raise yourself back up. Count two "steamboats" in each direction. *Goal*: beginners, ten repetitions; advanced, fifty repetitions.

THE SILENT SENSE: BALANCE

Balance is the encompassing cosmic metaphor for existence on every plane. On the earthly level, this silent sense is responsible for feelings of well-being, ease of movement, and the ability to orient our bodies in earth's three-dimensional spaces.

Balance, or equilibrium, in the human body is dependent upon the *vestibular apparatus*, a special sense organ in the skull called the *bony labyrinth*. This complex system of membranous tubes and ducts adjacent to our hearing organs is also connected to an information superhighway that takes sight data from our eyes and orientation and pressure feedback from our limbs into special processing reflex centers in the cerebellum at the base of our brain.

Injury or disease of the inner ear can cause a constant sense of dizziness, nausea, and a frustrating "drunken gait." Astronauts often suffer from nausea, sweating, and chills during their orientation to weightlessness, as the inner ear adapts to the changes of their new environment. Even seasickness is thought to stem from the clash of data coming into the brain from a moving environment.

POWER AGING THROUGH POWER BALANCING ACTS

The bottom line on balance and aging is that at the first signs of instability—isolated cases when you may be going down stairs, turning toward a noise, or stepping off an escalator—most people panic and assume that they are becoming feeble. It's usually seen as a negative sign of aging. Of course, falling is a fear that we all have, but one that is magnified when the elderly know that to slip and fall could result in the fracture of osteoporotic, weakened bones.

The good news is that balance is a skill that can be learned, relearned, and brought to a high degree of fine-tuning by simple practice at any age. In coaching people from seven to eighty-seven years old, I've found that most need to improve their balance.

A lifetime in shoes, walking on sidewalks, weakens the feet, creating muscular imbalances that can be crucial to equilibrium and efficient stride. Tension in the neck and shoulders often results in a stooped-over posture. And a spine pulled by various muscle imbalances can add to an unsteady gait as well.

Regardless of your age and present shape, the routine of practicing just a few of the balancing positions per day will keep your silent sense in focus. Breathe into your lower abdomen while you are in the positions. Moving from starting position to the actual balancing posture is also a beneficial exercise in what is called dynamic balance. That's the main ingredient of the poise that gymnasts and divers display in such abundance as they spin through the air.

But you don't have to be an Olympic gymnast to become skillful at the following exercises. With only a little effort, you can improve your sense of balance. And with it, a wonderful feeling of lightness that can sustain you, even in your most earthbound states of mind.

BALANCE BOOT CAMP

Before you start try the following diagnostic balance test: Stand on both feet, ankles together. Now close your eyes and stand on one foot only. Count slowly. How long can you go before you lose your balance and have to put the other foot down? After you practice your balance, you'll be surprised at how fast you improve.

It's easier to do these exercises without shoes. Spread your toes out as you are planting your foot on the floor and actually grip the floor with your toes. This will become second nature to you after a time and you will not have to think about it then. Also, practice in front of a mirror. Go slowly, without jerky movements. Relax, and breathe into your lower abdomen.

The Flamingo. Plant your foot firmly on the ground. With arms straight out at your sides, and back thigh and leg extended fully, lower your trunk until it is parallel to the floor. Stay for ten seconds without moving. Gradually increase to several minutes.

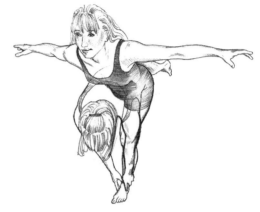

Flamingo Stretch. With one foot planted firmly on the ground, slowly reach forward and hold on to your ankle after you have achieved the posture of the Flamingo above. You may have to balance on your fingertips in the beginning as if you are a tripod. Don't let that you worry you in the least. No matter how shaky you are at first, you *will* improve. Start with a few seconds and build up to a few minutes. Change legs and repeat.

REACTION TIME

Reflex actions, the quick reactions to stimuli, are usually thought to be inborn. That is true to a certain degree, but many things can affect our reaction time, including alcohol, coffee, and even sugar. Lack of sleep, stress, medications, and illness are other factors that affect the timing and control of our reflexes.

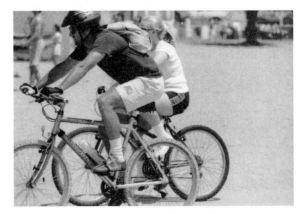

One common myth is the belief that reaction time must deteriorate severely with age. However, in my clinical experience, I've found that patients can improve balance, coordination, agility, and reflexes if they practice.

Think back to when you were a kid, climbing fences and walking on imaginary lines on the sidewalk. "Step on a crack, break your mother's back," we used to shout as we ran along, avoiding the sidewalk cracks at top speed. Everyone steps on a few at the beginning, especially if they're given a good shove. Do you see how kids practice reaction time and balance all the time as a natural part of playing?

Quickness and agility are responses that can be honed and improved with, you guessed it, practice. If you have ever seen a truly old, frail looking martial arts master pluck a fly out of the air without even a break in the conversation, you'd get the picture. Ping Pong players, magicians, pilots, and racing car drivers all work on their reflexes as part of their training.

But even if you never enter the Indy 500 or pull a rabbit out of a hat, the following exercises will keep you up to speed.

To start, you need to come up with a "cue." Take turns with a friend who should stand behind you, out of your line of vision. Your friend could clap his or her hands suddenly or even make a sound lie *ssss* for a cue to each exercise. If you live alone, you might pick a common word like *to*. Turn on the radio to any talk station and use that as a cue.

Fast hands. Place your fingers atop a desk or countertop as if you are playing the piano. At your cue, remove hands from the surface and close to a fist as quickly as possible. Get really competitive with yourself and try to become faster every time.

Fast feet. Stand relaxed, but ready, feet about shoulder width apart, knees slightly bent. At the sound, jump off the floor as quickly as possible with both feet at once. It doesn't have to be a big jump, just a fast jump.

Two hands are better than one. Have a friend try to touch the center of your palms while you try to close your hands on their fingers. Not fair if you move your hands up to catch their fingers, or if your hand is not open completely at the start. If you don't have someone around to play this with, then you could also try holding a dollar bill out in front of you with your fingertips. Let go, and try to catch the dollar bill before it hits the floor. If you use a larger denomination bill, you could call this one "balancing your budget."

Hand drumming. Make your hands fly on your lap, the tabletop, or the sofa cushions. Put on some good Latin music and go crazy. You could also watch *I Love Lucy* reruns and draw some inspiration from the episodes when Ricky lets loose down at the club. Try to finish up with ten seconds of fast-as-you-can drumming for a finale.

Foot drumming. Same principle as hand drumming. Make sure the floor is padded enough. Make your feet "sprint" in place for a finale. *Note*: You must do this one only after you are warmed up with five or ten minutes of mild aerobic activity such as walking briskly or pedalling an exercise bicycle, and avoid this one if your knees bother you. Be sure to stretch afterward.

REACHING FOR THE TRUTH: WHY BOTHER STRETCHING?

Ghandi once said that the key to long life was a supple spine. Indeed, flexibility in all phases of our lives becomes increasingly important as our lives become increasingly more complex.

Physiologically, maintaining our flexibility ensures that our joints and muscles function at their maximum potential throughout our lives. Flexibility is literally something that you must reach for. The penalty for ignoring it is rigid, inflexible joints and muscles that hurt.

Stretching also helps to maintain and maximize the explosive strength and power of a muscle. Think of a bow and arrow—the further you can draw back the bowstring, the farther and faster the arrow flies.

Reduced risk of injury and increased circulation to the area that's stretched are two more reasons for stretching. Flexibility movements help increase the range of motion in joints. All animals, even domesticated cats and dogs, stretch frequently: it's a primal urge, one that gives us creature comfort. Perhaps in our headlong rush to become "civilized" we have lost the importance of a few of our animal needs.

Even such simple activities as being able to sit and stand with correct posture are related to physical flexibility.

THE POWER STRETCHES

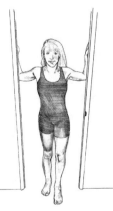

Hold each stretch for a minimum of thirty seconds. Take those seconds to breathe deeply and effortlessly. Do not go to the point of pain in doing any of these stretches.

Door stretch. See page 51. I love to do this stretch. It's simply wonderful to counterattack the ache that often occurs in-between the shoulder blades. Breathe slowly and hold the position for at least thirty seconds. Alternate feet and start again. I recommend this one at least once an hour to be done along

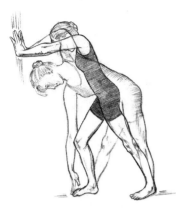

with a tall drink of pure water. It's a great stress-buster.

Calf and hamstring wall stretch. Hold the first position for thirty seconds, feeling the stretch in your calf. Then, slowly reach forward as shown and slide the palm of your hand down your shin, as far as it is comfortable. Feel the stretch, but don't make it hurt if this is a maiden voyage for your hamstrings.

Knee to chest stretch.

This one is to revital-

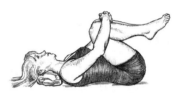

ize and relax the muscles of your lower back. Support your neck with a small pillow or a rolled-up hand towel. Grasp your shins with your hands and breathe slowly.

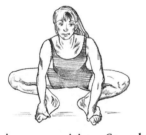

Groin stretch. Push against the inside of your knees with your elbows to make this one work. Placing your feet in a wider or narrower stance will slightly alter the intensity of this stretch.

Quad stretch. It's important to stretch the big muscles at the front of the leg and hip so that your back and pelvis can relax and support your upper body in the most maximum position. Stand tall and grasp the ankle of your outside foot.

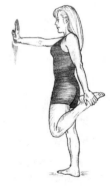

If you lean forward very slightly, you will feel more of a stretch to the front of your thigh. Hold for thirty seconds.

Pretzel stretch. An advanced stretch for the gluteus and lower paraspinal muscles. Sit on your sitting bones and visualize your back and trunk elongating and become taller as you do this one.

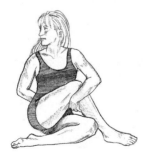

Start by resting one foot on the opposite knee at a 90-degree angle. Then put the straight leg's heel beside the other knee, as shown. *Note: Avoid doing this exercise if you currently have back pain that radiates down the back of your leg.*

Note: There are other stretches in Chapter 14 that are specifically for the back.

EXERCISE CHART FOR CHEATERS

FOOD	WEIGHT 1 OZ = 28,349 GRAMS GM	CALORIES KCAL	WALKING MIN	BICYCLING MIN	SWIMMING MIN	JOGGING MIN
Asparagus, cooked, 4 spears	60	10	2	2	1	1
Angel food cake, 1 pc (½ of 10" cake)	53	135	26	20	16	14
Apple, raw, 1 med (2½" diam)	150	87	17	13	10	9
Almonds, dried, salted, 12–15 nuts	15	93	18	14	11	9
Almond bar, chocolate, 1 bar (1¼ oz)	38	310	60	46	36	31
Blue Cheese (Roquefort) dressing	14	70	14	10	8	7
Bacon, lettuce, tomato sandwich						
—1 white toasted	148	282	54	42	34	28
Bologna with mayonnaise, sandwich						
1 slice; tsp	68	220	42	33	26	22
Beer, 8 oz glass	240	115	22	18	14	12
Bread (fresh & toasted) (white, rye,						
whole wheat, Italian, French), 1 slice	23	60	12	9	7	6
Bread, buttered, 1 slice, 1 pat	28	96	18	15	11	10
Biscuit, honey, 2" diam; 1 pat; 1 tsp	40	164	32	25	19	16
Bacon, crisp fried, 2 strips (20 strips/lb)	15	90	17	14	11	9
Banana split	300	594	114	89	71	59
Banana, 1 med	150	127	24	19	15	13
Beef TV dinner	310	350	67	52	42	35
Broccoli, 1 stalk (5½")	100	32	6	5	4	3
Cauliflower, cooked, drained, ⅛ cup	105	31	6	5	4	3
Corn, sweet, canned, ½ cup	128	85	16	13	10	9
Chicken TV dinner, fried	310	542	104	81	65	54

FOOD	WEIGHT 1 OZ = 28,349 GRAMS GM	CALORIES KCAL	WALKING MIN	BICYCLING MIN	SWIMMING MIN	JOGGING MIN
Chicken noodle soup	240	62	12	10	7	6
Caramel, 1 oz	30	118	23	18	14	12
Chocolate milk, teacup (6½ oz)	200	210	40	32	25	21
Coca-Cola, 8 oz glass	240	105	20	16	12	11
Coffee & sugar, 1 cup; 1 tsp	200	30	6	5	4	3
Chili con carne, no beans, 1 cup	250	334	64	50	40	33
Chicken breast, broiled, ½ breast (no bone)	72	105	20	16	13	11
Chicken breast, fried, ½ breast (no bone)	76	155	29	23	19	16
Cupcake with icing, 1 (2½" diam)	36	130	25	20	16	13
Cottage cheese, 1 round tbs	30	30	6	4	4	3
Cheese, American, 1 slice (1 oz)	30	112	22	17	13	11
Cheese, toasted sandwich	85	286	55	43	34	29
Cheeseburger	180	462	89	69	55	46
Doughnut, 1 average	32	125	24	19	15	13
Egg, fried or scrambled, 1 med; 1 tsp oil	53	108	21	16	13	11
Fruit cocktail, ½ cup, water pack	100	37	7	6	4	4
French dressing	14	57	11	9	7	6
Frankfurter (1 frank 8/lb pkg)	56	170	32	26	20	17
Grapefruit juice, ½ glass (4 oz)	120	47	9	7	6	5
Hamburger, cooked, 1 patty (3" diam x 1")	85	224	43	34	27	22
Hamburger	150	350	57	52	42	35
Hot dog with ketchup	110	258	50	39	31	26
Italian dressing	14	100	19	15	12	10
Ice cream—1 scoop	60	115	22	17	14	12
Ice cream bar, choc. coated, 1 bar	60	195	37	30	23	20

FOOD	WEIGHT 1 OZ = 28,349 GRAMS GM	CALORIES KCAL	WALKING MIN	BICYCLING MIN	SWIMMING MIN	JOGGING MIN
Lettuce, iceberg, ⅛ head (4¾" diam)	55	10	2	2	1	1
Low calorie dressing	14	15	3	2	2	1
Lobster, boiled with butter; 2 tbs butter	334	308	59	46	37	31
Mayonnaise, 1 tbs	14	100	19	15	12	10
Milk, whole, 8 oz glass	240	160	31	25	19	16
Martini, cocktail, 3½ oz	100	140	27	22	16	14
Meatloaf TV dinner	310	370	71	56	44	37
Mushrooms, fried, 4 med	70	78	15	12	9	8
Melba toast, unsalted, 1 thin slice	4	15	3	2	2	2
Milk, buttermilk, 8 oz glass	240	88	17	13	10	9
Orange, raw, 1 med (3" diam)	150	73	14	11	9	7
Orange juice, ½ glass (4 oz)	120	54	10	8	6	5
Pork chops, lean, 2 chops (3 oz cooked)	90	260	49	39	31	26
Peanuts, roasted, 6–8 nuts	15	86	17	13	10	9
Peanuts, dry roasted, 8–10 nuts	16	80	15	12	10	8
Pretzels, 3 ring, 4 (148/lb)	12	48	9	7	6	5
Popsicle	95	70	4	10	8	7
Pancake, 4" diam	45	105	20	16	12	11
Pancake & syrup, 4" diam; 2 tbs	85	204	39	31	24	20
Peach with cottage cheese; 2 med halves; 2 tbs cheese	156	105	20	16	13	10
Potato salad, ½ cup	100	99	19	15	12	10
Peanut butter and jelly; 1 rounded tbs; 1 level tbs	86	290	55	45	35	29
Pizza, sausage, ⅛ of 14" dia pie	75	195	38	29	23	20
Peas, green, cooked, ½ cup	80	58	11	9	7	6

FOOD	WEIGHT 1 OZ = 28,349 GRAMS GM	CALORIES KCAL	WALKING MIN	BICYCLING MIN	SWIMMING MIN	JOGGING MIN
Potato, baked with butter, 1 med; 2 pats	110	160	31	24	19	16
Raisin, dried; 1 tbs	10	30	6	4	4	3
Sunflower seeds, 30—40 nuts	15	84	16	13	10	8
Shrimp, French fried, 3½ oz	100	225	43	34	27	23
Tomato soup	245	90	17	14	11	9
Turkey, roasted, 2 slices; (3" x 3½")	80	160	31	24	19	16
Turkey, roasted with gravy, 2 slices; 2 tbs	115	240	46	36	29	24
Tomato, tuna salad, 1 med; 2 tbs	180	100	19	15	12	10
T-bone steak, broiled, 3 oz cooked	90	175	33	26	21	18
Waffle, plain, 5½" diam	120	345	66	52	41	35
Watermelon, 1 wedge (4" x 8")	10	30	6	4	4	3

SEPARATING FACT FROM FANTASY

You'll automatically lose endurance with age. Don't buy into this one. The secret to endurance is to work out aerobically. People lose endurance because they remain sedentary and muscles atrophy.

Eating meat builds bigger muscles. If that were true, elephants, whales, and gorillas would be 90-pound weaklings, because they're mostly vegetarian animals. Red meat is high in saturated fat, and most experts agree that high consumption of red meat is incompatible with a healthy cardiovascular system.

If you sweat a lot, you're out of shape. Actually, fit folks sweat more than their sedentary counterparts, but the sweat is more diluted.

You should feel fairly sore after a workout. At the beginning of a new exercise program, you may experience some muscle soreness, but it should subside within a week if you drink plenty of water and eat nutritious foods. If you feel muscle-sore after a particularly challenging hike or other hard workout, chances are you have pushed your envelope a little too hard. The soreness should subside within two to three days. *If you're really out of shape, it takes longer to see the results of exercising.* Not! Especially if you're doing weight training.

If you really want to lose weight, then go on a diet. Another myth that just keeps on going. It's physical activity that makes the big difference in weight loss. Dieting can actually decrease your metabolism because the body thinks there might be a famine going on, so it slows down to conserve energy. In contrast, exercise boosts your metabolism after the workout for several hours; and if you are weight training, you may be able to increase your metabolism by up to 15 percent, because lean body mass, like that of muscles, requires more nutrients than if it was still sedentary.

I'm too old to start lifting weights. I coached a man once who was ninety-eight years old. He wanted to lift weights because he had just moved to California and he wanted to look good in a muscle shirt when he was walking around town. He started to get stronger within the first week. By the second week, we were already increasing the size of the weights. He died when he was 101 years old—with highly improved shoulder muscles, I might add.

I'll never be able to improve my reaction time. Turn to the balance and reflex sections in this chapter. It's never too late to improve these skills and all it takes is a little practice. Okay, for some folks it will take a lot of practice, but it's earlier than you think to get into a regular exercise regime.

11 POWER EATING

What is food to one, is to others, bitter poison.
From the heart of this fountain of delight wells up some
bitter taste to choke them even amid the flowers.
But if one should guide his life by true principles, man's greatest
wealth is to live a little with contented mind;
for a little is never lacking.

—Lucretius (99–55 B.C.), *On the Nature of Things*

"Thy food shall be thy remedy." Hippocrates uttered these words to his medical students on a hillside in Greece some twenty-five hundred years ago. All medical students take the Hippocratic oath, and while it is a wonderful tribute to the highest of ethical standards, we have thrown the baby out with the bath water by ignoring Hippocrates' most profound teaching on food as a key component to health. As we focus more on "better living through pharmaceuticals" instead of treating food as our medicine, we are sickening ourselves to death. That's not to say that modern medical drugs do not have their place. Plenty of people with HIV are getting extra years because of protease inhibitors, antibiotics can reverse a pneumonia infection almost overnight, and millions of people have benefited from the discovery of supplemental insulin for diabetes. But it's time to get back to basics—and get back to the garden, because in spite of all the miraculous advancements in the medical world, in our personal world, many times when we open our mouth to put something in it, we're making life-shortening decisions that will take away years of joy.

It seems like there's a different story in the news every day about some new miracle food that will prevent cancer, and about yet another food that seems to cause it. We all know that we should be eating more fiber, and if reading this makes you want to scream and reach for a piece of chocolate cheesecake, at least read the next two sentences: Researchers now believe that at least one-third of all cancers are related to what we eat and some now state that up to nearly two-thirds of cancers are caused by what we eat. Also, eating the right foods can lower your risk of heart disease by about 50 percent. Is that enough to make you think just a *little* about what you're putting on your plate today?

The food you eat has a very powerful effect on your hormones. Food may be our best medicine, but eating it the way we do, it has become our most addictive drug. Chocolate bars, white bread, muffins, candies and pancakes with syrup, lemonade and soda, corn flakes and raisins—these all came out of the closet and into the "bad guy" limelight when author Barry Sears blew their cover in his best-seller *The Zone* in 1995. Sears says in his best-selling book that "glucose-rich carbohydrates like breads and pasta, virtually sprint from the liver back into the blood stream" in a runaway reaction that manipulates our insulin levels, jerking around our blood sugar, causing mood swings, energy drops, and lots of extra body fat. And with all that goes the walking time-bomb of plaque on our arteries that leads to heart disease.

Actually others have been saying it for decades, but without the wallop of Sears' research background to back it up. Take these words, for instance: "Most of what we eat is superfluous. Hence, we only live off a quarter of all we swallow. Doctors live off the other three-quarters." A little modern cynicism about our diets? This quip was inscribed on an ancient Egyptian papyrus from antiquity!

Perhaps it is our distrust of something as low-tech as food as a cure in our overly mechanized, high-tech society. But when it comes to food, the answers are really simple stuff: eat less, avoid red meat, eat five servings of fruits and vegetables every day. When you're thirsty, drink plenty of pure water. Cut out caffeine in coffee and cola drinks and drink green tea instead. There's a little caffeine in green tea, but it helps lower cholesterol, has anticancer and antibacterial properties, and helps improve the metabolism of fats. Avoid sugar, and allow yourself four glasses of red wine each week. And eat to heal yourself by focusing on antioxidant foods (more on that soon).

STAYING YOUNG THROUGH FOOD

Imagine a world where we can defeat the tyranny of time. Today there are 70,00 Americans over one hundred years of age. By the year 2006, there will be more than 160,000. By the year 2020, statisticians expect the ranks of the "over one hundred" club to swell up to 2 million. And as the science of antiaging gathers more and more momentum, there is every indication that these can be healthy, productive years.

It will require some effort on your part, and you'll need to learn new things about food and how to eat well. And you may have to accept that Mom may have fed you wrong. In my experience with patients, this can turn out to be one of the greatest stumbling blocks to changing poor food choices into good ones. It doesn't mean that you are rejecting your mother and all the love she fed you with. She did great considering that she didn't have the widespread access to facts that we have now. It's hard for some to give up the idea that bacon and eggs for breakfast, like Mom made every day of the week, are not healthy for your heart. And that washing your whole meal down with as much milk as possible may be the reason why you have allergies, gas, bloating, and indigestion so frequently. Or that the family pot roast recipe with all that fatty gravy could put you in the grave a lot sooner than you need to go there. Food is a very emotional topic, and it can be very confusing when it seems there is yet another new diet book on the market every week.

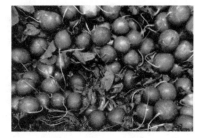

There are some basic guidelines to this eating thing, and you *can* learn what to do now. Statisticians are predicting that 5 percent of the baby boomers will live past one hundred years of age. George Burns said, "With some effort and a little luck, there is no reason why you can't live to be one hundred; once you've done that, you've got it made, because few people die over age one hundred." With any luck, you'll be up there, kicking up your heels at your one hundredth birthday party and glad that you made it in such good health and spirits.

THE BIGGEST TROUBLEMAKERS

"Free Radicals and the Electrons Who Love Them." If there ever was a talk show topic that would be of great interest to your cells, this would be the "sweeps week" supershow to grab all the ratings. All cells in the body produce free radicals. These are highly reactive molecules of oxygen that contain an odd number of electrons. In the world of molecular biology, any oxygen molecule that has an electron without a partner is an outlaw ready for a shootout. If two radicals react with each other, both are eliminated. If one free radical reacts with a regular oxygen molecule, another free radical is produced, because one of the normal oxygen's electrons is stolen, so to speak, by the first outlaw it encounters. This type of behavior keeps up until you have a chain reaction. Picture one of those old westerns when the barroom brawl breaks out, and you have a pretty good idea of how the place gets wrecked up.

Most oxygen molecules that have been stripped of an electron become highly destructive and reactive *superoxide anions* that react to form hydrogen peroxide and another oxygen molecule. The main effects of the highly reactive outlaws in that barroom brawl scene we described above is they damage the lipid (fatty) membrane of cell wall, alter the bonds of proteins, and raise havoc by altering the DNA genetic code. If the DNA code is not repaired, DNA replication can be inhibited.

EXAMPLES OF FREE RADICAL INJURY

Free radicals are involved in many adverse physiological mechanisms in the body, including cancer and the inflammation and aging of cells.

Chemical Injury. Toxic chemicals and drugs can fuel the conversion of their own ingredients into free radicals.

Inflammation. Toxic oxygen by-products are produced when the body's own white blood cells are activated by tissue damage, causing a cascade of reactions that draw other cells to the scene of the crime. The pain and inflammation of arthritis is one example of this kind of reaction.

Bacterial wars. Bacteria are literally eaten alive by the body's white blood cells and thereby killed. This is a good thing. However, free radicals are one of the toxic by-products eventually released from the white blood cells after the bacteria are melted down.

Radiation damage. This type of damaging free radical reaction is quite well documented. Tissue is damaged by irradiation and free radicals are produced. Therefore, avoid X-rays unless they are necessary for your doctor to diagnose your health problem and insist on protective shields for reproductive organs.

Over exposure to oxygen, ozone, and other gases. Lung damage results from exposure to high concentrations of gases.

Aging. Environmental exposure to free radicals, reduced availability of antioxidants, and decreased activity of the body enzymes that fight free radicals are all thought to contribute to aging. Evidence points to free radicals as contributing to cancer growth in cells and even the fatty plaques on blood vessels that we know to cause hardening of the arteries.

HOW DOES THE BODY GET RID OF FREE RADICALS?

Luckily, the body produces enzymes and proteins that act like biomolecular ninjas to shut a cell down when the barroom brawl breaks out. Superoxide dismutase, glutathione peroxidase, and catalase are three stellar performers as free radical assassins. Other substances, in the foods we eat or in supplements, are called "free radical scavengers" or *antioxidants* because they oppose the crazy oxygen molecule with only one electron. They act like a powerful braking system on the wild reactants, to keep them from hurtling out of control. This can give the cell time to either repair itself or program to self-destruct. Cancer is thought to occur when the cells do not shut down under the siege and keep on producing in the midst of the molecular mayhem.

One of the best antiaging strategies is to eat antioxidant and cruciferous foods in abundance. "Every tomato slice, every piece of cauliflower, every glass of orange juice contains hundreds of naturally occurring chemicals, some of which are believed to provide significant protection from many cancers," state Sidney J. Winawere, M.D., and Moshe Shike, M.D., physicians at the world-famous Memorial Sloan-Kettering Cancer Center in New York City. Their book *Cancer Free* is an absolute must-read for anyone who has or wants to prevent cancer. People who eat lots of fruits and vegetables have 50 percent less cancer than those who don't. Antioxidant foods are those high in vitamins A, C, and E as well as some "new" compounds that have been researched and isolated. Foods that are rich in these antioxidants combat free radicals in the body, preventing cancer from starting in the first place.

CRUCIFEROUS VEGETABLES

Cabbage

Cauliflower

Collard greens

Bok choy

Broccoli

Brussels sprouts

Kale

Kohlrabi

Mustard greens

Rutabaga

Turnips

Turnip greens

These vegetables are called *cruciferous* because their flowers resemble a cross. They contain a sulfur compound called *sulforaphane*, a powerful anti-oxidant that strengthens the body's defenses.

ANTIOXIDANTS IN FOODS

Allyic Sulfides and Quercitin. Garlic and onions contain these active enzymes that neutralize carcinogens.

Genistein. Found in greatest concentrations in soybeans. It helps block cancer's ability to grow new blood vessels around it; tumors simply cannot grow.

Selenium. Cuts cancer risk by over half. Found in garlic.

Lycopene. In tomatoes and red grapefruits, helps prevent prostate cancer and fatty plaque buildup on arteries.

Some common foods high in vitamin C: Oranges, lemons, grapefruits, limes, green and red peppers, cantaloupe, cherries, strawberries, papaya, and bean sprouts.

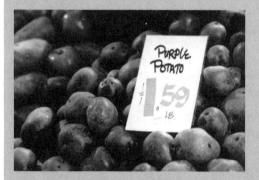

Some common foods high in beta carotene: Carrots, spinach, broccoli, sweet potatoes, yellow squash, apricots, papaya, kale, beet greens, mango, pumpkin, bok choy, turnip greens.

Foods high in vitamin E: Whole grains, nuts, vegetable oils, egg yolks, green leafy vegetables, dried beans.

Vitamin D. It doesn't act as an antioxidant, but is thought to enable the body to absorb calcium, which may inhibit colon cancer. Found in milk products, tuna, salmon, eggs, cod liver oil, egg yolk.

WHAT ARE YOU EATING NOW?

It can be quite shocking when we actually admit what we eat every day—especially the stuff we eat really fast, when nobody is looking. This is why the first thing I do with patients when we are trying to get a handle on the love handles and fight the good fight with the battle of the bulge is to have them write down every single thing they eat for an entire week. I tell them *not* to censor the list of food and drink they consume, or in what amounts, because I will be analyzing it, not judging them on it. One of those small spiral-bound notebooks works well; carry it with you in your pocket or purse and write down all your meals and snacks right after you eat.

It really is amazing when you see how much you actually eat every day. Be honest!

Write down if you ate a half pint of ice cream, standing up in front of the refrigerator, or half of your kid's sandwich. Don't forget to write down beverages too, and things you add to your cereal, or mayonnaise and salad dressing. Also, the number of cookies and the amount of meat or chicken or the size of the pizza slice you've just had. If you want to count calories, buy yourself one of those inexpensive drugstore pocket calorie counters and do it.

When you are eating junk food, you have to eat a lot of calories to be satisfied. Because the junk food is essentially empty of nutrients, your body's appetite control mechanism (called the *appestat*) does not respond to all the empty calories, so you eat more. For instance, I've known people who could put away a whole loaf of white bread at one sitting. (Ever done that with a couple of breadbaskets worth of bread in a restaurant while you're waiting for them to serve the entrée?) But eat two slices of home-baked dark, fermented rye bread and you're full. The difference here is possibly 1,000 calories for the white bread, and 200 calories for the whole grain bread that's full of fiber and other nutrients.

THE SOUR FACTS ON SUGAR AND REFINED CARBOHYDRATES

And while we're on the bread topic, did you know that the glucose from one slice of French bread goes into the bloodstream faster than that from a tablespoon of refined table sugar? A rating system based on the rise in blood glucose following ingestion of a particular food is called the "glycemic index." This information is important because the rise in blood sugar causes a big surge of insulin, which results in a reactive swing of the blood sugar down to levels even lower than the hunger point when the food was eaten. The result: onset of fatigue, mood swings, and a host of other hormonal changes in the body that are generally regarded as unhealthy. On page 134 you will find a list of a few items on the glycemic index, with a "value" scoring system.

Presence of salt in the meal increases the glycemic response. That's why corn flakes may rate higher than the white bread. Presence of fiber decreases it, as does fat. That's how oatmeal cookies came in at a 78 value: The fiber and the fat content will slow down the rate of absorbed glucose effect on the bloodstream. Legumes not only come in at the lowest end (check out the low rating for peanuts and soybeans), but they also flatten out the glycemic index response to the next meal eaten.

GLYCEMIC INDEX FOR SOME COMMON FOODS

Food	Mean Glycemic Index	
Corn flakes	115	Extremely high (100 or more)
White bread	100	
Mashed potatoes	100	
Corn chips	99	High (80–99)
Shredded wheat	97	
White sugar	89	
Rice	71–84	
Banana	84 (+ or -5)	
Oatmeal cookies	78	Moderate (40–79)
Orange juice	67	
Green peas	65	
Apple	53	
Kidney beans	45 (+ or -11)	
Soy beans, canned	22	Low (below 40)
Peanuts	15	

OF FAT AND FIBER

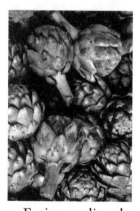

Did you know that an estimated 90 percent of Americans eat twice the amount of fat that's healthy? Yet according to a Harvard University study of more than 88,000 nurses, those who ate red meat every day had two to three times more colon cancer than those who ate it less than once a month, probably because of the saturated fat in red meat, which has been linked to cancer. And, after studying the eating habits of 51,000 men, researchers at Harvard University found that men with high-fat diets (up to 89 grams per day) had twice the rate of advanced prostate cancer of those who ate only 53 grams of fat per day.

Eating a diet that gets an average of 40 percent of its calories in fat puts us at greater risk for heart disease (the number-one cause of premature death in America). There's double trouble when a high-fat diet is combined with eating less than half the recommended healthy requirement for fiber from fruits and vegetables, as is true for most Americans. Fiber helps bind fat, preventing us from absorbing all of it and thus partly deactivating it. This in turn helps to keep us from becoming overweight. Keeping trim not only cuts your risk of heart disease, it cuts your risk of breast, uterine, and possibly ovarian cancer. Fiber has also been studied for its role in binding estrogen in the body. Because the estrogen is then eliminated by the body more effectively, that may explain why women who eat high-fiber diets have a lower risk of breast cancer. In 1989, scientists at New York Hospital–Cornell Medical Center discovered that adding fiber to the diet could shrink cancerous colon polyps that had already begun to form. And fiber may also play a role in decreasing stomach cancer.

CHOOSING A HEALTHY DIET

I know, it sounds like all the good stuff we like is bad stuff and there's nothing left. Don't give up. We're going to go step by step through the very basics right now, so that you can get on the right track. Actually, volume-wise, you're probably going to be eating *more* food than you have before, because you will be increasing your fiber intake. Yes, you may have to give up that steak or cheeseburger-a-day habit. But remember that you are the captain of your own ship. You alone are in control of the whole deal—your health, your life, and your future.

Don't be too hard on yourself. You can do it in degrees and at your own speed. In my experience with patients, I usually ask them to start by picking the worst piece of junk food that they consume—you know, the one you eat really fast when you're alone—and try eliminating that one thing each day for two weeks. Making better choices for yourself becomes easier and easier, because the pride and increase in self-esteem derived from making that first choice makes it easier to make another better choice when you're ready, and your personal success history then repeats itself. Making that one choice per day to replace the junk habit with a healthy alternative snack is a great start. After you make your decision, then slam-dunk that old snack into the garbage. As for alternatives, how about adding a crisp piece of fruit, or "light" popcorn, low-fat cheeses, or those already washed, cut, and peeled packages of veggies in the supermarket?

Give yourself a period of months to gradually make changes. It becomes easier. Anything worthwhile will take a little effort, so be gentle with yourself. Many report they make good progress trying out one new healthy recipe a week. As for red meat, you don't have to eliminate it all at once. For starters, try for one meatless day a week. Then work your way up to more days. Substitute broiled or steamed fish or try a stir-fry vegetable dish with tofu. Many supermarkets and health food stores stock veggie burgers and meatless hot dogs made out of soy protein. That'll work. When it comes to getting more fiber, you could start by having a pear or apple or melon wedges for an afternoon snack instead of a sugary, fat-filled one. You'll get up to 4 grams of fiber this way, almost one-sixth of your minimum daily recommended 25 grams. Try just half of a cup of a bran cereal for breakfast (9 grams of fiber) along with your pear, and with those two items alone, you've got half your daily fiber. Check out the charts that follow for fiber-rich foods and low-fat foods and you'll be on your way to making the healthy, antiaging choices that will keep you in good working order.

WHAT ABOUT VEGETARIANISM?

We discussed earlier about how the typical American diet has too much fat, too little fiber, and too many calories. That makes us overfed, undernourished, and overweight. The result is that we look and feel older than we should. Vegetarians are healthier than meat eaters, with less cancer, less than half of the heart disease, less diabetes, constipation, gall stones, and osteoporosis, according to study after study. Also, because of the ongoing commitment to a healthy lifestyle, vegetarians tend to smoke less, eat less fat, and exercise more, which of course lends itself to the rewards of greater health and all-round vigor.

Allow me to show my bias right up front: I am celebrating my twenty-sixth year of committed vegetarianism. At the beginning "the experts" agreed that I would never amount to much as an athlete on a vegetarian diet. "No stamina if you don't eat some steak for protein" were the familiar words from the chorus of naysayers. But my career only began to take off when I became vegetarian—and after achieving third in the world-ranking in the marathon, the critics of my lifestyle were fewer and farther between.

True, becoming vegetarian, while it will most likely make you leaner and may make you more energetic, will not release you from the big blood sugar swings that come from eating lots of refined carbohydrates. Barry Sears, author of *The Zone*, acknowledges the possible anticancer, antiobesity result of vegetarianism, but is less than enthusiastic about it because the focus is away from proteins and because of possible low levels of omega-3 fatty acids.

However, it is possible to make healthful protein choices within a vegetarian diet, but you may have to think about it at the beginning. And you can still get the important essential fatty acids from vegetarian sources. Flax seed and flax seed oil are a rich and wonderful natural source of EPA (omega-3 fatty acids) oils that help reduce cholesterol with all the anticancer and prostaglandin blocking action that helps prevent arthritis symptoms from flaring up. And all without the fishy aftertaste of fish oil capsules and sardine sandwiches. High fiber cookies, breads, and cereals chock full of nutritious and tasty flax seed meal are welcome addition to your daily fare. If you don't feel like hunting around for the flax meal or don't have the time or inclination to bake from scratch, you can order some really tasty flax seed goodies from Natural Ovens in Wisconsin. Contact them through their website, www.goodbread.com, or by calling 1-800-962-9536. I have a stack of 1,200 research articles on the benefits of flax seed dating back to 1928. It's probably one of the best kept secrets as far as super-foods are concerned.

If You Would Like to Eat More Veggies and Less Meat

If you would like to steer clear of meat more than you have in the past, here are a few suggestions to get you going. You don't have to become a total vegetarian, but experiencing more vegetarian-style eating can help you enjoy more of the health benefits of vegetarianism. For instance, in switching to soy for half their protein volunteers experienced a reduction of blood pressure of about 24 percent, the same as is achieved by most cholesterol-lowering drugs, but without the side effects, according to research published in the *New England Journal of Medicine*.

Start with one meatless day a week. You can buy veggie burgers and soy hot dogs at many supermarkets and most health food stores. It's not as hard as you may think. Try eating out in a Chinese or Thai restaurant. You could eat there every day of the week and never ask, "Where's the beef?" Or find a salad bar. Go easy on the dressing though—some salad bars have soup ladles in the vats of dressing, and I've noticed folks dishing up the equivalent of one cup of dressing onto their otherwise ideal and healthy 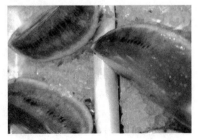 salad fixings. We're talking a 200-calorie salad with about 700 calories worth of dressing. Ouch!

Ask "Where did it grow?" In my experience with patients, I've found this to be the simplest way of demystifying what's good and what's not. Ask, "Where did it grow?" If you can't answer, then you're probably better off not eating it. For example: an apple. Where did it grow? That's easy, on an apple tree. Chocolate eclair. Where did it grow? You get the idea. Same goes for ingredients on labels. If you can't even pronounce it, then you're probably better off without it.

Want calcium? For your top choice of calcium rich foods, it's not milk. Surprised? Most people are. Per half-cup serving, here's how other sources of calcium stack up against milk:

Collard greens	188 mg.
Kale	187 mg.
Turnip greens	184 mg.
Oatmeal	163 mg.
Skim milk	151 mg.
Orange juice, calcium	150 mg.
Cottage Cheese, low-fat	78 mg.

An ounce of cheddar comes in at 218 milligrams of calcium, but most fat-phobes avoid it because it's not only a saturated fat, which can contribute to higher cholesterol levels, but with 8 grams of fat per one-inch cube of cheese, it tips the scale at 72 saturated fat calories per serving. And, there are always calcium supplements. For a discussion on which are the most absorbable, please turn to Chapter 13.

Magnesium, the mighty mineral. Only 25 percent of all Americans get the recommended daily allowance of this mineral, and some experts think that the RDA on it is too low anyway. Magnesium seems to protect the heart from abnormal arterial spasms and deters clot formation by inhibiting thromboxane, a substance that makes blood platelets sticky. A Harvard study linked magnesium deficiencies to high blood pressure. New research has magnesium stepping into the spotlight for its role as a possible inhibitor of insulin resistance. That new research will be of benefit to solving the vexing riddle of diabetes. As if that wasn't enough, this mighty mineral has been shown to boost the "good guy" kind of cholesterol (HDL) while suppressing the blood fats known as triglycerides. Helping us to keep strong bones and fight free radicals is also part of the resumé held by magnesium. Whole grains, legumes, nuts, and seeds are loaded with magnesium. If bran cereal, pumpkin seeds, almonds, cashews, or peanuts are not on your daily menu, you may consider taking a 300 milligram supplement. *Note:* If you have kidney problems or severe heart problems, consult your doctor before taking these or any other supplements.

Reach for beans over beef. Meat substitutes like a four-ounce serving of tofu, a half-cup of beans, or two tablespoons of seeds like sunflower seeds are all ways to get protein without eating red meat. Tempeh, a fermented soy product, is delicious and nutritious. It's great in stir fry or in a sandwich. One of my favorite lunches is sauteed tempeh over a baked portabello mushroom on 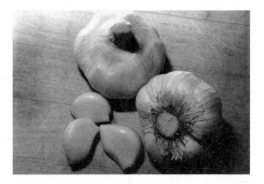 fresh, home-made rye bread, with tomato, lettuce, sprouts, and crushed pine nuts. Baked tofu also works well. Use the firmest type you can get for baking. Simply brush lightly with olive or canola oil, sprinkle with crushed garlic, and allow to bake about 40 minutes at 375 degrees Fahrenheit. Or mix tofu in with a stir-fry vegetable dish. I like to use the silken type of tofu when making smoothies. I add a frozen banana and frozen berries, a dash of some real vanilla extract, and purée on high speed.

Travel the world. You don't have to actually get on a plane and go somewhere, but you can *eat* internationally and the variety in your diet will be a blessing. Start in Mexico with chili with tofu one night (freeze the tofu first for a chewier consistency), then opt for Chinese stir-fry veggies over brown rice the next. Go to the Far East for curried rice and lentils, back to the United States for veggie tofu burgers and hot dogs, or a hearty bean soup with vegetarian cheese melted on the top for another main dish and you'll get most of the way through the week. You can cook up an omelet one night if you plan to eat eggs, or use an egg substitute. Pad-Thai noodles with a spicy peanut sauce makes for another tasty entrée and you can throw in leftover baked tofu that's sauteed in sake first. I have a quiche recipe in which I puree tofu and soy cheese, add fresh cloves of garlic and jalapeño peppers, and then pour into a homemade pie crust and bake. Experimenting is a lot of fun. There are also some wonderful vegetarian cookbooks in the bookstores and libraries that will keep you cookin'.

Hold the mayo. Eating more vegetarian style is fun and healthy, but you still need to watch your fat intake. Mayonnaise, french fries, doughnuts, corn chips, and chocolate bars are meatless, but they are still not the best choice that you can make for yourself. Avoid the sugary, fatty snacks like Cheez-Whiz, beer nuts, and cookies, as well as overloads of salad dressing, fried anything, and cream cheese.

DEVELOP A HEALTHY RELATIONSHIP WITH FOOD

"Thank you, they look lovely, but I'm not hungry," I said to the hostess, who was pressing me to take a plate of rich hors d'oeuvres. "What on earth did hunger ever have to do with eating!" she sputtered. Indeed . . .

Emotions like anger, depression, boredom, loneliness, fear, frustration, and low self-esteem may often be the trigger that gets us to open the refrigerator door, searching the shelves for something to relieve our uncomfortable feelings. It all looks so inviting in the light, especially late at night—that's why I take the light bulb out. Go ahead, reach in and unscrew it. Things just don't look as inviting without that familiar glow.

The two key components of keeping a healthy body weight are, first of all, the calories we consume, and second, the calories we use. You will enjoy the Exercise Chart for Cheaters in Chapter 10. Did you know that if you did not alter your eating habits, but went on a 3-mile brisk walk every day, you'd lose about one pound of fat every ten days? Most people lose about a pound a week when they try this. Think of it. Eat the same, lose a pound a week this week, a pound next week—that's four and a half pounds a month, and over twenty-five pounds in six months, if you have that much to lose!! This is a real calculation. Here's why: You burn approximately 100 calories per mile (300 per day for the 3 miles) and every ten days you'll reach 3,000 calories burned, which is roughly the number of calories stored in one pound of human body fat.

This is mentally and emotionally a great way to go, because that walk every day does wonders for your stress-reduction and self-esteem. You feel in control. You are a person who takes care of yourself and takes responsibility for your own health. With this ammunition under your belt (and you'll be tightening that belt each week), it's easier to make better choices for yourself in the food department. What follows is a list of some better choices. Treat it like one of those big menus in a Chinese restaurant—some items from each column will likely end up on the end of your fork. Armed with the knowledge of how you can do better for yourself, you'll find yourself making the shift toward healthier eating that will help you become leaner, feel more energetic, and slow down the aging clock.

LOW-FAT SNACKS

Choose these more often
   Breadsticks
   Finn Crisp
   Hardtack
   Matzo
   Popcorn with no butter or oil
   Rye Crisp
   Wasa Brod
   Zwieback toast

FRESH FRUITS

Each item contains about 15 grams of carbohydrate, 2 grams of fiber, and only 60 calories.
   Apple, raw
   Apple sauce, unsweetened (½ cup)
   Apricots, raw (4 apricots)
   Banana (½ of a 9-inch one)
   Cantaloupe, cubed (1 cup)
   Cherries (12 raw)
   Grapefruit (one half)
   Mango (one half)
   Nectarine, 1½" in diameter
   Orange (one whole)
   Papaya (1 cup)
   Peach, 2¾" in diameter
   Pear, 2¾" in diameter
   Pineapple, raw (¾ cup)
   Pomegranate (1 cup)
   Raspberries, raw (1 cup)
   Strawberries, raw, whole (1¼ cup)
   Watermelon, in cubes (1¼ cup)

FRESH VEGETABLES

Each item contains about 5 grams of carbohydrate, 2 grams of protein, 25 calories, and 2 to 3 grams of fiber. A serving is ½ cup.

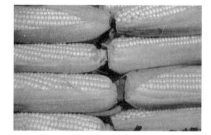

Artichoke, ½ medium
Asparagus
Beans (string beans, green, yellow)
Bean sprouts
Beets
Broccoli
Brussels sprouts
Cooked cabbage
Cauliflower
Eggplant
Greens from turnips, collard, or mustard
Kohlrabi
Leeks
Mushrooms, cooked
Okra
Onions
Pea Pods
Peppers (green, yellow, or red)
Spinach, cooked
Summer squash (yellow)
Tomato, one large fresh one
Turnips
Water chestnuts
Zucchini

HIGH FIBER FOODS

These can be eaten in abundant, guilt-free quantities.
Cabbage
Celery

Cucumber
Bok choy
Endive
Escarole
Green onions
Lettuce
Spinach
Horseradish
Hot peppers
Mushrooms
Radishes
Romaine
Zucchini

HIGH-FAT FOODS TO BE AVOIDED

Note: You need fats and carbohydrates to live, but if you overeat on the fat or carbohydrate side of the equation (as most people do), the excess calories in your diet will end up on your hips, thighs, belly, and arteries.

Food	Serving size	Grams of fat
Almonds	¼ cup	32
Avocado	half	15
Bacon	3 slices	21
Butter	1 tbsp.	12
Cashews	¼ cup	32
Clam chowder	1 cup	10
Cold cuts	2.5 slices	21
Cream, half & half	¼ cup	7
Cream cheese	1 oz.	10
Cream soups	1 cup	6–10
Cheese	1 oz.	7–10
Coconut	1 oz.	5 (shredded and unsweetened)
Ice Cream	1 cup	14 for regular, 24 for rich
Margarine	1 tbsp.	12

Food	Serving size	Grams of fat
Mayonnaise	1 tbsp.	11
Milk, whole	1 cup	9
Milk, evaporated	1 cup	9
Peanuts	¼ cup	48
Pecans	¼ cup	48
Ricotta Cheese	½ cup	16
Sausage	1 sausage	22
Salad dressing	1 tbsp.	7
Sour cream	2 tbsp.	6
Spare ribs (pork)	7 oz.	77
Steak	10 oz.	89
Tofutti	1 cup	28
Walnuts	¼ cup	20
Whipped cream	¼ cup	11

What's low fat and good for you? Fish, chicken and turkey without the skin, tofu, tempeh, low- or no-fat cottage cheese, and salads with sparing amounts of dressing. Vegetables and fruits of all kinds. Eggs in moderation. Clear-broth soups. Breadsticks, matzo, oysters, oyster crackers. Vegetables stir-fried with tofu.

Ever wonder what your snacks are really like? There's lots of fat hidden in those snacks. Listed below is the fat content of some of America's favorites. Yes, I know that "one piece" *could* mean that you just don't cut the pan of brownies into sections, but these figures are for one medium piece, as deemed medium by usual restaurant sizes and *not* the traditionally more generous portions one might give oneself while dining in private. When it comes to pie, one slice means one-eighth of the pie.

Food	Serving size	Grams of fat
Brownies	1 piece	15
Chocolate cake	1 piece	11
Cookies (most store-bought cookies)	4 cookies	12
Potato chips	1 small bag	12
Crackers	1 cracker	1 (Does anyone ever eat just one?)
Croissant	1	13
Doughnut	1	10

Food	Serving size	Grams of fat
French fries	21	15 (This is considered a small order of fries.)
Muffin	1	9
Onion rings	3	11
Pancakes	2	10
Pie, fruit filled	1 piece	15
Pie, pumpkin/pecan	1 piece	17 (That's without whipped cream on it.)

WHAT YOU CAN EAT INSTEAD

- Buy fat-free potato or corn chips
- Need a "crunch"? Eat a pretzel.
- Got a craving to snack? Have a big fat dill pickle.
- You'd rather die than not have your favorite snack? Buy the smallest bag possible and ration it.
- Like cheese? You can get it with 50 percent less fat or even fat-free.
- Substitute soy hot dogs for real hot dogs, even kids can't tell the difference. And you won't be getting the nitrates and nitrites (food preservatives that have been associated with increased risk of stomach cancer).
- Instead of high-fat salad dressing, substitute reduced-fat or fat-free.
- Use fresh fruit or cut-up veggies as snacks. Make a nonfat yogurt dip yourself using nonfat yogurt, vinegar, mustard, and garlic.
- Have a big cup of herbal tea.
- Sip on broth. At a health food store, you can buy veggie bouillon that's sodium-reduced, and it's delicious.
- Don't scream for ice cream—go for nonfat frozen yogurt.
- When you go to the movies, bring your own air-popped popcorn to munch.
- Eat a bran muffin to satisfy the cake craving.
- Take a nap instead.

BELIEVE IT

- If you have to ask how many calories it has, you can't afford it.
- Never food shop when you're hungry.
- Never eat stand-up meals in front of the refrigerator.

- Don't skip meals.
- Act like you're already trim—stand up straight and pull in your stomach.
- If you don't buy it and keep it in the house, you won't eat it.
- Buy smaller packages of your favorite comfort foods.
- Give away your "fat wardrobe" to charity so there will be no turning back.
- Don't expect to "oink out."
- You really *can* stretch your stomach by overeating all the time. And shrink it by eating less.

DON'T BELIEVE IT FOR A SECOND!

- Eating after midnight helps you sleep.
- Cheesecake is just packed with vitamins.
- Dessert helps settle a heavy meal.
- If you eat it real fast, and nobody sees you, it doesn't count.
- Chocolate bars are chock-full of milk protein and energy.
- You'll get extra points if you clean your plate.
- It's not me—the scale must be broken.

WHAT ARE THEY DOING FOR ME TODAY?

Proteins. All living things are made up of the same twenty-two amino acids considered to be the building blocks of protein. Proteins are made up of those amino acids linked in various ways. Proteins play a structural role in all body tissues, and they are the most abundant substance in our body after water. Bones, muscles, cartilage, skin organs, arteries, and hair are all protein structures. The unseen elements of the body such as antibodies, hormones, collagen, and enzymes all depend on various proteins as well. Hemoglobin is the blood protein that transports oxygen through our systems. Food sources of protein are: meat, dairy, tofu, tempeh, soy, and grain. Excess protein consumption is linked to age-associated processes like osteoporosis and kidney problems. High-protein diets typically result in fewer grains and vegetables eaten and have been found to be linked to colon cancer. Protein deficiency may result in weakness, lowered resistance to

"Desserts" is "Stressed" spelled backwards.

infection, depression, and lack of vitality. Did you know that three and a half ounces of tofu or a half-cup of navy beans has as much protein as one ounce of tuna or cheese or one medium egg? Tofu, a plant protein made from soy, is equal in quality to animal sources, with no cholesterol. To figure out your minimum daily protein requirement (according to the National Research Council) divide your body weight by two. For instance, if you are 140 pounds, your daily recommended protein intake is approximately 70 grams. Of course, body size, height to weight ratio, and activity levels all influence nutritional requirements.

Carbohydrates. The word carbohydrate tells us about the composition: *car*bon, *oxy*gen, and *hydr*ogen. Carbohydrates are the main source of energy for everything the body does. Without carbohydrates, the body cannot metabolize fat properly. Carbohydrates are also important for the formation of nucleic acids, connective tissues, and nerve tissues. The body digests carbohydrates from food and converts them into the blood sugar known as glucose. *Complex carbohydrates* (the good guys) are the high-fiber starches found abundantly in grains, fruits, vegetables, and legumes. The fiber in complex carbohydrates acts like a brake to keep glucose from flooding into the blood stream. *Simple carbohydrates* (the bad guys) are the sugary foods and refined white flour foods with no fiber that lack the essential nutrients of complex carbohydrates, and are often called "empty calories" because they rapidly convert to glucose. This gives a big energy jolt to the body, but ends up crashing us further down than when we started. Headaches, dizziness, mental depression, or irritability are often associated with these sudden drops. Food sources to be avoided: corn flakes, white bread, white sugar, corn syrup, pastries, cookies, candies.

The fiber in complex carbohydrate foods protects us from many medical problems and helps keep our bodies from aging and breaking down. Constipation, obesity, colon cancer, diabetes, cardiovascular disease, hemorrhoids, diverticulosis (a painful disorder of the large intestine), and high blood cholesterol levels are all associated with diets that are lacking in fiber.

Fats. Fats are called *lipids* in the biochemical world, but, under any name, they are the most concentrated source of energy in our bodies. How concentrated are they? When oxidized by our systems, they give off twice as many calories per gram of either carbohydrates or protein. Fat plays a vital role in keeping our bodies heated. Fat is beneficial in transporting the fat-soluble vitamins A, D, E, and K, and an important constituent of hormones. Fat gives nutrients to our skin and scalp and protects our internal organs from trauma, insulating us from cold and shielding sensitive areas of the body. The mammary glands of a woman are protected by fat deposits on the chest. The liver and heart are held in place by fat deposits.

So here's the bad news on fat:

We eat too much of it. As a result of high-fat, low-fiber diets, most Americans have excess fat deposits on their bellies and thighs, and arteries. High-fat diets are linked to innumerable human diseases: heart disease, cancer, diabetes, and obesity, for starters. Most experts agree that no more than 30 percent of our diet should be composed of fat intake. Others fix on no more than 20 percent. I like to use the lower number, simply because in my experience with patients, a certain "food amnesia" tends to occur when calculating the french fries eaten or the size of the piece of cheesecake consumed, and the 20 percent goal is then more limiting. Most Americans consume more than 40 percent of their food intake as fat.

Are there good fats you can eat? Fats are classified according to the length of their chemical attachments, because that affects the character, absorption, and effect they have. The most healthful fats for us are found in fish and most plants. Because these

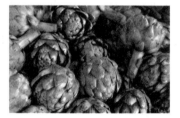

fats have chemical attachments missing, they are called *unsaturated fats*. A trick for easily identifying these nutritional good guys is simply to observe them at room temperature. If they are liquid, they're usually unsaturated. Olive oil, corn, canola, safflower, and vegetable oils fit this description. The exception is coconut or palm oil, which is saturated. Margarine or vegetable shortenings are solid at room temperatures, but they have been chemically altered.

When only one attachment point is missing, we call those *monounsaturated fats*. When a bunch of attachments are missing in the chemical chain, they are named *polyunsaturated fats*.

And when the chemical bonds of the chain are basically all taken, we call those fats *saturated fats*. Butter, animal fat, like the fat you see around a steak, cheese, eggs, and milk, as well as the coconut and palm oils mentioned earlier, are all examples of saturated fats, and they are solid at room temperature. If you'd like a memory helper on this, remember that we belong to the animal kingdom, so the fat that you can pinch around your waist is solid at room temperature and it's saturated. In case you are ever on a quiz show, those chubby-producing fat deposits of ours are made up of triglycerides, which are three fatty acids linked to a glycerol. Animal food products also contain cholesterol. These need to be limited to not more than 10 percent of our diets. Excesses here can lead to fat deposits on our arteries and the rest of our bodies.

THINGS THAT AGE YOU FAST

Red Meat. The high-tech feed given to animals by U.S. farmers contains synthetic hormones, antibiotics, and dioxin, a deadly toxin used industrially. Red meat adds cholesterol and saturated fat to the diet. It's an abundant source of protein, but if it's smoked, salt-cured, or barbecued, then nitrites, nitrates, and other carcinogen-producing substances are part of the meat-eating package.

Secret: fish; low-fat dairy products like cottage cheese or reduced-fat hard cheeses; plant proteins like tofu or tempeh from soy; legumes, beans, and grains eaten together.

Fat. Eat less of it. Overweight adds years to a body and face, not to mention your arteries.

Overeating. A toned, firm body without excess fat on it looks and feels younger. Most people eat dinner as if they expected to drop dead of malnutrition within the half-hour. Don't overeat and make time to exercise on the days when you do overeat.

Sugar. I heard on a radio show one time that the White House got more mail on a proposed ban on saccharin than on the whole Vietnam War. Forget about the artificial sweeteners in food and sodas; Americans consume gallons of diet soft drinks, but that can't be the answer, because we're still an overweight nation. The artificially sweetened products may just feed the unhealthy cravings and addictions to sweet tastes. And sodas are high in phosphorous and caffeine, both of which can contribute to osteoporosis, the crippling deformation of bones.

Secret: Cut way back on sugar consumption. To do this, you will have to read labels, because sugar is the number-one food additive in everything from catsup to cereal. Your taste buds will gradually make the switch. Fruits are the natural way to go, because the fiber acts like a brake on absorbing the sweetness. If you're thirsty, how about drinking some water instead of soda? Flavor it with a wedge of lemon or lime or a fresh mint leaf. You need eight to ten glasses of pure water a day.

Salt. It is unlikely that one could develop a sodium deficiency living in America, because salt is the number-two food additive, a close second to sugar. Excess sodium is linked to high blood pressure, fluid retention, and increased rate of conversion of dietary refined carbohydrates into blood glucose (*not* a plus for our insulin levels). And from the shallow, vanity angle, when you look in the mirror in the morning, it may not be immediately life-threatening to see those big, puffy bags under your eyes, but it can sure make you *feel* old.

Secret: Get rid of the salt shaker on your table. Enough already with the salt! Substitute Veg-it, a tasty herbal powder that you can shake on food. It's great on rice, vegetables, baked potatoes, and in soups. Try cayenne pepper, herbs, garlic, roasted sesame seeds, lemon juice, and some of the no-salt alternatives you can find in a health food store. I like to flavor food, soup, salads, and sauces with liquid aged garlic (Kyolic) extract—the smell has been removed, so there's no garlic breath to worry about, and the latest studies say it prevents cancer. Is this a bargain or what? You can buy it in health food stores.

Alcohol. Alcohol consumed in moderation, no more than four glasses of wine a week, is known to provide some antiaging protection to the body because of phyto-chemicals that work to help a heart-healthy program of diet and exercise. People who moderately consume alcoholic beverages like wine and beer tend to live longer than complete teetotalers. However, alcohol is a drug, it's highly addictive, and is responsible for about 50 percent of all traffic fatalities, as well as premature death due to heart, liver, pancreatic, and other diseases when consumed in excess. Cancer, diabetes, cirrhosis of the liver, dementia, and nerve disorders are all linked directly to chronic alcohol abuse. Alcohol is also a known trigger for hot flashes during menopause.

Secret: It's a wonderful sign of healthier times that it is now trendy *not* to drink. I love to order a Virgin Bloody Mary when I'm in a restaurant—it's basically spicy tomato juice with a stalk of celery in it for a flourish. Tonic water with a wedge of lime, sparkling apple cider, sparkling water, and fruit juice cocktails are all healthy alternatives to alcoholic drinks. And you'll be avoiding the empty calories of alcoholic beverages, because mixed drinks and the like can add up to couple of hundred calories to your daily intake. If you drink as a stress-reliever, try working out instead.

Caffeine. If you've read this far, you'll know that I have little good to say about caffeine. And I'm so sorry, because I used to love a good cup of coffee first thing in the morning—it was the gasoline that got me going when I was in my early twenties. But then I learned about all the bad effects it has on the body, so I quit. There were some whopper headaches and fatigue for a few days, but it was worth it. Most experts agree that caffeine can be consumed in moderation, but it does have some aspects that need to be considered.

Caffeine is in coffee, tea, cola drinks, many over-the-counter stimulants, some headache medications, diet pills, and, of course, chocolate. I've seen caffeine cleverly disguised on labels of "all natural" vitamin and protein powder products as "kola or cacao nut extract." Don't be fooled. Read your labels. Even some non-cola-colored soft drinks like Mountain Dew have about 54 milligrams of caffeine—that's more than a cup of brewed tea. Caffeine's hit list of deleterious effects looks like this:

Constipation. Caffeine is a diuretic, so it dehydrates the body.

Fatigue. The energy drop after the initial boost causes fatigue.

Infertility. Harvard University School of Public Health compared 3,833 women who had recently given birth to 1,050 with infertility problems. The new mothers were the ones who consumed less caffeine. Those who reached for more than two cups of coffee per day or more than four cans of cola per day had greater risk for tubal damage or endometriosis.

Hearing loss. Caffeine has an effect similar to nicotine's in constricting blood vessels, and some experts link them both to hearing loss.

Heart arrhythmias. If you're susceptible to arrhythmias, avoid caffeine.

PMS. The anxiety and mood sings of premenstrual syndrome can be intensified by caffeine. Of course, that's just when you're probably most likely to crave chocolate, which is loaded with caffeine. Premenstrual breast tenderness is often relieved when caffeine is curbed and 1200 units of vitamin E is supplemented.

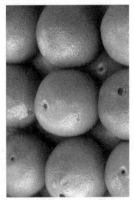

Sleep. Caffeine is a well-known thief of sleep.

Tinnitus. In my experience with patients, cutting caffeine cuts the ringing sensations in the ears.

Try green tea. It does contain a minimual amount of caffeine, but it has been given credit for reducing digestive and lung cancer risks. It's a good substitute for coffee.

12

KEEPING OUR SENSES SPECIAL

Where'er you walk, cool gales shall fan the glade,
Trees, where you sit, shall crowd into a shade:
Where'er you tread, the blushing flow'rs shall rise,
And all things flourish where you turn your eyes.

—Alexander Pope (1688–1744)

Here we will sit, and let the sounds of music
Creep in our ears; soft stillness and the night
Become the touches of sweet harmony.

—William Shakespeare (1564–1616),
The Merchant of Venice

YOUR VISION

"Windows to the world" and "windows of the soul" are two wonderful descriptions for our eyes. Many species on earth have eyes of all sorts, from the compound eyes and antennae of the smallest insect, to the relatively small and seldom-used eyes on the head of the largest whale.

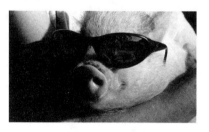

In the human species, sight is our dominant sense. We react to and process literally millions of bits of information every day with our eyes. We are cautioned to brush and floss our teeth, keep our ears clean, and spend several hours a week exercising our bodies, but curiously, we practice few, if any procedures to care for our valuable sense of sight.

Have your arms seemed a little too short lately? You know what I mean—all of a sudden it is simply more comfortable to read when you are holding the page a little farther away. It happens to nine out of ten of us. As time goes by, vision fades a little. Most people keep good vision well into older age, but serious eye diseases are generally painless and symptoms don't usually manifest themselves until it's too late to get help. To set your sights on the future, read on and learn how to protect those peepers of yours.

EYE ON AWARENESS

Experts rarely agree on everything, but when it comes to your eyes, they're all reading off the same page: The most important thing you can do for your vision is to get regular eye exams. Half of all blindness can be prevented. More than 10 million Americans over the age of twenty-five have some loss of vision, and many of them don't even know it. If you've had no problems in the past, and you're over the age of forty, then go at least every three years to an ophthamologist. If you already wear glasses or contact lenses, or have a personal or family history of diabetes, hypertension, or glaucoma, your doctor will recommend a more frequent schedule of checkups. In the meantime, here are some of the things you need to look out for. I don't want to nag you about getting those regular eye exams, so please read over the next section carefully.

Vision changes. Here's why your arms may suddenly be feeling too short: As we age, the lenses in our eyes stiffen. The less flexible they are, the more difficult it is to focus on something close, like the page you are reading now. This is known as farsightedness, because you can see far, but you can't see close—technically *presbyopia*, from the Greek word *presby* for old and *opia* for eye. Correcting this problem is very easy, either with glasses or contact lenses. The shape of our eyeballs may also change as we age, with the eye going from round to a more flattened out oval, and then our far vision may also need correcting. If you do need your near and far vision corrected, the good news is that bifocals no longer have that "window pane," divided look. With the newer blended lenses, only you and your ophthamologist will know for sure. Even contact lenses are now made as bifocal lenses.

Glaucoma. An estimated 1 to 2 percent of Americans over age forty have glaucoma right now, and 25 percent of these cases are undetected. That's important, because untreated glaucoma that begins at ages forty to forty-five will probably cause complete blindness by age sixty to sixty-five.

What is it? Glaucoma is a group of eye diseases caused by an increase in the pressure of the fluid inside the eyeball, which can choke off and destroy the optic nerve. There may not be any symptoms until it's quite advanced, which could be too late for many. Yet early diagnosis and treatment is successful in most cases. There are two major types of glaucoma.

Chronic open angle glaucoma accounts for about 90 percent of all glaucoma cases. This type stems from a gradual buildup of pressure in the eye. There are usually no symptoms in the early stages. However, sufferers have difficulty adjusting to the light in darkened rooms and slowly lose peripheral vision over the years, resulting in tunnel vision (they can only see what's right in front of them). In the later stages, they see "halos" around lights. This kind of glaucoma is usually in both eyes. People of African decent, nearsighted individuals, diabetics, people with high blood pressure, or those who find themselves changing their eyeglass prescriptions frequently may be at higher risk.

Successful treatment involves special eye drops or laser treatment to open up the eye's drainage canals. In most cases, early diagnosis and treatment will preserve vision throughout your life.

Acute closed angle glaucoma comes on rapidly, but luckily, it has symptoms: Severe eye pain, blurry loss of vision with "halos" seen around lights, red eyes, and dilated pupils are the big tip-offs here. Farsighted people and those of Asian descent are at greater risk for this. It's treatable with medication, but it's important to get treatment immediately, because permanent visual loss can occur within two to five days after symptoms begin.

COMMON VISION PROBLEMS

Cataracts. Cataracts, a gradual cloudiness of the lens of the eye, usually occurs in both eyes over time and causes blurry, hazy vision and light sensitivity. Sometimes you can actually see the cloudiness yourself when you look in the mirror. Most people over the age of sixty have some degree of opaqueness of the lens of the eye, and if you live a long time, you're more likely to have cataract surgery than any other.

Cataracts used to mean blindness and, many decades ago, cataract surgery was risky. Because of old-fashioned sutures, the patient was required to stay perfectly still for a week after surgery with the head weighted down with sandbags.

But today, modern suturing and new laser procedures have reduced surgery to a 30-minute outpatient procedure. Thousands of people each year have their sight miraculously restored with the new plastic implanted lenses. The rest of the good news is that cataract surgery is the one of the most successful of all types of medical surgeries performed.

Cigarette smoking can increase your risk of getting cataracts by 63 percent, according to a Harvard Medical School study of 120,000 nurses. If you still need another reason to quit the nicotine habit, put on your glasses and read this one twice. Exposure to sunlight also quickens the formation of cataracts, so wear a hat and UVA/UVB blocking sunglasses when you're outside or driving. Remember that a good deal of sun- 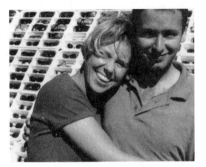 light can strike the eye from the side of your head, so wraparound sunglasses are a good idea.

Antioxidant vitamins are also a good bet here, according to the Harvard Nurses Health Study. Also, eating three or more servings of fruits and vegetables every day may help prevent cataract formation.

Macular degeneration. The central part of the retina, called the macular region, includes a dense concentration of rods and cones that allows us to read and do close-up work. In age-related macular degeneration, photoreceptors in the colored membrane of the retina break down. The end result can be a fibrous scar, which causes loss of the central section of vision.

Risk factors besides age (over fifty) include: being white, a family history of the disease, a history of cigarette smoking, and being female. (There's only a slight female predominance, though.)

Gradual, increasing central vision loss in both eyes implies macular degeneration. Sometimes laser surgery can stabilize the deterioration process. The hope is that you probably won't get the condition until after sixty years of age, and by then there may be a preventive strategy based on antioxidants. Lutein, an antioxidant found abundantly in green vegetables like collard greens and spinach, is found in high concentrations in the macular area of the eye.

Diabetic retinopathy and proliferative retinopathy. The longer a person has diabetes, the greater his or her chance of experiencing some kind of eye damage. And in the age group twenty to sixty-five, these problems are the leading cause of blindness among American adults. Because of circulation changes caused by diabetes, the blood vessels deep in the eye tend to leak, and the retina can become detached or scarred.

Laser treatments can now treat the blood vessels, but only those who get their eyes examined regularly will be able to benefit from treatment. If you have diabetes, it is essential that you have your eyes dilated and examined at least once a year.

You can try to avoid adult-onset diabetes by keeping trim, exercising, limiting alcohol, eating a more vegetarian diet. Turn to chapters 10 and 11 for more strategies.

Flashing floaters. These sudden "spots of light" in the eye could mean a detached retina. This is a 911 emergency situation. Get medical attention immediately.

Fuzzy bugs. Small specks, or tiny clouds or "fuzzy bugs," that you see from time to time in your line of vision are particles floating around inside the fluid of your eye. They cast a shadow on the retina. They're normal and most people start noticing them more after age forty.

AN EYE-CATCHING GLOSSARY

We talked earlier about the importance of getting regular eye examinations. The next question is: To whom should you go? Here's an easy rule of thumb for remembering the *Who's Who* of eye specialists: generally, the longer the name, the more education and training they've had.

Ophthamologists. These are M.D.s who have at least four years of college, plus four years of medical school, followed by one year of a medical internship. Then, a complete hospital residency program of at least three years of specialized eye care is required. Ophthamologists prescribe glasses, contact lenses, and drugs for diseases of the eye. Some, but not all, perform surgery.

Optometrists. After four years of college, they attend four years of optometry school and are specialists in the physical properties of the eye and corrective lenses (glasses and contact lenses). But are they not licensed to prescribe drugs in some states, or to perform surgery.

Opticians. Up to two years of training in lens technology is required. Once an ophthamologist or optometrist has prescribed corrective lenses, the optician is normally the next step for you to get the prescription filled.

CALISTHENICS FOR YOUR EYES

We consider working out the rest of our bodies, so why not strengthen our eyes while we're at it? These exercises are not meant to get you to throw away your glasses or contacts, but they are good for your eyes and are a lot less work than going to the gym or doing sit ups on the living room floor. And they feel good.

Palming. This one is like a yawn and stretch for your pupils. Close your eyes and cup your hands over them—not touching or pressing on your eyeballs. Stay like that for a slow count to ten. Then open your eyes. The idea is to give your eyes a break with the darkness and then wake them up as you remove your hands. It is very relaxing and refreshing, especially when you are under stress. Five minute breaks like this, several times a day, are a wonderful stress management technique. Think lovely thoughts as you rest your elbows on your desk and breathe effortlessly during this time.

Focus, please. Think of this one as a bicep curl for your eye reflexes—important for everyone, particularly in racquet sports like tennis, squash, and racquetball. I learned it from a man who was an active teaching tennis pro at eighty-six years young. Take a golf ball and turn its label toward you. Focus on the label while holding the ball at arm's length. Now move the ball in a circle in front of you, never letting that label get out of focus. Make circles of all sizes in both directions.

Next, while still focusing on the label, move the ball toward you and away from you, in an arc. This does wonders for practicing the focus range and reaction reflex of your eyes. Start with one minute and increase to ten minutes daily. You could keep the golf ball next to the TV remote control and practice during the commercial breaks without even breaking a sweat.

Fluttering. Tilt your head back slightly and close your eyes. Then open your eyes and "flutter blink" them for a count of five seconds. It helps lubricate your eyes and rest them. Repeat two to three times throughout the day. This exercise is of particular benefit to computer users, people who read a lot, and those involved in endurance activities such as bike riding and distance running. In the case of endurance activities, the exerciser stares for long periods of time as a result of the beneficial biochemical changes in our blood composition from the exertion. These changes produce a gentle euphoria that promotes staring, which dries the external eye tissues.

When studying, reading, or doing close work. Every ten to fifteen minutes, look away from your work and focus on an object in the distance. In a Harvard study, the amount of myopia, or nearsightedness, among students increased each year they spent at graduate school. The good news is that after graduate school, the eyes can correct themselves. As a literate society, we spend so much time in close work that our far vision (our relaxed vision) suffers.

SETTING YOUR SIGHT ON THE FUTURE

The key to keeping your eyes sharp is prevention and early detection of problems. Here are some suggestions for setting your sight on the future.

Get your eyes examined. This at the top of the list for a reason—it can save your sight.

Protect your eyes from sunlight. Wear sunglasses that block both UVA and UVB light. It may help reduce your risk of cataracts. Wearing a hat in addition will help shield your eyes from the damaging effects of the sun.

Get some sleep. The eyes are the first to show the strain of sleep deprivation. Most of us get a lot less than we need for optimum health.

Stop smoking. It increases your risk of cataracts and decreases your chances of living. Nicotine also reduces blood supply to the eye.

Wear goggles. Use sport goggles for racquet sports. Whether you swim in a chlorinated pool, a freshwater lake, or the ocean, you are exposed to bacteria that can infect your eyes and from which goggles will protect you. Make sure you wear safety goggles for any work that could endanger your eyes. Scraping off old paint, mowing the lawn, and pruning your rose bushes put your eyes at risk if they are unprotected.

Avoid excess alcohol and caffeine. These substances decrease circulation of blood to the eye.

Eat your veggies and consider taking antioxidants. Zinc, glutathione, vitamins A, B2 (riboflavin) C, D, E, and beta-carotene are cataract and macular degeneration fighters. The bilberry fruit, rich in anthrocyanidins, has traditionally been used for eye health in Europe. Lutein and zeaxanthin are antioxidants strongly linked with reduced risk of macular degeneration, and eating five or more weekly servings of leafy green vegetables (rich in these ingredients), such as collard greens and spinach has been shown to offer protection. Calcium has been linked with improving nearsightedness. Glutathione, found in asparagus, avocado, watermelon, and oranges, is known to help protect against cataract formation. Selenium and zinc deficiencies are linked with cataracts. Vitamin E has a favorable effect as a macular protectant. Fish oils have been shown to reduce pressure on the fluids of the eyes in preliminary studies, thus possibly helping prevent glaucoma. Choline and inositol, ingredients found in lecithin, are also used by natural practitioners for the health of eye tissues. Taurine, an amino acid important for eye tissue, is manufactured by the body from the amino acid cysteine and vitamin B6, and may improve eye health. Cats, who make even less taurine than humans, may become blind on taurine-deficient diets, but the visual impairment can be reversed if the deficiency is corrected in time. In 1982, Dr. M. J. Voaden and his colleagues found retinitis pigmentosa patients to have abnormally low levels of taurine and published his findings in the *British Journal of Opthamology*. The amino acid cysteine and vitamin B6 form taurine in the body. Taurine is naturally abundant in animal and fish protein.

Pain, unusual redness, vision changes, foreign objects, or chemicals in the eye. All warrant an immediate trip to the doctor.

EYE OPERATIONS THROUGHOUT HISTORY

Ancient documents reveal that ophthalmic surgery was one of the most advanced areas of medicine in the ancient world. The Babylonians seem to have developed eye surgery long before the Greeks or the Romans. During the rule of King Hammurabi of Babylon, in 1800 B.C., cataract surgery was described in the legal code: "If a physician performed a major operation on a nobleman with a bronze lance and has saved a nobleman's life, or opened up the eye-socket of a nobleman with a bronze lance and has saved the nobleman's eye, he shall receive ten shekels of silver." A commoner's eye was worth five shekels; a slave's, two shekels. For a surgery to require legislation, it had to be a fairly common occurrence. Two thousand years later, the medical writings of Roman Cornelius Celsus described cataract surgery in great and gory detail. With a plain bronze needle syringe, the surgeon would push the cataract out of the way and the patient felt only minimal pain—if the procedure was done precisely.

An interesting note on Hammurabi's legislative code: If a surgeon destroyed the sight of a patient's eye, the law stated that his hand be chopped off.

YOUR HEARING

When a person with poor vision asks for our assistance, we leap to their aid, glad to be able to help, proud of ourselves for being there at the right time. But too often when a person with poor hearing asks us to repeat things over and over again, we become irritable and annoyed, thinking "Oh, never mind" to ourselves and ready to forget the whole thing.

Why? Probably because with the unsighted person, we feel like a hero—we've done our good deed for the day. We are humbled by their willingness to carry on regardless as we mentally change places with them and wonder if we would have the same courage and optimism on a daily basis if we were blind.

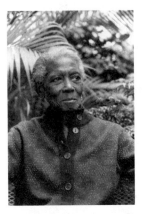

But with a hearing impaired person, it is different. Perhaps in repeating our own words, we realize how banal our comments really are. We feel foolish, embarrassed, or sometimes ashamed of our mumbled innuendos that the hearing impaired person asks be repeated, loudly.

Indeed, hearing is a very emotional subject. Dr. Philip Zimbardo, a Stanford University psychologist writing in *Science* magazine (June 25, 1981), found that when told under hypnosis that they had a hearing disability, otherwise normal, healthy subjects exhibited paranoid tendencies.

Fear, embarrassment, and vanity are major reasons why people with hearing loss do not seek help when they need it. The same type of vanity that prevents people from wearing glasses when they need them is multiplied when it comes to seeking help for their hearing and isolation from the rest of the world may be the result.

I have one patient, who, at ninety-eight years of age, *refuses* to use a hearing aid because she says, "That's for old ladies." The exasperating frustration experienced by the rest of the family as a result of this stubbornness would be impossible to describe.

The fact is that nearly 60 percent of the people surveyed by the University of California, San Francisco, School of Medicine, noticed symptoms before they were forty years old. Pilots, motorcycle riders, rock musicians, garment industry workers, construction workers, assembly line workers, airline ground crews, and gardeners (from those noisy leaf blowers) are some of those who experience job-related hearing loss and damage.

Diseases such as measles, mumps, multiple sclerosis, viral or bacterial infections, and adverse reactions to aspirin and antibiotics are additional causes of hearing loss. The changes in air pressure from constant air travel can be another factor in aural damage. During the physical exam of new patients, I am still surprised to discover the number of patients who experience hearing loss simply because their ears are impacted with wax. When the wax is removed, they hear clearly, sometimes for the first time in forty or more years!

OUR HUMAN STEREO SOUND SYSTEM

Traveling through the atmosphere on air molecules, sound vibrations reach our outer ear and are funneled toward the cone-shaped membrane stretched across the end of the ear canal and tethered to one of three tiny bones in the middle ear. The *hammer, anvil,* and *stirrup* bones, so named because of their shapes, transmit vibrations to the fluid inside another structure, the *cochlea*. If you can picture a tiny snail shell filled with fluid, then you have the idea. Now add about 50,000 tiny hairs growing inside that snail shell. The vibrating fluid inside the cochlea transmit the vibrations further, stimulating the hairlike structures so that impulses are then transmitted to the brain via the auditory nerve. The vestibular nerve, actually a division of the auditory nerve that we use for balancing, is also located nearby.

TIME AND OUR STEREO SYSTEM

Hearing loss is associated with aging because the ear drum tends to stiffen over time. The small bones of the ear may also undergo some changes such as calcium deposits at their junction points, and the tiny hair cells of the cochlea may become damaged from, for instance, loud rock music, leaf blowers, some prescription medications, or infections.

Age-related hearing loss is named *presbycusis*, from the Greek word *presby*, meaning old, plus the word *cusis* meaning ear. In those under the age of fifty, the most common cause of hearing loss is from the damaging effect of loud noises.

Think of your ears as a parking meter. The damage adds up eventually. If you avoid continuous exposure to excessive noise, the meter will tick along more slowly. If you're exposing your ears to daily amounts of sound over 80 decibels, then your auditory parking meter is going to run out of time a lot sooner. The majority of damage is done to the permanent cilia cells and, once they are destroyed, they do not grow back.

Scientists at Albert Einstein School of Medicine in New York have shown that retinoic acid encourages new growth of damaged hair cells in rats, but human studies will take a while. In this area, birds, sharks, and frogs are way ahead of us: They regrow hair cells naturally after there has been damage. But then again, they're usually not the groupies who get the good seats in front of the amplifiers at rock concerts.

FOR WHOM THE DECIBEL TOLLS

Here are some common sounds that we might encounter on a daily basis, with their decibel ratings. The lowest sound a human being can detect would be zero decibels. But the scale goes up in intensity in a logarithmic manner similar to that of the Richter earthquake scale: 20 decibels is 10 times louder than 0; 40 decibels is 100 times louder than 0; 60 decibels is 1,000 times louder.

THE DAILY ZONE

0 decibels	the lowest sound that a human ear can hear
30 decibels	the sound of your fingers rubbing together next to your ear
40 decibels	a quiet room
50 decibels	leaves rustling in a soft wind
60 decibels	normal talking between people with normal hearing
70 decibels	a busy restaurant, noisy traffic. Continuous exposure to noise at this level may begin to affect your hearing in a negative way.

THE DANGER ZONE

80 decibels	Subway train coming into the station, noisy city traffic. Over eight hours a day and it's unhealthful for your ears.
90 decibels	Power lawn mower, leaf blower, snow blower, kitchen blender, vacuum cleaner, a power drill. In less than eight hours, you can have damage.
100 decibels	Chain saw, stereo headphones, a symphony orchestra in the big finale. Even two hours at this level is dangerous for your ears.
120 decibels	Rock concert, a thunder boom, a jackhammer—your ears are blasted immediately. There will be temporary hearing loss that may return, and some permanent damage. Continual exposure to these levels of sound will kill off the hair cells of the ear.
140 decibels	Rock concert if you're in front of the speakers, a gunshot, a cannon firing, a firecracker exploding, a jet plane if you're next to it on the runway outside. Any exposure causes pain and damage. Your ear hairs are basically fried at these levels.

180 decibels   Rocket launching pad. Hearing loss is irreversible and inevitable at this range. Practical information to have before you plan your next moon mission!

WHAT THE EXPERTS ARE LISTENING FOR

There are two types of hearing loss. First, that which is caused by malfunction of the cochlea or the auditory nerve, which is usually called "nerve deafness." And second, that caused by impairment of the mechanisms for transmitting sound into the cochlea, which is usually identified as "conduction deafness." To determine the type of hearing disabilities, a simple earphone connected to an electronic oscillator is used. Known as an *audiometer,* it is able to emit pure tones and vibrations from very low to very high frequencies, based on what calibration of sound a normal person could hear. For instance, if the tone must be increased in loudness to 30 decibels above normal to be heard, the person is said to have hearing loss of 30 decibels for that particular tone.

Presbycusis or age-related hearing loss becomes most apparent in the higher pitches of our hearing range. Men tend to experience more hearing loss in the higher ranges than women, and researchers speculate that may be as a result of increased lifelong exposure to heavy machinery in a work environment.

Some examples of high-frequency sounds in the English language are: *s,f,t,sh,th,* and *ch.* In the world of computer speech recognition that converts the spoken word to written words or computer commands, there is a classic example of "mis-hearing" the following sentence: "You can't wreck a nice beach" versus the sentence "You can't recognize speech." Even people who can hear well could have trouble discerning between the two statements. Now imagine someone who has difficulty hearing the high frequency sounds. Perhaps it will sound like, "You can red a nigh bee." This is exactly how a person with an uncorrected hearing loss becomes isolated from social interaction.

BREAKING THE SILENCE BARRIER

I had a grade school teacher who used to write the following quotation on the blackboard at the beginning of each class and then wait for us to settle down: "Silence is golden, let's get rich quick." However, there are a lot of people out there for whom the silence is more than a few stops short of golden.

Most people avoid having their hearing checked because of vanity. Remember the ninety-eight-year-old woman I described earlier who wouldn't get a hearing aid that would correct her problem because she said "it's for old ladies"? As a result of that stance, she'll never hear the laughter of her great-great-grandson or participate in a meaningful conversation with her grandchildren. Even television turned up full blast is hard for her to understand, so she lives her life as a socially isolated victim of her own stubbornness. Like many others smitten with pride, she has been misdiagnosed with dementia—it's not that she can't recall what was said it's that she never heard it in the first place.

The National Institute of Health estimates one in ten Americans has some form of hearing impairment that prevents understanding normal speech and conducting normal conversation. An estimated 28 million actually suffer hearing loss: as the sixties flower children (and rock-concert survivors) reach senior age those numbers will rise. In a survey by the National Institutes of Health, 58 percent of those surveyed over the age of sixty-five said that they had a hearing disability, but only 8 percent of that group used a hearing aid.

There's a strange reverse side to this scenario. Because of recent advances in technology, some people who were previously unsuitable for electronic hearing correction can now benefit from a hearing aid after all. "It sounds hard to believe," says Gloria Frias, a California physical therapist who is herself hearing impaired. "But these people are so well integrated into the nonhearing social environment that they choose not to get a hearing aid that would allow them to hear again, because they would then have to reintegrate into the hearing world. They are very comfortable within the safety of their own nonhearing world, with the friends who share their disability."

WHAT'S NEW IN SOUND SYSTEMS?

Analog circuitry that's programmed digitally to customize each hearing aid to an individual's requirement is like having your own personal "graphic equalizer" built in. Older model hearing aids worked on amplifying all sound frequencies and the devices could not be fine-tuned to fit individual requirements.

If you think that you may have some hearing loss, don't wait years until you get some help. The sooner you go, the sooner you can get help. Some hearing loss is simply due to impacted wax. Ringing in the ears and dizziness may be controlled with diet and medication. Other conditions could benefit from surgery or correction with one of the new powerful hearing aids that can fit inconspicuously inside your ear.

In the meantime, listen up and let's go over some ways that you can protect your hearing for the decades to come.

NOW HEAR THIS!

Protecting your hearing for the long haul is a lot like the other strategies we'll discuss in the book: Prevention is key.

Get your hearing tested every few years unless you have a personal or family history of hearing disability, and then once a year is prudent.

Protect yourself against loud noises. Wear ear plugs if you are exposing yourself to loud sounds like motorcycles, concerts, or power tools. The squishy foam ones that you buy in drugstores work well: They're washable and inexpensive enough to be disposable. They're also wonderful when traveling to ensure a good night's sleep.

Turn down the sound. Keep your stereo in the lesser volume ranges. I saw a documentary on a native tribe in Africa that spoke only in whispers. Their hearing acuity was measured in the superhuman levels.

Your portable stereo may be a sneaky hearing thief. Earphones transmit sound so directly into the ear that sudden changes in volume that often occur in music can cause damage.

Avoid flying if you are suffering from a sinus infection or a cold. The eustachian tubes that lead to your ears can become blocked and the changes in air pressure can lead to a tubal pressure situation that could cause painful damage to your eardrum. You may consider using a nasal decongestant, trying to yawn, sipping water, or chewing gum to equalize the pressure.

Don't drink and fly. Alcohol swells the mucous membranes in the eustachian tubes and can help create painful ear pressure problems as the plane descends.

Quit smoking. Nicotine reduces blood flow to the ears and thereby slows healing to the ears when there has been damage from loud noises.

Kick the caffeine habit. Caffeine works in a manner similar to nicotine by constricting blood vessels, thereby decreasing blood flow and, with it, the chance to heal from damage.

Easy on the aspirin. Aspirin overload may cause your ears to ring.

Review your medication. Some antibiotics can cause damage to your hearing. Ask your doctor or pharmacist if your medication could be the cause of a hearing loss.

Don't freeze or fry them. A lot of skin cancer develops on the tops of ears because it's not an obvious place to apply sunblock. Also, when you're outdoors in the winter, be very mindful of frostbite—I can tell you from experience that it happens very easily when you're outside enjoying the slopes. It hurts!

Go easy on the cotton swabs. I've seen same nasty scrapes inside patients' ears from overenthusiastic cotton swab action. My mother always told me that the only thing that you should put in your ear is your elbow. She was right, because sticking small things in your ear—hairpins, cotton swabs, etc—only pushes the wax further in toward the eardrum. If you have enthusiasm to clean the wax out of your ears, buy a wax removal kit at any drugstore. Otherwise, leave it to the professionals!

Get in shape. Are you wondering what losing your spare tire could possibly have to do with your hearing? Wonder no more. The same artery-clogging fatty diet that is bad for your cardiovascular system is also bad news for your ears. Arterial plaquing can reduce blood supply to your ears and eventually choke off your hearing.

Food for your ears. A low-fat, high-fiber diet and exercise help to reduce the formation of arterial plaques that can reduce blood circulation to the ears.

WHEN TO CHECK IT OUT

Symptoms of hearing impairment can happen at any age. Here's when to get checked:

- If you hear a ringing or buzzing in your ears
- If you are frequently asking people to speak up
- If telephone conversations seem difficult to follow
- If you experience ear pain of any kind
- If you feel dizzy
- If you find yourself leaning forward in meetings to hear others

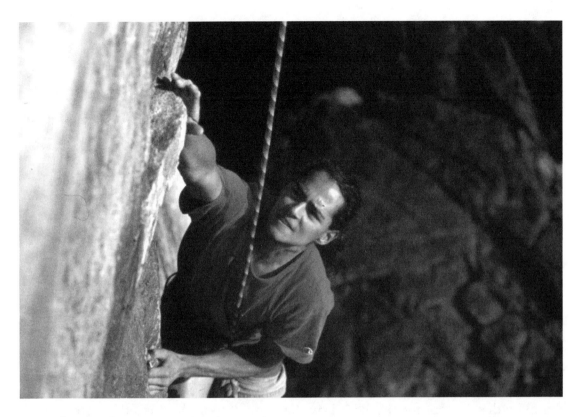

- If you miss conversation in a noisy area
- If family or friends suggest you have your hearing checked

Has all this come in loud and clear? Good. Because if you are good to your ears, they will bring a lifetime of sweet sounds.

CHAPTER

13

KEEPING YOUR BEAUTIFUL BONES

I knew a woman, lovely in her bones
When small birds sighed, she would sigh back at them;
Ah, when she moved, she moved more ways than one:
The shapes a bright container can contain!

—Theodore Roethke (1908–1963), "I Knew a Woman"

*W*hen one of my patients, age thirty, wondered whether she should be concerned about osteoporosis after her fifty-five-year-old mother fell and broke her hip, I had to say yes. The tendency toward brittle bones is inherited. But before you skimp on that present for Mother's Day this year, keep in the mind that osteoporosis can be prevented.

According to the National Osteoporosis Foundation, more than 25 million Americans—80 percent of them women—have osteoporosis. This loss of bone tissue affects more women than men because women are usually thinner, with smaller bones to begin with, and they live longer than men so there is more time to develop it.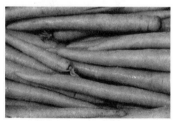

Approximately 1.3 million fractures per year are directly attributable to osteo-porosis with estimated costs, medical and social, at $7.5 billion annually. Osteoporo-sis is considered a disease of epidemic proportions affecting one-third of all American women, resulting in a 20 to 40 percent loss of bone mass by age sixty-five. This con-tinuing bone loss causes the incidence of hip fractures to double every five years after age sixty. By the age of seventy, some experts estimate that 40 percent of U.S. women will experience a fracture due to osteoporosis.

Additionally, when the vertebral bones of the upper spine become demineralized

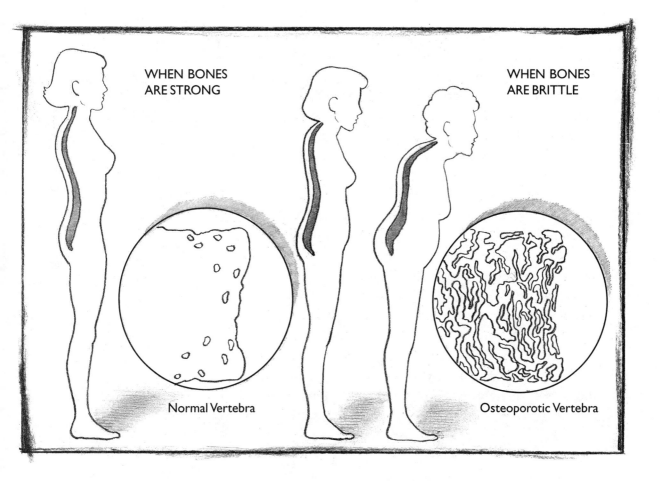

WHEN BONES
ARE STRONG

WHEN BONES
ARE BRITTLE

Normal Vertebra

Osteoporotic Vertebra

and fracture, you lose height and your spine starts curving forward into a "dowager's hump." Average loss of height by the age of eighty-five is three inches. By age seventy, women will have lost 25 to 50 percent of their skeletal mass if they do not work to prevent it. Some nine out of ten women are affected by osteoporosis by the age of seventy.

Bone is composed of a tough organic substance that is greatly strengthened by deposits of calcium salts. The organic matrix of bone is 90 to 95 percent collagen fibers. The bone ingredients are mainly calcium and phosphate. Magnesium, sodium, potassium, and carbonate are also present in bones as are many other minerals like strontium, uranium, and plutonium. Did you know that nine of the fourteen major radioactive products of the hydrogen bomb can be found in bone tissue? Lead, gold, and other heavy metal molecules are also found in bone.

Bones in babies and children are relatively soft. Estrogen causes bones to build and grow as girls reach puberty. That's why there's a rapid growth rate in teenage years when estrogen is being produced in abundance. Bone is constantly changing, with new cells being added and old ones being recycled all the time. As estrogen and progesterone production by the ovaries winds down before menopause, the deficiency reduces the building activities of bone. Then bone matrix decreases and so does the rate of deposit of bone calcium and phosphate. Without the vigorous deposition of minerals and building of the matrix, the architecture of the bones weakens and becomes porous. Bone density is reduced. *Osteo* is a Greek word that means bone; *poros* means passage or opening, like the word "pore."

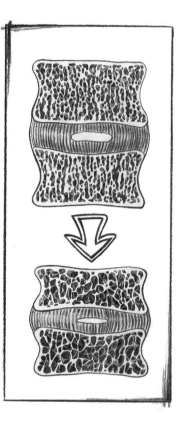

You could think of your bones as being like a bank. You make a lot of deposits when you're a teenager, but as you near menopause, you start making more withdrawals than deposits. To reverse this trend, read on and learn how to keep your bones out of the poor house.

OSTEOPOROSIS: CAUSES AND PREVENTION

How do you know if you have osteoporosis? Chances are you won't notice it until your total height decreases. I measure the height of my elderly patients on each visit. X-rays can show bone loss, but not until there's been a 30 to 40 percent loss of bone already. CAT scans, bone scans, and other specialized radiographic techniques can also show bone density changes. However, the best test with the least amount of radiation is called dual energy X-ray absorptimetry, or DEXA, and examinations of the hip or spine take about five to fifteen minutes. Single-energy-X-ray absorptiometry measures the bones of the wrist or heel. If you think that you may already have it, ask your doctor for a DEXA test, available at most large hospitals. Your best bet is to study the risk factors, and avoid them.

BONE ROBBERS

- Caffeine
- High-protein, red meat diet
- Excessive fiber—it binds calcium, making it unavailable for absorption
- Alcohol
- Physical inactivity
- Smoking
- Low-calcium diet
- High salt intake
- Certain prescription drugs like corticosteroids
- Prolonged dieting or fasting
- Inadequate intake of vitamin C
- Vitamin D deficiency

If you have more than two of these biological factors you may be at risk of developing osteoporosis.

- You're a fair-skinned, thin, short female with freckles
- A family history of osteoporosis
- Early menopause
- Scoliosis
- Never had children
- Northern European or Asian ancestry
- You are approaching or past menopause
- You are a heavy smoker
- You are a heavy drinker

HERE'S THE GOOD NEWS . . .

Osteoporosis is preventable. Sure, the *tendency* toward developing brittle bones is genetic, but there are many lifestyle factors that you can control so that you don't have to become one of these gloomy statistics.

Exercise

Exercise is now recognized as one of the biggest weapons against osteoporosis. Weight-bearing exercise, like rigorous walking or stair climbing, can help maintain and even increase bone mass. Better yet, try pumping iron with handheld weights like barbells and dumbbells. See the exercises at the end of the chapter.

Thirty minutes of moderate daily exercise helps shift your risk for not only osteoporosis, but also heart disease, according to the American College of Sports Medicine. Yet nearly three out of four women aren't meeting that minimum, according to the Centers for Disease Control and Prevention. In one study, a group of seventy-year-old osteoporotic women simply pushed against a wall or clasped their hands and pushed their wrists together in three workouts a week for five months. There was a 3.8 percent increase in the wrist bones in the exercise group. The nonexercisers in the study lost 1.9 percent of their bone mass during the same time period.

Vegetarian Diet

I was really surprised to see the research on this one, because most critics of vegetarian diets target the typically lower protein ratios of a veggie lifestyle. However, in two studies involving postmenopausal vegetarian women, greater bone loss was found in women who consumed meat. Additionally, high-protein diets have been related to bone loss in several studies. So you may think twice about ordering steak if you're concerned about keeping your bones strong. You can cut down on your protein intake from animal sources. Tofu, tempeh (soy products), beans, grains, and legumes are alternate sources of protein. Turn to Chapter 11 for tips on how to eat more vegetarian foods.

Caffeine and Other Calcium Thieves

If you drink more than four cups of coffee a day, you need to know about the research that shows that risk of hip fracture is three times more likely in women who consume large amounts of caffeine. Studies also warn about possible links between caffeine and a host of other problems, including fibrocystic breast disease, elevated cholesterol levels, intensified PMS symptoms, heart disease, cancer, and insomnia.

How do you ease off the caffeine? First of all, recognize the things that add caffeine into your day.

CONVICTED OF CAFFEINE

Coffee (5-ounce cup)

Drip	115 mg.
Percolated	80 mg.
Instant	68–98 mg.
Decaf	4 mg.

Tea (5-ounce cup)

Tetley	64 mg.
Lipton	52 mg.
Constant Comment	29 mg.

Soft Drinks

Mountain Dew	54 mg.
Diet Coke/Coke	46 mg.
Pepsi	38 mg.
Diet Pepsi	36 mg.

Chocolate (1 ounce)

Dark Chocolate	24 mg.
Milk Chocolate	4 mg.

Nonprescription Drugs

Maximum strength No Doz	200 mg.
Vivarin	200 mg.
Excedrin Extra Strength	65 mg.
Anacin/Anacin Max Strength	32 mg.

THINGS TO AVOID TO MAINTAIN BONE MASS

Alcohol. Alcoholics, both men and women, are at higher risk for bone loss.

Diuretics. Many women get hooked on these to relieve bloating and PMS, but every day you take diuretics capriciously, you are flushing valuable bone minerals down the toilet. Instead, drinking more water, at least eight to ten glasses a day, and taking your vitamins and minerals will help prevent premenstrual bloating without the unwanted side effects of diuretics.

Protein. There is significantly less osteoporosis in developing countries. Why? Because people in industrialized countries tend to eat too much protein. How much are you supposed to eat? Review Chapter 11 and get the skinny on protein. Animal protein like steak is high in phosphorus, which has a negative effect on calcium.

Carbonated beverages. The phosphates in soda interfere with the absorption of calcium and vitamin D. Given the amount of diet colas consumed by many adolescents, osteoporosis is considered by some to be a pediatric problem.

Smoking. If you smoke you're at great risk for osteoporosis.

Salt intake. A diet high in sodium upsets other mineral balances in the body and this has a negative effect on calcium.

HOW TO BUILD BEAUTIFUL BONES

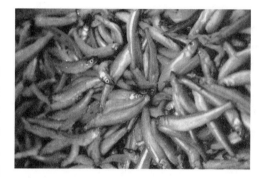

While food is the preferable way to consume daily calcium, few women get the minimum daily requirement of 1,000 milligrams per day from their diets. Think that drinking milk is the best way to get your calcium? Think again. Despite the millions of dollars spent to convince us otherwise, here are the facts on how much of this important mineral can be found in other foods. Note that skim milk is way down the list! Other dairy products like cheese fare better, but remember that it's important to watch your intake of saturated animal fats, which are high in dairy foods and contribute to elevated cholesterol levels.

CALCIUM CONTENT OF SELECTED FOODS*

Sardines, 3 oz.	371 mg.
Swiss cheese, 1 oz.	272 mg.
Tofu, firm, ½ cup	258 mg.
Cheddar cheese, 1 oz.	218 mg.
Collard greens, ½ cup	188 mg.
Kale, ½ cup	187 mg.
Turnip greens, ½ cup	184 mg.
Rhubarb, cooked ½ cup	174 mg.
Fruit yogurt, ½ cup	172 mg.
Salmon, canned 3 oz.	167 mg.
Oatmeal (instant, fortified, 1 packet)	163 mg.
Skim milk, ½ cup	151 mg.
Orange juice, calcium added	150 mg.
Molasses, blackstrap, 1 tbsp.	137 mg.
Low-fat cottage cheese, ½ cup	78 mg.

*From *Composition of Foods Handbook*, no. 8 (Washington, D.C.: ARS USDA, 1976–86).

Vitamin C. The bone matrix is 90 to 95 percent collagen fibers. Vitamin C is essential for activating the enzyme *hydroxylase*, which is an integral ingredient of collagen. You can get the healthy 1,000 milligrams daily of vitamin C by eating oranges, but you'd have to eat fourteen whole oranges and that would leave room for little else! I recommend 1,000 milligrams of vitamin C per day to my patients at risk for osteoporosis.

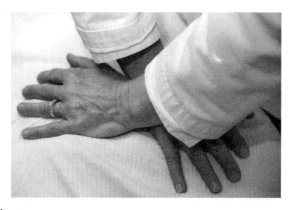

Calcium supplements. Calcium citrate is the preferred form of calcium. It's best absorbed when in small amounts throughout the day. *Calcium carbonate* can be tough on your stomach. My patients seem to digest calcium citrate much better, even when they take it between meals, whereas calcium carbonate seems to cause digestive difficulties. *Calcium lactate* and *calcium gluconate* are other forms you'll see on the market, but they're usually a lot more expensive and not readily available in stores. Be sure to look on the bottle for *elemental calcium*. Check the label to see how many tablets you have to take to get your daily requirement. Read carefully, because a favorite trick is to list the number at the top of the nutrition information as in "Six tablets supply. . . ." That's important information, because you might have to take eight or nine calcium gluconate tablets, for instance to get the same amount of elemental calcium in calcium citrate.

GETTING THE LEAD OUT

Consumers have been warned about the possibility of calcium supplements that contain lead in a recent edition of *Nutrition Action Healthletter* (December, 1993). Calcium supplements containing bone meal (from animals), dolomite (from rocks), and calcium carbonate (from oyster shells) have all been implicated. Powdered bone meal is often a supplement choice because it is so inexpensive. Lead is stored in the bones, its effects are cumulative and toxic, and it should be avoided.

The National Osteoporosis Foundation recommends the following levels of calcium each day:

ADULT WOMEN

Pregnant, lactating, age 24 and under	1,200 to 1,500 mg.
Pregnant, lactating, over 24	1,200 mg.
25 to 49 years (before menopause)	1,000 mg.
50 to 64 years, taking estrogen supplements	1,000 mg.
50 to 64 years, without extra estrogen	1,500 mg.
65 and over	1,500 mg.

ADULT MEN

25 to 64 years	1,000 mg.
65 and over	1,500 mg.

Many people ask if they can take antacids for their daily calcium. Calcium in food needs the strong hydrochloric acid of the stomach in order for it to be absorbed by the body in the digestive system. Antacids contain calcium, but its name says it all: it's an *antacid*; its job is to neutralize stomach acids and this buffering action will cut down on absorption. The calcium then basically passes inert through your system.

Vitamin D. The recommended daily amount is 400 International Units (IU). Vitamin D is essential for calcium absorption. Exposure to sunlight can help the body produce this "sunshine vitamin," but just fifteen minutes on bare skin is needed per day in the summer and up to an hour on bare skin in the winter when the rays of the sun strike our planet at a greater angle. Ultraviolet light will not penetrate most clothing, and the more tan you are, the longer the exposure needed to gain the benefit.

However, in view of the fact that more than 90 percent of all signs of premature aging of the skin is linked to exposure to the sun, do you really want to go out without sunscreen? And how practical is it to sunbathe for an hour in the winter? Vitamin D is available at any health food store.

DHEA. For a full description of this adrenal body hormone, see Chapter 22. The decline of DHEA in the body has been linked with thinning of bone density, among other negative effects of aging. You can get a baseline check on your DHEA levels with a simple blood test. DHEA is available at your local health food store. But before you start taking supplements, make a decision with your doctor based on the facts, because once you begin, it's a commitment to your endocrine system to maintain levels. DHEA is not something you take when you happen to remember it.

Boron. Recent studies by the U.S. Department of Agriculture on postmenopausal women showed that the bone-building minerals calcium and magnesium were excreted *less* in women who had only 3 milligrams of boron supplement added to their diet for forty-eight days. Additionally, the women taking boron experienced dramatically elevated levels of serum estrogen. Most vegetables and fruits have some boron, but prunes and apricots are especially good sources.

THE MEDICAL APPROACH TO BONE DENSITY

Taking drugs to combat osteoporosis is not the first approach I recommend to patients, because prevention is the key. However, here are the possibilities.

Hormone replacement therapy (HRT). It's usually the image of a stooped-over older woman that makes us worry about osteoporosis. Estrogen replacement therapy has been the main medical means of protecting women against osteoporosis. It has been shown to reduce the risk of hip fractures by 50 percent over the long term.

However, there is still considerable controversy over whether or not HRT increases the risk of breast cancer. For a more detailed discussion of the risk factors, please turn to Chapter 22, get an idea of what's involved, and then make a decision with your doctor on what's best for you. Proponents of natural progesterone creams believe that they can help reduce the risk of osteoporosis without the breast cancer issue.

Calcitonin. This is a thyroid hormone that is important in bone and calcium metabolism. For osteoporotic women who are unwilling or unable to have HRT, calcitonin is an FDA-approved treatment which involves either injections every forty-eight hours or a nasal spray.

Sodium alendronate. This is the generic name for a drug called Fosamax. It is a biphosphonate drug that has been shown to decrease bone loss. However, there are some serious side effects and not everyone is a candidate for the drug, proving that, as usual, there's no free lunch.

ARCHITECTURE FOR YOUR BONES

The three most fractured bones due to osteoporosis are in the wrist, the spine, and the hip. Here are some exercises to help strengthen those key areas.

WRIST WORKERS

Chair Dips. See page 115.

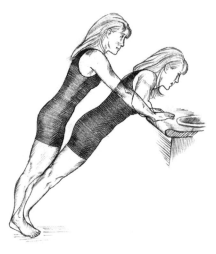

Wrist roll-ups. Use a broom handle and screw an eye-hook into the middle of it. Thread a small piece of rope through it and you'll have yourself a fancy piece of exercise equipment. Attach a small weight on the end of the rope and roll up the rope as shown. Slowly allow the weight to roll back down to the starting position. If it gets too easy to do it three times in a row, then add a heavier weight.

Push-ups from the bathroom sink. This one is great because it helps prepare you for the sensation of taking your body weight on your hands and wrists. Think of it as "falling practice." The movement here is to start with your arms extended, hands resting on the edge of the sink. Do not lock your elbows. Lower yourself a little by bending your elbows and then push yourself away from the sink in a forceful manner, so that your hands actually leave the sink. Repeat. As you get stronger, you will be rhythmically pushing and "catching" yourself on the sink in one graceful, repeated motion.

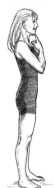

KEEPING YOUR SPINE IN LINE

Posture perfect—keep your chin in. Remember all the commands for a military posture—Stomach in! Chest out!

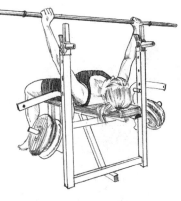

Back straight! Eyes straight ahead! Forget it. All you need to know is to keep your chin slightly tucked in. Try it, and you will feel your body naturally aligning itself. *Wall push with the spine.* You'll look like you're trying to hold the wall up! That's the idea, if you're doing it correctly. Stand as shown, facing away from a wall with feet shoulder width apart and try to push against the wall. Keep your chin tucked in. Hold for about five minutes. This is a good exercise to do during commercial breaks.

Bench press. Not only does this exercise help put pressure on the thoracic (upper) vertebrae to help the bones stay strong, but it helps build cleavage by developing the pectoral muscles. Lie on your back on a weight bench and lower the bar slowly. Extend your arms to raise the bar back

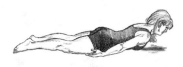

to the starting position, but do not lock your elbows. Repeat. The weight you use should be light enough for you to be able to do three sets of ten lifts each.

Back extensors. Starting position: Lie face down on the floor with a rolled towel under your pelvis. Raise trunk off the floor slowly. Lower and repeat. Beginner's goal: five repetitions; advanced: three sets of ten.

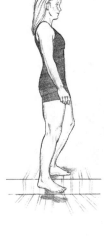

KEEPING YOUR HIPS SHIP SHAPE

Glute extensors. See page 116

Stair climber. Starting position: as shown. Keep the dangling leg straight, with the toes flexed upward. Now, slowly lower your body on the standing foot, until you can just touch the stair below with the heel. Straighten the standing leg as shown and repeat. If you stand up very straight, you will be using your thigh muscles the most. If you lean over, you will feel the exertion in the gluteus muscles.

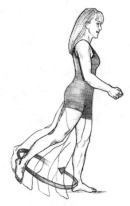

Hip circles. Hold on to the back of a chair. Now, with the toes pointed inward, move your thigh and leg away from the body

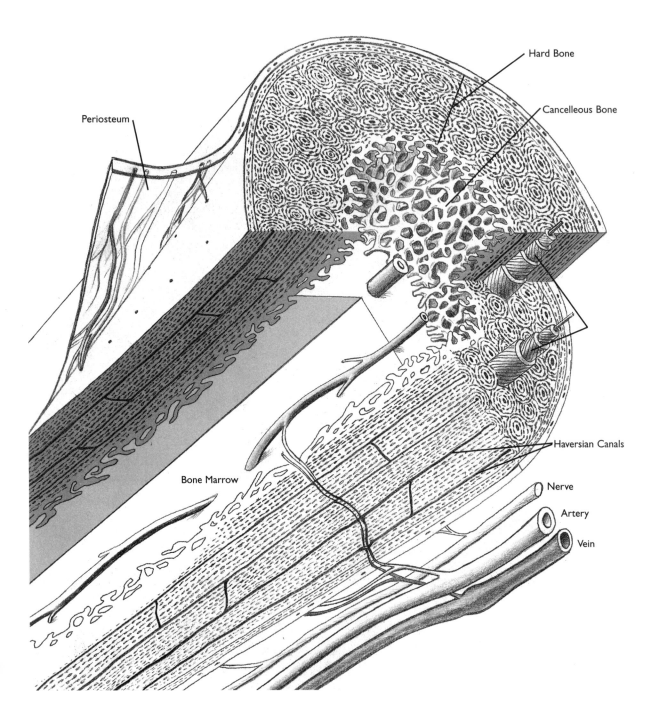

Periosteum

Hard Bone

Cancelleous Bone

Haversian Canals

Nerve

Artery

Vein

Bone Marrow

in a circular motion. Try to make the circle as big as you can. As you get stronger, you won't need to hold on to anything and you will be able to accomplish big circles with your foot with excellent balance. Try to build up to fifty of these a day.

DOWN TO THE BONE

Long after the rest of us has turned to dust, bone remains. Bone is the architectural framework that supports our body. Muscles attach to bone and give us movement. Bones protect our brain and internal organs. Deep down in the center of long bones like those in our thighs and calves, bone marrow cells produce most of the body's red blood cells, the platelets that allow blood to clot, and some of the body's immune system white cells as well.

As babies we start off life with about 350 bones, but by adulthood, many of those have fused, so we have 206.

14 BACKBONE OF HEALTH: HOW TO KEEP YOUR SPINE IN LINE

But at my back I always hear
Time's winged chariot hurrying near;
And yonder all before us lie
Deserts of vast eternity.

—Andrew Marvell (1621–1678),
"To His Coy Mistress"

WHAT'S IN A BACK?

The back, mighty and strong, is able to resist even the powerful force of the earth's gravity. But when weak, it reduces us to bent-over creatures—impairing our ability to stand erect, walk, or even breathe correctly.

The bony architecture of the back consists of twenty-four oddly shaped bones, called *vertebrae*, stacked up one on top of the other. Sandwiched in between the bones are tough, rubbery pads that have a liquid center and are called *discs*. The vertebrae are stacked up on a thick triangular bone named the *sacrum*, from which some tiny "tail bones" are linked, called collectively the *coccyx*.

A strong web of ligaments holds the whole thing together, facet joints on either side of the back bones help guide and align the spine, and bony arches in the middle of each vertebra form the boundaries of the spinal canal, which protects the all-important spinal cord. Spinal nerves exit the spinal cord at each vertebral level, and pass through a space between each bone of the spine, branching out to serve the muscles, organs, and tissues of the body. It's quite an amazingly complex structure: all the bones, the twenty-three rubbery discs, and all the ligaments, tendons, nerves, blood, and lymphatic vessels that work together.

The back, with its large, flat, five layers of muscle, is the source of great power in the body. Yet, even though it is capable of enormous strength, if you've ever strained your back, you know just how debilitating it can be. "Oh, my aching back!" is a complaint heard all too often, and usually because of a complete unawareness of how to strengthen it.

Stability of the back prevents injuries to many different body parts, including feet, knees, neck, and shoulders. It is important to every movement in the body. When you consider that back muscles protect our spinal column and central nervous system, you shouldn't need any more motivation to develop the area. Building your back is like an insurance policy on your spine, and you will be rewarded with a sinewy grace that can be yours as long as you live.

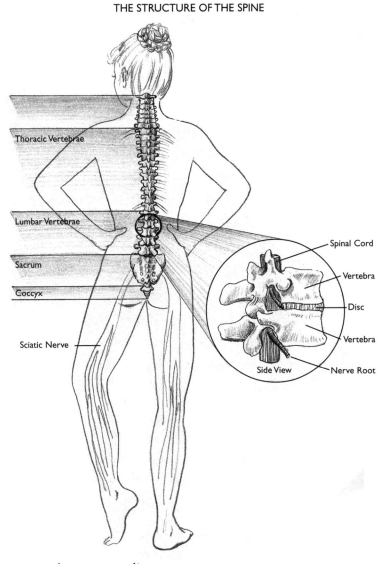

THE STRUCTURE OF THE SPINE

Thoracic Vertebrae

Lumbar Vertebrae

Sacrum

Coccyx

Sciatic Nerve

Spinal Cord

Vertebra

Disc

Vertebra

Side View

Nerve Root

WHY BACKS HURT

Most athletic injuries, as well as most injuries to the back that everyday working people get, are preventable. Back pain will be experienced by almost everyone at some time; back pain is second only to the common cold as a cause of days lost from work each year. Yet 80 to 85 percent of all back pain is from muscle imbalances that can be corrected and prevented. But to learn this, we have to take a step back and look at the big picture of how you live your life and use your body.

RATE YOURSELF ON THIS CHECKLIST

Back pain is the major cause of disability in people under the age of forty-five. In those over forty-five, it ranks third. Think about the following questions. Based on my experience with patients, these questions will help you identify the cause or causes for your back pain now and even help predict and prevent future back pain.

1. Do you sit a lot on your job?
2. Does your job require standing for hours at a time or manual labor?
3. Are you more than ten pounds over your ideal weight?
4. Does your regular day include exercise?
5. Do you drive lot?
6. Do you spend more than one hour a day watching TV?
7. Do you spend more than five minutes a day using the telephone?
8. Do you drink less than 100 ounces of water a day? (That's ten big glasses full.)
9. Do you feel that your job or your home life is stressful?
10. Do you slouch over your desk or when you're standing?
11. Do your joints and muscles feel "stiff" in the morning?
12. Do you wish that your bed was better for your back?
13. Have you ever had a backache before?
14. Do you sometimes avoid certain activities, like dancing, sex, tennis, or golf because of your back?
15. Do you wear high heels or tight jeans?
16. Do you sleep on your stomach?
17. Does your purse or brief case weigh more than one pound?
18. Are you at risk for osteoporosis? (The checklist is in Chapter 13)
19. Do you smoke?
20. Does your stomach stick out when you are standing normally?

If you have answered yes to any of these questions, read on, and we'll go step by step through what you need to know to help your back.

WHAT THE CHECKLIST MEANS FOR YOUR BACK

1. If you sit a lot on your job, chances are you are slumping over your desk, sitting in a chair that is not ergonomically designed to support your back, and putting strain on your sacroiliac joint. Fold up a towel or a sweatshirt until it makes a roll about the length of your hand and the width of your fist. Put that in the small of your back at the office, in your car or truck, or whenever you are sitting for a long period of time. I have a long wool scarf I wear to the symphony and then roll up to support my back with during the performance. Also, if you can raise your knees up slightly when sitting, it will take some stress from your lower back. Try this: Use a thick telephone book on the floor under your desk to rest your feet on. Just another handy use for those Yellow Pages.

2. If you are standing, are you in the best posture? If you are doing manual labor, are you lifting correctly? Always lift objects by squatting down and then keeping the load close to your body as you use your legs and thighs to lift up. Never bend over from the waist to lift something. Carry objects close to your trunk and above your waist. Use a shopping cart or a backpack and think about how you could lighten the load. Avoid reaching over your head to get things from shelves; use a ladder or a stool.

3. Think how tired it would make you feel if you had to carry around a ten or twenty or thirty pound weight suspended from your belt. That's how your back feels when you gain weight. We call it "anterior carriage" on medical reports sometimes, and even if that sounds less harsh and blaming than saying you have a big belly, either way, it's still a tremendous strain on the vertebrae in your lower back.

4. If you are not exercising on a regular basis, you are most likely overweight and also more likely to have stress buildup in your muscles, especially those muscles along the length of your spine. Perhaps you store your stress in between your shoulder blades or in the muscles in the back of your neck. It all adds up over the years unless you do something to relieve it and balance the muscles of your back. Additionally, you need to maintain strong abdominal muscles to maintain a pain-free back. Do you have to do abdominal exercises every day? My rule is this: only do abdominal exercise on the days you eat.

5. Driving is typically not a fun experience for your back. I remember driving cross-country a few times. You get out of the car to buy gas and feel like that car seat is going to have to be surgically removed from your backside! A good lumbar

support is essential for back health when you're driving. Also, adjust the seat properly so that you are not hunched over the steering wheel. Additionally, try pointing your toes inward when you are driving; it gives your lower back and hip muscles a break.

6. Most people "sit" on their lower back on a overstuffed sofa with no back support. That's bad enough for your spine, but watch television for over an hour a day, and you turn into a "couch potato." Studies show that people who watch in excess of an hour of television a day are 20 percent more obese than those who don't. I think all the food ads are partly to blame!

7. Crooking the telephone into your ear when you speak on the telephone strains the vertebrae of your neck and causes tremendous stress on the joints. On an X-ray you can actually see the buildup of bone on the neck of a person who spends a great deal of time on the phone, for example, real estate agents, attorneys, and office workers. Buy and use a telephone headset. It will do wonders for your neck and avoid a lot of headaches caused by muscle tension.

8. In my experience with patients, the ones who don't drink enough water experience more stress in their bodies, have more rigid muscle spasms, and a poorer quality of skin than those who are well hydrated. It's only common sense. Water is an essential nutrient for the body. Chronic muscle spasms lead to back problems, and more than 80 percent of all back problems are due to muscle imbalances. So drink up!!

9. "If people have peace of mind, pain is not uncontrollable," says best-selling author and medical pioneer Dr. Bernie Siegel. "I would challenge any doctor to show me someone who has their life in order, and you can't control their pain." Everyone carries their stress in a different body part. If it's in your back, then keep reading, and let's get to the back exercises and what you can do right now to feel better. If the stress is really eating you up lately, may I suggest the stress-busters regime in Chapter 5.

10. Monitor yourself. Practice good posture and use an office chair that offers proper support that can position you correctly and comfortably.

11. If your joints and muscles feel stiff and achy in the mornings, you may have a form of osteoarthritis, which is basically the wear and tear legacy of our joints. There's a lot you can do to help yourself. Arthritis is discussed in Chapter 15.

12. We spend up to one-third of our lives in bed, sleeping on our backs. If your bed is tired and saggy, it's time to change it, before you become the same. A bed

should be firm, but still have enough padding so that you when you lie on your side, your ribs and hips are supported and there's no gap between you and the bed. A big piece of plywood under the whole mattress is one way to put some life back in your bed.

While we're at it, water beds are terrible for your back. Yes, I know, they're lots of fun, but it's the biomechanical equivalent of sleeping in a hammock, which is okay for a short nap at Club Med when you're in between two palm trees, but incompatible with good back health. The best sleeping position? On your back, with a pillow under your knees.

13. I have patients who come into the office with back pain, and when I ask them how long it's been bothering them, you'd be surprised at the number of people who will say "Well, Doc, it's been hurting me on and off for about twenty or thirty years." When your back talks to you, it's a good idea to listen. Especially since back pain can also be a referred pain from an internal organ and is therefore an important clue to a potentially more serious illness, like ovarian or prostate cancer. Pain anywhere in the body is your body telling you that there is problem. Listen.

14. If you are avoiding certain activities, like dancing, sex, tennis, or golf, because your back hurts, it's time to get some help. Read number 13 over again, and I'll meet you in the next section, "What to Do When Pain Strikes."

15. If you wear high heels, your back is going to tell you about it sooner or later. Aside from causing bunions in your feet, high heels put stress on the lower back by causing an exaggerated curvature of the spine, or "sway back" position, that can result in weakening and straining the lower vertebrae, resulting in debilitating wear and tear on the facet joints and discs of the back.

Yes, I know, I know—high heels are sexy and you have some great ones in your closet that have cost you a bundle. Then wear them on only two occasions: for stepping out of the limousine and walking those few steps to the opera/restaurant/symphony; in bed.

As for tight jeans, they are a problem for your back because they prevent you from bending your knees properly when lifting an object or even from sitting correctly. The end result? Back strain.

16. Don't sleep on your stomach. This can create some nasty neck problems, because your neck is twisted for hours at a time. For one patient who could not seem to kick this habit, I had his wife sew tennis balls into the front of his pajamas, so

that when he rolled over in the night, the tennis balls would nudge into him and remind him to turn back. It worked.

17. If you have a heavy purse, dump out half the stuff you carry around "just in case" and switch to a backpack. Lighten your load and be aware of what you hang on your shoulders.

18. If you are at risk for osteoporosis, read Chapter 13 first, and then come back for the rest of this chapter.

19. Smoking and back pain have been linked in a number of studies. Smoking reduces blood flow to back muscles and to the tissues surrounding the discs, all of which increases the rate of aging of those tissues. If you need another reason to quit, here it is.

20. Weak abdominal muscles deprive your back of much needed support. Even if you are not overweight, if you do not strengthen your muscles and flatten your abdomen, you are putting yourself at greater risk for back problems.

WHAT TO DO WHEN PAIN STRIKES.

When it comes to back pain, we're talking about an equal opportunity employer, because sooner or later most people experience pain and discomfort. Most back pain, including the severe kind, can be helped without surgery. In fact, the National Institutes of Health guidelines have stated that even when surgery is indicated and performed, 50 percent of the patients experience more pain after the surgery! Here's what to do when you first experience back pain:

YOU MUST SEE A DOCTOR WITHOUT DELAY IF . . .

1. You've had a car accident, a bicycle accident, or any other traumatic impact injury like falling off a roof and your back hurts.

2. You've hurt your back and you have bowel or bladder loss of control or sexual dysfunction.

3. You have back pain and there is tingling or numbness or loss of strength in your legs or the lower part of your body.

4. You have back pain and you can't walk on your heels or up on your toes.

5. Your back pain wakes you up at night. (If you are over fifty, organic disease that refers pain to the back could be the warning signal here.)

6. You are having neck pain or back pain, and you have a high fever or chills.
7. You have back or neck pain or back pain that runs down your arm or down your leg.
8. You have a backache with weight loss, severe fatigue, great thirst, or increased urination.
9. Your back pain is only relieved by taking painkillers.

CHIROPRACTIC CARE

Anyone who has experienced the abnormal and painful transmission of nerve energy in their back will agree: Back pain is not good for your general well-being, to say the least. The myriad of relationships between the spinal column and the nervous system is important. Chiropractic is a system of health care based on the premise that

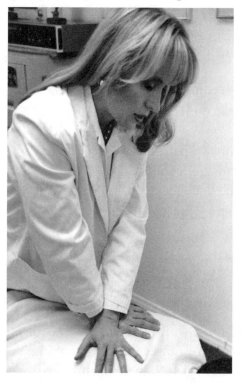

the relationship between the body's structure and function in the human body is a significant health factor. The normal transmission of nerve energy is essential to our health and human performance, which is why so many Olympic and professional athletes use chiropractic care to keep their spines in line and help prevent injury.

After a physical examination, one of the primary forms of treatment by a doctor of chiropractic is spinal adjustment. They use their hands to apply mild force to parts of the spine in order to adjust it back into place. Physiotherapeutic treatment such as ultrasound; electrical muscle stimulation to support healing and reduce pain; traction on specially padded chiropractic tables; massage; heat, cold, or exercise therapies and supports may also be used. Drugs or surgery are not used by chiropractors. Instead, a program of rest, diet, exercise, and postural retraining are often incorporated into the patient's daily regime.

According to the National Institutes of Health, chiropractic care is the most effective care for back pain, while drugs and surgery are successful for only 5 percent of back problems. The *Manga Report*, a study published by the government of Ontario, noted that patients who had chiropractic care had more effective relief and returned to work more quickly than workers who had other treatments. This repeated the findings of an earlier study done by the Rand Corporation, the West Coast technology and science think tank. The study found that patients who received chiropractic care fared better than those who made other choices.

OTHER TYPES OF PRACTIONERS

Osteopaths. Their training is almost identical to an M.D.'s, but osteopaths also receive some limited-focus training on spinal adjustments. They are licensed to prescribe drugs and use surgery.

Orthopedic surgeons. The name says it best. They are highly trained to perform surgery and specialize in the treatment of bones and joints, including fractures and diseases. They may prescribe drugs, casts, braces, or physical therapy for back problems.

Physiatrist. A physiatrist is an M.D. who specializes in physical medicine, designing physical therapy programs in order to instruct physical therapists who actually do the therapy.

Neurosurgeon. Surgery and treatment of the brain, spinal cord, and nerves of the body are the domain of this medical specialist. Damage from trauma or tumors that affect the brain or spinal cord is often a focus.

General practitioners. Family practice M.D.'s who may prescribe pain medication for your back and refer you to a specialist.

THERAPISTS

Physical, occupational, and kinesiotherapists. All must work under an M.D.'s direction to carry out the prescription for patient treatment of physical and mental impairments. Physical therapy modalities such as ice, heat, whirlpool treatments, massage, and electrical stimulation may be used to try to reduce symptoms along with exercise and patient training in daily activities and mechanical aids such as splints, braces, and crutches. These therapists are not licensed to diagnose, prescribe drugs, or perform chiropractic spinal adjustments.

Massage therapists. A message therapist may work under a medical doctor's direction, but many do not. By law, massage therapists are required to undergo training, certification, and health exams.

THE WORK AND SAVE BACK PROGRAM

When you learn how to work out your back correctly, you'll save yourself a lot of trouble later on. That's why I call this the "work and save" program. By working out, your muscles get stronger, your tendons and ligaments are restored to flexibility, and you can save yourself from a case of the "sore back blues." If you feel any pain or numbness or tingling when you are doing these exercises, stop. Don't force any of the exercises and stay within your pain-free ranges of motion. This is important to remember, because many of us have that "no pain, no gain" mentality that is *not* a sign of intelligent life when it comes to exercising and backache.

Note: Get evaluated by a doctor before you begin this or any exercise program. If your pain is associated with fever, chills, numbness, tingling, bowel or bladder problems, a traumatic accident, or leg or head pain, it's an emergency. See a doctor immediately.

GETTING STARTED

1. Change into loose, comfortable clothes. Tight jeans, for instance, don't allow you to bend your knees properly and lift objects correctly or do the exercises for the best biomechanical safety.
2. Warm up by walking or riding a bicycle or using a treadmill or stairstepper for five to ten minutes.
3. Use common sense: Move only in the pain-free ranges of motion. Don't force anything. If it hurts or causes tingling in your arms or legs to do a certain exercise or movement, then don't do it.
4. Do the exercise movements in a slow, controlled way without bouncing or jerking. It's always a good idea to avoid causing another injury while you're still doing the active rehabilitation for the first injury!

5. Remember to breathe when you are doing the exercises. Many people end up holding their breath, and this is always a bad idea.

KEEPING YOUR SPINE IN LINE

Relief Position. Lie on your back the floor. Bend your knees at a 90-degree angle with your calves up on a chair or sofa and a small rolled up towel under your neck. This position can often give relief to an aching back. I like to do this one as a stressbuster exercise. When sleeping, putting a pillow under your knees may give you relief also.

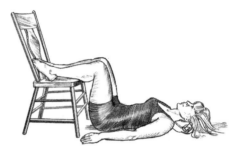

Knee to chest stretch. See page 121.

Pretzel stretch. See page 121.

Knee sways. Wait until you have a month of the other exercises behind you before attempting this one. Lie on your back with both of your knees bent and your feet together. Slowly allow both legs to move to one side while you keep your shoulders pressed against the floor. Return to the starting position and repeat on the other side. Repeat three times.

Door stretch. See pages 51 and 120.

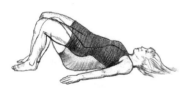

Pelvic tilt. Lie on your back with your knees bent. Press the small of your back into the floor. Hold for ten seconds. Now lift your pelvis off the floor and hold for ten seconds. Return to the starting position and repeat. Remember to breathe!

WORK THOSE ABS!

Abominable abdominal muscles are a big liability for your back. If your stomach sticks out when you are standing normally, when you are not consciously trying to suck your stomach in, you need to give your back a chance and strengthen those abs. Strong abdominal muscles are the key to a healthy back.

Abdominal crunch. Lie on your back with your knees bent and your neck supported by a small rolled up towel under your neck. Fold your arms across your chest. Now

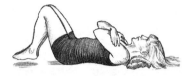

press the small of your back into the floor and raise the soles of your feet one inch off the floor. Just one inch! Hold it for a few seconds, rest, and try again. Eventually, you will be able to hold your feet one inch off the floor for one minute. This is hard to do, so don't start out making one minute your goal on the first day. If you can only do one second, that's okay, be happy— you'll get stronger each day and your stomach *will* get flatter.

Cat arch. This is a unique movement because it stretches your upper back while working your abdominal muscles. Distribute your weight evenly on all fours. Now pull in your abdominal muscles and round your back. Hold for ten seconds. Repeat ten times.

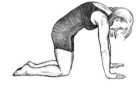

MORE BACK-STRENGTHENING STRETCHES

Standing quad stretch. See page 121.

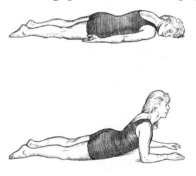

Cobra stretch. This one feels so good after you have done abdominal work. It may also be a relief-giving position when your back is achy, but do the motion very slowly. Turn your head to one side and lie face down on the floor with your arms at your side. Strive for slow, effortless breathing for about five minutes. Then, inch your elbows up until they are directly under your shoulders and rest your weight on your arms. Now slowly use your shoulder and arms muscles to push your upper body up to the position shown. Keep your eyes and head level to the ground. Hold for up to thirty seconds. *Note:* If you feel any sharp pain with this or any other exercise, then stop. Always move within the pain-free ranges of motion.

Arm and leg raise. This one helps to strengthen your back muscles, from top to bottom. Lie on your stomach with a large rolled up towel under your hips. Stretch

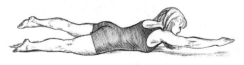

both arms out in front of you. Now lift one arm and the opposite leg off the floor by twelve inches. Return to the starting position and repeat on the other arm and leg.

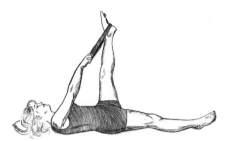

Lying hamstring with a belt stretch. Flexibility in the strong back and thigh muscles helps balance your body and keep your spine in line. Lie on your back with your neck supported by a small rolled up towel. Press the small of your back into the floor. Breathe and count slowly to ten. Now straighten out one leg and slowly raise it as shown. Don't lock your knee and hold for ten seconds. Return to the starting position and repeat with the other leg. Do this once the first day and work for yourself up to ten times comfortably. If you feel pain while straightening your leg, then stop.

WHEN TO REST, WHEN TO FORGET ABOUT RESTING

Staying in bed too long can actually weaken the muscles of your back. In my experience with patients, I usually set a limit of forty-eight hours bed rest and then only if the pain is very bad as a result of a car accident or disc injury. Even then, I advise the person to get up and walk around for half an hour every three hours. Sitting is generally the worst for back pain as it puts extra pressure on your spine, particularly in the lower back. That goes for sitting up in bed, too. If you feel like reading or watching television, then lie on your side with a pillow between your knees.

WHEN TO ICE, WHEN TO USE HEAT

Here's the rule for injuries in general, back included.

Use ice for the first forty-eight hours after an injury. To do this, apply a cold pack, a bag of crushed ice, to the affected area. Every two hours, you may apply the ice for twenty minutes. I find that a big bag of frozen peas works well. And unlike those fancy and expensive gel packs, you can eat them for lunch afterward.

Use heat after that. If your back is hurt from a car accident or from a fall or trauma to your back, then don't use heat at all. A hot water bottle wrapped up in a wet T-shirt can do wonders, and a hot water bottle is cheap. Heating pads are dangerous because it is dry heat, and people tend to fall asleep on it. That's how you can cook a muscle and really get into some trouble. Only use heat for twenty minutes maximum, and never use it in combination with creams or lotions such as Ben Gay.

WHEN TO WEAR A SUPPORT

The best support for your back is a set of strong abdominal muscles. But, until you get those abdominals in shape, a store-bought support can give some relief for a few days after a painful back episode. Ask your doctor to recommend one. Wearing a support belt while lifting objects is a very good idea, but wearing one indefinitely could result in weakening the very muscles you are trying to strengthen.

CORRECT LIFTING POSTURE

First of all, don't lift it if it looks too heavy. Get someone to help you. Bend your knees, *not* your waist. Tighten your abdominal muscles, use your leg muscles to help you lift, and keep the package close to your body. *Never bend over from the waist.*

STAND ON BOTH FEET!

This sounds so simple, but it is hard for most people to do: Stand on two feet. Most people stand on one foot, letting their hips sag and slouching forward. You could take a healthy person and probably *cause* back problems if you forced him or her to stay in that posture all day. Sound familiar? While we're at it, good posture is very valuable as it prevents strain on the back and neck. Furthermore, good posture allows you to emit a personal statement to the world that you are a person of power and commitment. Ever see royalty slouch? You may not notice your posture, but others do— and if you ask any child or comedian to imitate an old person, they will stoop over and shuffle.

Correct posture is actually quite easy. Forget the military commands: Stomach in, chest out, shoulders back, etc. That's making it way more complicated than necessary. Simply remember to keep your chin in. That's it.

GLOSSARY OF SOME COMMON BACK AILMENTS

Muscle spasms. The back muscles can be sprained or strained just like other muscles in the body. This most commonly happens when the muscles are weak, imbalanced, fatigued, or strained because of sudden lifting or twisting.

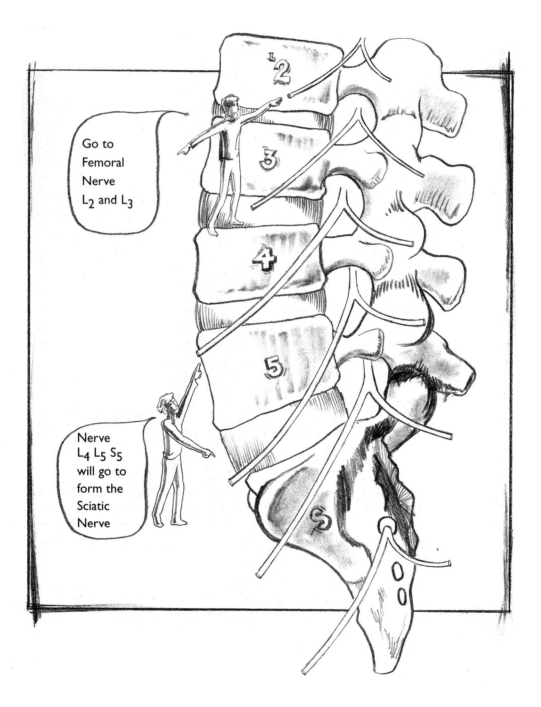

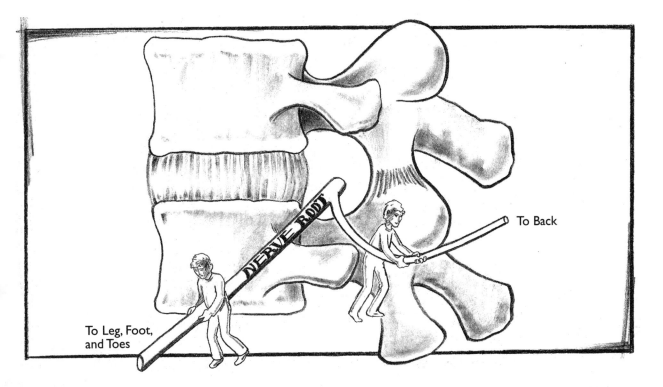

Herniated disc. The discs in our back are like tough jelly doughnuts. Small micro tears may occur in the disc over the years, but if they are big enough, then the jelly in the center (the nucleus pulposus) will leak out and the substance may impinge on one of the spinal nerves. It hurts and the pain may refer down the back of the leg all the way to the foot. After the leak, the disc will flatten out. The shrinkage may cause problems with the fibers, ligaments, and the facet joints directly above and below the injured disc.

Osteoporosis. Turn to Chapter 13 for a discussion about osteoporosis. The spine is very susceptible to special problems that occur as a result of bone loss—if you've ever seen an older person, usually a woman, with a large hump on her back, that is due to the fact that the vertebra have likely crushed and then formed a wedge shape. Osteoporosis is preventable, yet if a woman does nothing about preventing bone loss, she may lose more than three inches in height by the time she is in her early seventies.

Facet joint problems. The facet joints of the back help the vertebrae to glide in their ranges of motion. The facets also share some of the weight load with the discs. However, when the discs flatten out due to injury, or the facet joints change because of wear and tear, they can put painful pressure on spinal nerves. That's another reason why maintaining your spine in proper alignment is so important.

Spondylosis. This is the medical term for degenerative arthritis, or osteoarthritis of the vertebrae and related tissues. It may cause pressure on the nerve roots of the spine that results in pain in the arms or legs.

Spondylolisthesis. This is the term used to describe the condition of one vertebra slipping forward on another one. Most commonly, it is the result of a small fracture of the *pars*, a bridging part of the vertebrae. Defects in the back bones, disc damage, or congenital factors may be other reasons for the slippage.

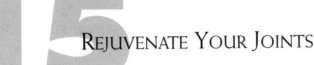

15 REJUVENATE YOUR JOINTS

Where I was born and where and how I have lived is unimportant.
It is what I have done with where I have been that should be of interest.

—Georgia O'Keefe (1887–1986)

$\mathcal{M}$illions of fans around the world thrill to the excitement of Sunday afternoons and a football game on TV. For the thousands of fans in the stadium, there's an added excitement as they feel the stadium structure actually shake with the collective roar when the home team scores a touchdown during the final moments of a championship game.

But what the ecstatic fans *don't* see is what the professional football heroes experience after the game. Most viewers would fantasize about the parties and general rumpus-raising that must go on. I thought so too until I attended a postgame celebration of the then–Los Angeles Raiders team after they won the championship on the way to the Superbowl. At the time, I was a personal fitness coach to a handful of professional athletes, including some members of the team.

I drove up to the opulent home of one of the players and was greeted by a few of the NFL wives and girlfriends who were busy in the kitchen. Some were preparing dozens of cloth ice bags full of crushed ice—the kind of ice bag you see in the movies when the leading actor has a hangover—and piling them on the kitchen counters. Others were cutting up fresh pineapple and loading up platters with it. (Pineapple is something I recommend to athletes after gruelling competitions of any kind: It contains proteolytic enzymes, which seem to help the body dispose of inflamed or damaged tissue in the body.)

By and by, the players lumbered in. Depending on their age and previous history of injury, they grabbed the ice bags, and hunks of pineapple, and collapsed on the furniture or on the floor. The rookies bounced in and either had no need for the ice bags, or were able to fake a "no pain" attitude better than the others. The older players shouted rude remarks to the younger ones. The big screen TV was on, but nobody was watching it. Nobody was moving much unless it was to change position of the ice packs. It looked like a scene from "M*A*S*H," except all of the characters were over 250 pounds of solid muscle. And this was the team that had *won*! I could only imagine what the post-game celebration would have been like in the encampment of the losing team.

Years after anyone has remembered the win-loss record or who even won the Superbowl that year, these NFL veterans will suffer the physical legacy of all their years of football: worn out and arthritically damaged knees, elbows, shoulders, and hips. Dr. James St. Ville, a Phoenix-based orthopaedic surgeon, among others, is replacing the joints of the graying ranks of those players from the era before megasalaries. "Without the surgery, I would be in a wheelchair," said former pro football star Fred Enke in a magazine interview. Enke, now seventy-one, could set off the metal detectors at any airport: He sports two titanium knees, one titanium shoulder, and a titanium left hip. Dr. St. Ville has helped out more than 150 ex-NFL players since 1992, donating an estimated $2.5 million dollars in services. Ron Gardin, who played defensive back for the Colts in the early 1970s, stated in a magazine interview: "It's just a slow, degenerating process that most athletes don't understand until many years down the line."

IS IT ARTHRITIS OR RHEUMATISM?

The word *arthritis* comes from the Greek word *arthron*, which means "joint." The ending *itis* on a word means inflammation. So there you have it: Arthritis is inflammation of a joint, usually accompanied by pain, swelling, and, frequently, changes in the structure of the joint.

Arthritis is not just one disease, though. It's a term that describes about a hundred joint conditions, syndromes, and rheumatic diseases. When I was growing up in Canada, nobody ever had arthritis. If anything hurt, it was always blamed on the same thing: "Oh, it's just my rheumatism acting up on me again." It always sounded like a pet dog that was scratching up the carpet or something. A sore back, a charley horse in your leg, a sprained ankle, that soft black gushy spot on your head that just got hit by a baseball—it didn't matter what you went to the doctor for, it was always the same diagnosis: "You've just got some rheumatism. Take two aspirin, lose another ten pounds, and you'll live another ten years." That was the anthem of Dr. White, the small-town doctor who treated everyone we knew.

Rheumatism is a general term for acute and chronic conditions that have the symptoms of inflammation, soreness, and stiffness. So far this sounds just like the arthritis definition. However, the definition of rheumatism extends to pain in the muscles, joints, and associated soft tissue structures like ligaments and tendons, while arthritis is generally used to define joint inflammations only. *Rheumatoid arthritis* is a fish of a different stripe and it describes a progressive disease that affects the whole body.

WHO HAS ARTHRITIS AND HOW DO YOU GET IT?

Various studies show that joint disease is very common and that 1 to 5 percent of the American population under forty-five, and 15 to 85 percent of older individuals suffer from some type of arthritis. Mostly this is osteoarthritis (the wear-and-tear kind) or rheumatoid arthritis (the inflammatory kind).

Osteoarthritis (OA) is the most common type of arthritis. Basically, it's the result of stress in the weight-bearing joints of the body: vertebrae, hips, and knees. Symptoms are influenced by the cumulative stresses the joints have experienced throughout your life. An estimated 16 million Americans—mostly women—suffer from the condition.

The age of a person can be told simply by evaluating key stress points on X-ray. I explain this to patients by relating that it's like wrinkles on the inside. Everyone gets them sooner or later after age forty. However, when you get a radiographic evaluation of a problem area and you're told that you have *degenerative joint dis-*

CARTILAGE DEGENERATION

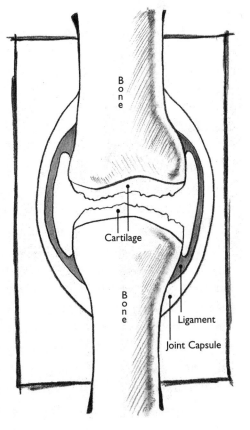

Bone

Cartilage

Bone

Ligament

Joint Capsule

ease (DJD), it sounds really bad. It's that "degenerating" tone of the whole thing. It's awful to think that you're sitting there, your doctor is pointing to various areas of the body, and there you are degenerating before his or her very eyes. But DJD is only another name for osteoarthritis.

It is essentially a wear-and-tear condition. The football stars of yesteryear that we met earlier are suffering from DJD in joints injured seriously over and over again during their football careers, but about 85 percent of the population over the age of seventy has some form of DJD. Fortunately, there are no symptoms in most people.

For the rest of us aging warriors, there *are* symptoms: stiffness in the morning, swelling and tenderness of the joints after working out, noisy "crackling" of the joints, decreased range of motion of the joints affected (knees, hips and back, and fingers), and generalized pain. If there is DJD in the back, the growth of calcium deposits called osteophytes can impinge on neck or low back spinal nerves. This is a fairly painful condition, but it can respond well to chiropractic care and home exercises. (See Chapter 14 on back care for a more detailed discussion on your nonsurgical options.)

What's Going On?

There are two main theories of how and why DJD develops: the biomechanical and the biochemical. The *biomechanical theory* says that repeated wear and tear on the joints leads to joints that don't line up exactly right. Due to the slower metabolism of an aging individual, the cartilage cells don't keep up maintenance work, the bones start to get soft around the joints, and the cartilage cells called chondrocytes eventually get ground out and die. Enzymes are then released which cause the cartilage to develop cracks and break down. Calcium deposits are laid down at the ends of the bones instead, which reduce mobility and cause discomfort.

The biochemical theory blames the whole mess on aging chondrocytes that emit destructive enzymes that lead to over production of the synovial lubricating fluid. The resulting inflammation and puffiness around the joint makes the body release inflammatory mediators: immune cells that try to stop the process. When these valiant white blood cells die, they release even more enzymes that kill off the chondrocytes and set off free radicals. The cartilage then cracks and flakes (just like it did in the biomechanical theory). Calcium deposits replace the long gone cartilage areas.

Both theories are probably correct depending on the person.

RHEUMATOID ARTHRITIS (RA)

About 1 percent of the world's population and more than 7 million Americans are thought to suffer from rheumatoid arthritis. Women are three times more likely to have it than men. Additionally, it is initially most prevalent in women in their thirties and forties.

RA is mostly a severe form of synovial fluid inflammation. Synovial fluid is produced by the chondrocytes (cartilage cells). Some fortunate individuals have few or no symptoms. Others experience destruction and fusion of the joints, and the skin, eyes, heart, lungs, and other organs may be affected as well. There are some chromosomal markers in certain people that are linked with susceptibility to this disease.

WHY DOES RA HAPPEN?

Most scientists believe RA is an autoimmune disease because 80 percent of people with RA have an antibody circulating around in them called *RF factor*, which stands for rheumatoid factor and which is directed against a part of the sufferer's immune system. In addition, diseases such as the virus-caused Epstein-Barr, life stress, toxic emotions, and a host of other events, including food allergies, have been linked to RA.

We could get very technical going through the various mechanisms for (cartilage) destruction, but the results are mostly from the body's immune system working against itself. Symptoms include localized swelling, redness and pain around the affected joints, and stiffness in the morning or after periods of inactivity. Sometimes the joints are damaged and distorted by the immune system reactions. In some people after a preliminary bout, the rheumatoid arthritis subsides and there is quiet behavior by the immune system for long periods of time. In unfortunate others, the process escalates to a crippling early death from the bleeding that is caused by the long-term use of aspirin, by infections from the lengthy reliance of steroid drugs, and from starchy deposits in various organs.

Every year, approximately 10 percent of the patients with RA achieve a spontaneous remission which can last for weeks, months, years, or forever.

OTHER TYPES OF ARTHRITIS

Gout is a type of arthritis resulting from deposits of uric acid crystals in joints, most often in the big toe. The excruciating pain of gout is experienced by about 2 million

Americans, mostly men who are overweight, over-eaters of red meat and rich food and who, are under-exercised. Ankylosing spondylitis, and inflammatory arthritis, mostly affects the back, particularly the sacloiliac joint at the bottom of the spine. Some unexpected contributors to arthritis include: common skin infections, lupus, Lyme's disease, psoriasis, tuberculosis, scleroderma, systemic lupus erythematosus, and sexually transmitted diseases such as syphilis and gonorrhea. Even some chronic inflammatory bowel disorders can also cause arthritis.

I am *not* recommending that you stop taking your arthritis drugs or discontinue your medical treatment for the symptoms of your arthritis. These natural therapies are presented as an addition to your present regime and not as an alternative to it. Talk to your doctor and get his or her approval before you try any of these natural therapies.

This is important, because if the natural remedies are of benefit to you, then you will be in a great position to keep the conversation open with your doctor and discuss the possibility of reducing your medication. It's always important for you to be part of the solution in consultation with your doctor. That way, you empower yourself to the highest body-mind healing connection.

POSITIVE OUTCOMES

All drugs have side effects and that is why you need to be continually monitored by your doctor when you are taking medication. I have osteoarthritis as the result of a car accident that ended my twenty-year running career. I tried the drug route at one point, but was unable to continue taking the painkillers and antiinflammatory medications because I found the side effects like stomach pain and nausea to be far worse than the symptoms that were being treated in the first place. The idea of surgery was discussed with my orthopedic surgeon, and I dreaded the idea of it, but I was in enough pain to agree to it. It was difficult to accept that I had gone from running twenty or thirty miles before breakfast to someone who took ten minutes to get from the bed to the bathroom in the morning.

Very fortunately, before my scheduled knee surgery, I met a man who had developed the *Myopulse*, a remarkable physical therapy modality that had me canceling those surgical orders at 4:45 P.M. the night before—after one treatment. With a combination of exercise, supplements, and a maximizing mindset, I was able to progress from barely being able to walk the length of my block without pain, to the point where I can now hike vigorously in the mountains near my home several days a week, ride up those same trails on my mountain bike on the other days, and use my rest days to work out on my cross-country ski machine or stairclimber—all without the dreaded knee surgery. I had those surgical orders framed. It still makes me smile and count my

blessings when I look at the wall. To find the name of a health care practitioner near you who uses the Myopulse you can call Electro Medical, Inc., at (800) 367-7246.

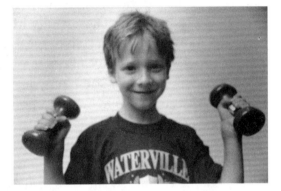

The most positive outcome is going to be the one which maximizes *your* potential. You may not be able to prevent rheumatoid arthritis or osteoarthritis, but you may be able to find the most healthful ways to prevent your arthritis from controlling you.

And you may be able to prevent further wear and tear on your joints and get a grip on dealing effectively with your pain.

It's an ongoing process. I still surf the Internet, eager to learn new information. I can't run anymore, and went through a mourning process for that because it had given me a lot of joy and dreams-come-true happiness to become a champion athlete. But I am grateful that I had the opportunity to learn so many new things, to heal my life, and now to help others to a more active way of living.

An exceptional person and patient of mine taught me many magnificent lessons. When Heidi Von Beltz, Hollywood stunt woman and actress, was paralyzed from the neck down as a result of a movie set accident, she refused to accept the daunting diagnosis of a life in a wheelchair. During the time we worked together, Heidi regained the use of her upper body and progressed to the point of standing up, supported only by leg braces. Her inspirational motto: Be happy for the things you *can* do instead of moping about things you *can't* do! She went on to author a book full of wit and humor about her journey titled *My Soul Purpose*. Before we launch into the natural therapies, here's another "Heidi-ism" you may enjoy: "We're all wired for electricity, but it's still up to you to plug in your own lamp."

NATURAL ARTHRITIS STRATEGIES

The word *doctor* comes from the latin word *docere* which means "to teach." However, more often than not, the greatest teaching that occurs in my office is from my patients. Of the natural therapies that will be reviewed below, those listed are the ones that have been the most successful with the patients in my practice and that yield to the criteria of having respectable research data.

Win the battle of the bulge. Take ten pounds off your midsection, which will equal about thirty pounds less stress on your knees when you stand, seventy pounds when you walk or run, and one hundred pounds when you sprint down the stairs. Aching backs also benefit from reducing the weight around your midsection. Your hip bones will be grateful to you as well if you can keep your weight within the normal range for your height. Some researchers have shown that that keeping excess weight off your body can reduce your risk of developing osteoarthritis in the hands by up to three times. A University of Michigan School of Public Health study followed 1,300 residents of Tecumseh, Michigan, for twenty-three years and noted the link between between overweight and osteoarthritis. Obesity also leads to immune system problems that may well be a trigger for RA.

I have seen firsthand how losing weight helps osteoarthritis patients lose their pain in the knees and hips and back. It's like magic. And unlike drugs, the side effects of weight loss are all good—you look and feel wonderful! If you would like to win the battle of the bulge once and for all, turn to Chapters 10 and 11 right now, and get started today!

Exorcise your pain with exercise. In our high-tech world, it is refreshing to see that something as low tech as exercise can be more effective than high-priced drugs in relieving the pain of arthritis. Losing weight and exercise go hand in hand. More importantly, it puts you in an active role in your own recovery. It feels good to be doing something about your aches and pains, and this in turn activates a powerful belief system in your body that brings you toward healing and regeneration. Additionally, inactivity may heighten pain and stiffness in both RA and OA. Movement of the joint stimulates the natural lubricant, hyaluronan (HA), which enables joints to move freely.

Gentle, rhythmic exercises like water aerobics and walking are a good place to start. If you just walked back and forth in the shallow end of a pool you'd get a good workout. Water exercising is good because the buoyancy of the pool takes pressure off your joints (you weigh only one-tenth your land weight), and the swishing around in the water is like getting a free massage every time you work out.

I've found pool exercises most effective with the use of a water flotation belt. This allows you to float vertically in the pool and increases the variety of workouts you can do in a pool. All without even getting your hair wet. A water aerobics class is also fun, and the camaraderie and commitment is contagious.

T'ai chi is another wonderful activity that de-stresses you, improves your balance, and can be done at any age. A martial arts studio, YMCA, or library bulletin board are all places that might guide you toward a class near you.

Bicycling is another great non–joint pounding exercise for your body, whether it's in your living room in front of the TV or out in the real world. It's highly recommended for wounded knees because it strengthens the important and powerful thigh muscles that help to stabilize the knee joint.

Weight lifting is great for arthritis sufferers. Start with light weights and either join a class or invest in some personal instruction from a certified trainer for a few sessions so that you learn how to do the exercises correctly. Emphasize strengthening exercises for your abdominal muscles to ease back pain and thigh muscles for knee and hip pain. For a description of back exercises that might be helpful, turn to Chapter 14.

Stretching is another time-tested pain reliever. There's always a yoga class going on somewhere in the big cities. I've found classes when I'm traveling by simply looking in the Yellow Pages. Stretching helps improve your range of motion in the joints and it is a very potent de-stressor.

The idea is to increase your strength and flexibility, which will take stress off the joints. *Eat well.* Aside from being a very good sign of self-respect, eating well can only help the overall health of your body and once again activate the powerful body-mind connection that is paramount to healing and regeneration. Many studies have shown the link between healthful eating and relief of many ailments, especially from RA. Scandinavian studies showed that RA patients improved their symptoms dramatically within only thirty days on a vegetarian diet. Nathan Pritikin, the low-fat diet pioneer, documented 90 percent reduction of RA symptoms in the hands, wrists, and fingers and 50 percent reduction of RA symptoms in the knees and hips of those who ate very low-fat diets.

The healing comfort of warmth. A warm bath first thing in the morning can do wonders for your range of motion, flexibility, and absence of pain throughout the day. I find that one to two cups of epsom salts in the bath water is the magic ingredient. The idea of de-stressing before the day really gets going is, well, de-stressing. Epsom salts contain magnesium sulfate, which is absorbed through the skin in minute amounts. Sulfur is the main ingredient in the healing waters of the great spas around the world.

Taking an epsom salt bath can give you many of the rejuvenating features of the healing spa waters without the hefty price tag. A two-liter carton of epsom salts goes for about two dollars at a drugstore nearest you.

Warm compresses, in the form of a hot water bottle wrapped up in a damp T-shirt, are another favorite. The great things about hot water bottles are that a) they are cheap and b) they run out of heat in about ten minutes, which is, coincidentally, the maximum time that you should have heat on the area. Wait an hour before reapplying the heat, because too much heat causes overcongestion of the area and that's counterproductive. Patients commonly ask me about heating pads, but I usually advise that you throw these out. The reason? The heat makes you sleepy, you drift off into dreamland for a few hours, and then wake up with a nasty, overheated joint and cooked muscles. So stick to the hot water bottle. An important note of caution: Do not use heat with any of the over-the-counter analgesic lotions like Ben Gay, etc. You could burn and blister you skin.

When to use ice. When you know that you have overworked a joint, then ice is useful after the workout as a safety precaution. For instance, I just finished a longer that usual hike in the mountains, so I have an ice gel pack on my knee right now as I write this. I'll keep it on for fifteen to twenty minutes, and do it probably twice more until the evening. It doesn't hurt right now, and I don't expect that it will, but I guess you could say that I want to be respectful that my knee gave me a little extra enjoyment today. So I'm icing it just in case it needs it.

Call in the free radical fighters. Scientists know that the cartilage damage from free radicals equals part of the damage of OA. At best, supplementing your diet with the antioxidant vitamins A, C, and E may help the joints defend themselves and help you heal existing damage. At worst, you may live longer; protect yourself from cancer, cataracts, and heart disease; and at the very least enjoy the placebo effect of being proactive against your arthritis rather than reactive to it. Tests of the placebo effect with arthritis medicines show that even among the patients getting the phony pill 30 percent report significant relief from taking the so called "medication." That much of a result may be what you need to get your arthritis to go into a long period of abatement.

Consider a general vitamin and mineral supplement as an "insurance policy." The B complex of vitamins including folic acid; the antioxidants like vitamins A, C, and E mentioned above; and the key minerals like calcium and magnesium are all important for those who suffer from arthritis. Studies point to the low levels of these nutrients in patients with RA in particular. Vitamin D, calcium, and magnesium are all essential for RA patients and especially for women, who often develop osteoporosis over time in the bones adjacent to the affected joints.

For a more complete discussion of antioxidants, vitamins, and minerals and what levels work in the body, turn to Chapter 11.

Omega-3 fatty acids. Flax seed and flax seed oil, cold water fish such as anchovies, bluefish, halibut, herring, and sardines packed in water, and Atlantic ocean mackerel are all good sources of omega-3 fatty acids. Contained in the omega-3 fatty acids is the important eicosapentaenoic acid (EPA). Researchers have found that women who eat fish two or more times a week were 43 percent less likely to develop RA than those who eat fish once a week or less often. Most of the researchers indicate that eating eight ounces of the cold water fish five times a week is preferable to animal meats for those with RA.

I have OA rather than RA, but have found that the EPA supplements have decreased the pain and inflammation in my knees to the point where I have started jogging on a treadmill after thirteen years of no running whatsoever. I've been taking 1,000 milligrams of flax seed oil for one month now, and my symptoms have gradually improved each week. It took me about seven days before I noticed a difference. This is, of course, the anecdotal story of one person, but I offer it as hope that taking a food concentrate with no side effects other than reducing my risk of heart attack seems preferable to taking a prescription drug. Note: Do not take omega-3 oils in supplement form if you are already taking a blood-thinner type of medication. Check first with your doctor.

Prevent injuries that could lead to OA. This means wrist, elbow, and knee guards for in-line sidewalk skating, shin guards for soccer, and knee and elbow guards for racquetball and handball. You get the idea. Wear the right stuff and you'll reduce the injuries that could set off a lifetime of pain.

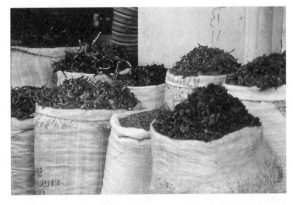

Drink plenty of water. Most of us are dehydrated. Water is probably one of the most overlooked essential nutrients we need. Do you drink eight to ten glasses of pure water every day? Cartilage cells, muscles, skin, blood and collagen tissues, synovial fluid—they all need lots of water to maintain maximum health. And it's cheap.

Therapeutic massage. World-class athletes get regular massage as part of their training and recovery. Why not you? The gentle stroking of the skin, such as the effleurage movements of Swedish massage, are known to stimulate oxytocin, a natural hormone that works to relax the body and quell stress hormone production. Tense, taut bodies feel more pain.

Beat the arthritis blues with red hot chili peppers. Capsaiscin is derived from red hot chili peppers. It's being used more and more in creams that help relieve the pain of sore joints in a kind of "hair of the dog" mechanism. When you feel the hot sensation after rubbing the cream into the affected part, the capsaiscin causes a reaction in nerve cells and reduces their pain transmitting capability. It's not a cure, but the relief is nice. *Note:* Avoid getting the capsaiscin cream into your eyes or other mucous membranes. Also *do not use heat* over the area after you have used the cream. Heat and cream together can cause serious damage to tissue.

Activate your body-mind connection. The best is saved for last. As noted above, tensed up, stressed out bodies feel pain more. Relaxation is the key learning for pain control of all kinds, especially for those with arthritis. For some stress buster ideas that might work for you, turn to Chapter 5. Doesn't music and meditation sound more wonderful than misery and moping? The mind-body connection has been proven over and over again to be the most powerful force in healing our lives, healing our pain. Best of all, it's free and the side effects are a more joyous life. Doesn't get better than that, does it?

SOME FREQUENTLY ASKED QUESTIONS ABOUT JOINTS

Q: What causes the clicking and "snappy" sounds in my joints when I move around? Should I worry about it?
A: The medical term for the harmless extra sounds in joints is *crepitus*. The clicking sound is usually nothing to worry about. It could be due to small fragments of cartilage or bone that are loose in the joint capsule or some roughened cartilage rubbing. Loose fragments may be reabsorbed by the body after some time. "Snappy" sounds could be a slightly lax tendon snapping back into it's groove after a period of inactivity, like after sitting in a movie theater for several hours. Grating or grinding noises in the knees are more serious, because they could be an indicator of a condition like chondromalacia patella (the knee's cartilage is roughened and wearing away) or a torn

meniscus (a shock-absorbing structure of the knee that gets damaged with twisting injuries). If you experience pain with any clicking, snapping, or grinding, consult a specialist.

Otherwise, creaking sounds need not be a barrier to performance. I have some athletic friends who get up out of a chair and sound like the Tin Man in need of a lube job. Then they lace up their sneakers, walk out the door, and beat the whole world.

Q. Why does my knee suddenly buckle when I'm walking, especially going down stairs?
A. It's possible that you have a torn cartilage fragment that is wedging itself in the knee joint and causing the locking. You could also have a torn or very lax anterior cruciate ligament (which runs from the middle of the knee joint to the front of the knee) that is no longer able to prevent the knee joint from excessive forward motion as you descend the stairs. It's a serious enough problem for you to consult a specialist.

Q. Does regular vigorous running mean that I will increase my chances of developing OA?
A. A study of 451 runners fifty to seventy-two years old with an average of twelve years of running under their belts were compared to a sedentary group of 330 controls. After eight years, the couch potatoes were compared to the runners. The rate of disability was several times lower in the runners than in the controls. Runners were also considerably less likely to have died during the study period.

Not surprisingly, the runners were leaner, reported fewer joint symptoms, and had fewer medical problems and took fewer medications to begin with. I smiled when I read the cautionary statement by the authors: "Increased physical activity could be the self-selected result of good health, rather than good health the result of physical activity." However, regardless of that "lawyer's disclaimer" the issue of whether or not OA was directly linked to running was not proven in this study. So lace up your sneakers and keep on going for it!

Q. What if I already have osteoarthritis in my knees? Shouldn't I be resting them? My doctor already said that I have degeneration and my knees hurt.
A. In a study published by the *Journal of the American Medical Association* in 1997, regular aerobic exercise and weight training were shown to increase mobility and

decrease pain in 439 people with knee degeneration. Score another bull's eye for the "use it or lose it" anthem. If you've just overworked you knees, then take it easy for a day or two by doing an aerobic activity, like swimming, that won't be so hard on your knees. But keep moving, because natural joint lubricants are stimulated by exercise.

Q. Are the nonsteroidal antiinflammatory drugs I'm taking for my osteoarthritis going to be bad in the long run? They do seem to help the pain.
A. All drugs have side effects. At the beginning, they take care of the pain, and that feels pretty good. However, the side effects may include bleeding of the stomach and intestines, liver damage, and long-term cartilage damage.

Q. Cartilage damage? I thought that these drugs were great for arthritis.
A. In a study of 186 arthritis patients in Norway, the fifty-eight patients taking the drug Indocin had more rapid hip destruction than the 128 patients who were not taking NSAIDs. Dr. Julian Whitaker, M.D., stated in *Health & Healing* (August 1996): "Doctors routinely prescribe steroids such as prednisone for acute flare-ups in rheumatoid arthritis patients. While the steroids are very powerful for reducing inflammation, their long-term side effects far outweigh this short-term benefit. Steroids can bring on heart disease, diabetes, eye problems, and severe osteoporosis, as well as facial and body changes. Continual steroid therapy is neither desirable nor safe."

Ask your doctor to recommend exercises, weight training, and aerobic activities that will help you be in charge of your treatment. Dr. Whitaker also noted that one-fifth of all suspected adverse drug reactions reported to the FDA have to do with NSAIDs.

As a competitive athlete in the marathon, and like most others competing at the world-class level, I tried NSAIDs at the beginning of my career. I found the side effects like stomach pain and nausea to be worse than the original injury. So from a "been there, done that" standpoint, it seemed more logical to find more natural ways to deal with the pain.

Q. What about glucosamine sulfate for osteoarthritis?
A. A healthy joint is constantly repairing and updating the cartilage that lines the ends of the bones. In an arthritic joint, the repair does not keep up the pace of the destruction. Pain, swelling, and further destruction can result.

Glucosamine sulfate is a substance that is made by cartilage cells called chondrocytes. It helps give cartilage resiliency and shock absorption. Extra supplementation of glucosamine sulfate has been shown to be quite effective in some preliminary clinical studies to help the pain and swelling of joints damaged by osteoarthritis. I tried 1,500 milligrams a day myself for about a month and didn't see a big difference, even after doubling it to 3,000 milligrams. However, I have seen dramatic results in others taking only 1,000 to 1,500 milligrams a day. Glucosamine sulfate is available in health food stores.

Q. How long do replacement joints last?
A. It depends on the joint and the amount of stress you subject it to. I've seen patients with hip replacements from thirty years ago and there's no sign of a replacement being needed. And I've seen knee replacements revised with a new prosthesis after eight years. Your surgeon will be able to indicate your prognosis.

Q. What can I do about my feet? They ache at the end of the day now. My doctor said that I'm getting bunions and, because my mom and grandmother have them, that I'm just next in line.
A. The word *bunion* is believed to have its roots from the Latin word *bunio*, meaning turnip. They've been described in medical articles for several hundred years, which is a small consolation when you're trying to fit your bunions into shoes. Actually, that's a big part of the problem. Shoes. Make that high heels. High heels are bunion-makers because they force all the weight of the body forward and bunch the toes together. Heredity does play some role in how susceptible your joint may be to degenerative changes as well. But before you line up for surgery, you may consider these options.

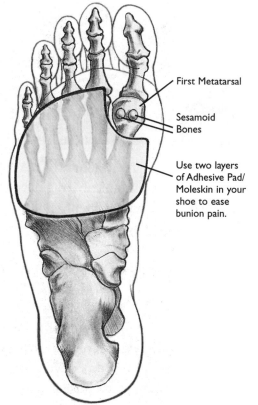

First Metatarsal

Sesamoid Bones

Use two layers of Adhesive Pad/ Moleskin in your shoe to ease bunion pain.

Try sticking feet in cold water at the end of the day to decrease inflammation. You could simply sit on the edge of the bathtub and let the

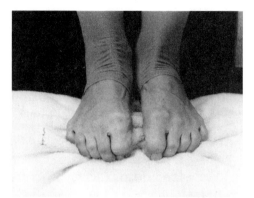

cold water run from the tap. When I was competing in marathons, I used to stick my feet in a small shallow pan of tomato juice after a twenty-mile run. I've never seen any studies on it, but you're welcome to try it.

Try switching to low-heeled shoes with cushioning and some arch support. This helps distribute weight more evenly over the foot.

Chiropractic adjustment of the bones of the feet can also bring welcome relief.

Try strengthening your feet with this towel toe-crunch: Sit in a low chair, spread a towel out in front of you, and try gathering it with your toes. When it gets too easy, place a book on the towel.

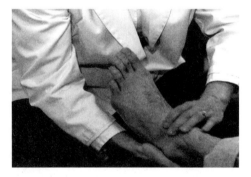

In my experience with patients, I've had great success treating painful bunions by designing and fitting a functional orthotic for the feet. No, I'm not talking about the kind where you stick your feet in a foam box. After evaluating the patient's gait and preforming a biomechanical analysis of the feet and lower legs, a plaster cast is made of the foot in its optimum anatomical position, while the patient is relaxing on the treatment table. A high-tech prosthetic device that fully supports and corrects the anatomical irregularities of the foot is then made. These lightweight, padded devices then fit in shoes. I've had several pairs made for both athletic and casual shoes. They feel great.

WHAT TO LOOK FOR IN THE FUTURE

Synvisc. This is a new option from Canada for patients suffering from osteoarthritis. Scientists have engineered a thicker version of the body's own hyaluronan, the joint's natural lubricant, and perfected it as a gel that can be injected into any joint. It is not considered a drug, because it is the body's own lubricant and it acts as a mechanical assist the joint rather than a chemical one. When the clear gel is injected into the joint to replace lost lubricant, less pain, less stiffness, greater ease of movement, and eventual return to normal activity can result for six months or longer. It is manufactured in Quebec and has been in clinical use for several years.

Cartilage cloning. A very small piece of cartilage from the patient is removed and then grown in a laboratory. Later, this cartilage is injected into the joint with a thin surgical tool called an arthroscope. Early Swedish studies in 1994 had a good success rate, but the surgery at this point is limited to fresh injuries in patients under the age of fifty. By preventing the further destruction of cartilage, osteoarthritis would be prevented, but not reversed.

In the big stakes world of horse racing, million-dollar equine athletes with acute cartilage damage have been repaired with harvested and lab-grown cartilage that has growth factors added. To complete the potion, fibrinogen, a body protein that helps glue the chondrocytes in place one they are injected, is added. The racehorses have returned to the track within six to eight months. Observers are betting that the procedure will be widely available to the human sector in a few more years.

BEATING THE ARTHRITIS BLUES

We'd all like to have and keep perfect bodies forever, but it doesn't always happen. Both kinds of arthritis can be serious, but our attitudes can either enhance or decrease our bodies' ability to deal with it. Ultimately, we decide in our minds whether our symptoms are more or less severe. Will you wake up to a good attitude tomorrow morning or not? If you are limited in doing one activity for that day, will you chose to do another that will keep you active anyway? Will you choose to become part of the solution to your arthritis rather than heaping all the responsibility on your doctor or the people who will look after you?

I hope you have learned some helpful things in this chapter. May our joints rejoice with the new information that is being gathered right now all over the world.

Until then, it's up to us, but then again, it always has been.

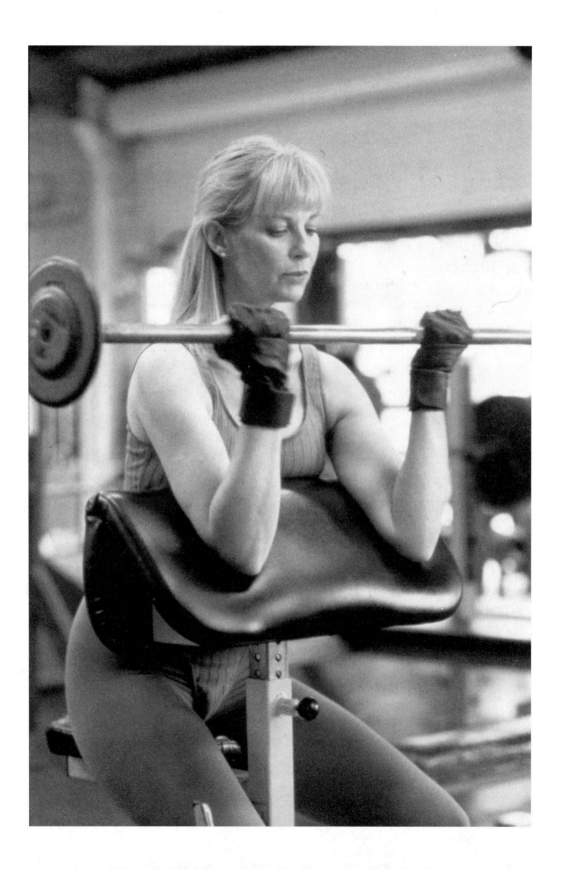

16

GETTING TO THE HEART OF THE MATTER: CARDIOVASCULAR HEALTH

A merry heart doeth good like a medicine.

—Proverbs 17:22

$\mathscr{P}$oets and incurable romantics throughout history have always believed that the heart is what rules us. Now, exercise physiologists and scientists are confirming that belief. A heart attack strikes like a thunderbolt, and it can change your whole life in just one thunderbolt second. In America last year, it changed more than 1 million people from living to dead. Another 800,000 underwent expensive procedures to bypass or reopen clogged, blocked arteries that supply the heart. The words "expensive procedure" don't even get close to the fact that hundreds of thousands of people are doing everything up to and including open heart surgery in an attempt to live a few years longer. The American Heart Association estimates that treating heart disease and all the related cardiovascular problems that occur, including stroke, cost $117 billion in 1995.

The next time you see a football stadium packed with fans, divide the stadium in half. All those on one side will die of some form of cardiovascular disease. That's what the statistics show: over half of all Americans. Yet most heart attacks and cardiovascular disease are preventable—if you make simple lifestyle changes.

WHAT'S IN A HEARTBEAT?

The human heart is a pumping muscle with four chambers. Frog hearts have only three chambers and insects can have half a dozen. I include this extra information from time to time, because you never know when a piece of anatomy trivia might win you the grand prize on a TV game show!

The heart has a big job—to deliver refreshed, oxygenated blood containing nutrients to every cell in the body, through over 60,000 miles of blood vessels and tissue fluids. In our hearts we have three types of muscle tissue that are specialized to perform in different ways. The reception, or reservoir, areas of the heart are called the right and left *atrium*. These chambers receive blood from the great veins of the body. The *ventricles* are the remaining two chambers of the heart, again one on the right side and one on the left side. The ventricles provide the main pumping force that propels the blood through the lungs and the arteries of the body.

The atrium and the ventricles each have a different type of muscle cell so that they can perform their work. Basically, they contract just like a skeletal muscle in, for instance, your arm or leg, except that the contraction is much longer for the heart muscle. The relative size of cardiac muscle cells is smaller than that of skeletal muscles, but cardiac cells have a special design feature called "T tubules"—flow tubes for essential calcium ions that have a capacity twenty-five times greater than the tubules of skeletal muscle.

Special muscle fibers allow transmission of electrical impulses through the heart to regulate the rhythm of contraction.

WHAT CAUSES THE SOUND OF A HEARTBEAT?

When blood flows into the left ventricle chamber and reaches a certain pressure, it actually pushes the valves open with a rush, like horsemen charging through the castle doors. After the initial rush, the valvular doors swing shut again. Boom! We have sound vibration that travels in all directions through the chest. We call it a heartbeat.

Each minute, even when we are at rest, our beating hearts pump more than thirty times their weight in blood. That's more than 1,800 gallons of blood a day. Age, gender, body temperature, use of tobacco and other drugs, stress, obesity, diabetes, and elevated blood fats as well as our level of physical activity all influence the rate of heartbeat. A newborn baby has a naturally high heartbeat (more than 100 beats per minute), and women have slightly higher heart rates than men. The average heart rate is sixty to one hundred beats per minute. Endurance athletes, with their highly trained hearts, can have rates as low as twenty-eight beats per minute.

The heart is so well made that it pumps without stopping for our entire lives. Exercise is important to keep the heart functioning properly because physical activity gets the heart in shape just like any other muscle. When it is more energy efficient, it beats more slowly. You could think of the longer interval between beats as a well-deserved rest.

WHAT IS HIGH BLOOD PRESSURE?

High blood pressure, or hypertension, is a major concern because it can contribute to strokes, heart attacks, and other cardiovascular diseases. Blood pressure is caused by the heart muscle contracting. When those aforementioned horsemen rush through the castle doors, the force with which they move is like the force of blood when it pushes out of the heart and into the arteries and veins.

It is normal and desirable for the rush of blood to meet with some counter-resistance, or pressure, from the blood already in the system. But too much pressure against stiff and narrowed arteries full of plaque causes trouble. Hypertension has three lethal effects:

1. It makes the heart work too hard, which can lead to diseases of the blood vessels in the heart, or of the heart muscle itself, resulting in a heart attack.
2. The high pressure can rupture a major blood vessel in the brain, which will cause an arterial spasm (stroke).
3. Very high blood pressure almost always causes multiple hemorrhages in the kidneys. The kidney damage eventually results in kidney failure and death.

HOW DO WE MONITOR BLOOD PRESSURE?

The body has built-in nerve cells installed in blood vessels. These pressure-sensitive cells sense changes in blood pressure and transmit that data to the brain. The heart must then speed up or slow down. A variety of hormones and chemical reactions can be set in motion, according to the data received.

Blood pressure may be monitored externally by using a blood pressure cuff and a stethoscope, and is recorded using two numbers:

- Systolic pressure is the first number mentioned and it represents the pressure of blood in your arteries when the heart is pumping.
- Diastolic pressure is the second number and represents the pressure in the arteries in between heartbeats, when the heart ventricles are filling up with blood, getting ready for the next contraction.

Generally, a systolic blood pressure greater than 135 to 140 mm.Hg and a diastolic blood pressure more than 95 mm.Hg under resting conditions is considered elevated. This pressure would be read as "135 over 90"; when you get your blood pressure taken the systolic number is given "over" the diastolic.

Taking your own blood pressure is easy to do. You can buy a kit in most drugstores for about $20. Blood pressure does vary according to the time of day, by whether you've just eaten, or just exercised, or even from the stress of having your blood pressure taken. According to the American Heart Association, your doctor should base a diagnosis of high blood pressure on at least three elevated readings taken a few days apart while you are sitting and standing.

As for those coin-operated drugstore blood pressure machines, they aren't always that accurate, so don't rely on them for a diagnosis of high blood pressure. Of course, if you think that you have high blood pressure, see a doctor.

HEART ACHES

A *stroke* happens when there is a sudden shut-off in blood going to the brain. This may happen when blood is forced through narrow, hardened arteries, or when a piece of the hardened artery breaks off and gets stuck somewhere. People who have had a stroke may suffer from paralysis on one side of their body, visual disturbances, slurring of words, or difficulty speaking depending on which part of the brain was oxygen-deprived by the clot. An artery that spasms may also cause a stroke.

A blood vessel can also develop a weak spot and balloon out like piece of bubble gum until it bursts. That's an *aneurysm.* You may have a congenital defect, or it can result from high blood pressure and other heart problems.

If the heart has to pump against stiff arteries for decades, then the ventricle chambers can become so enlarged that their walls are too thick to let in blood. In turn, the blood cannot be pumped out. Sooner or later, the heart throws in the towel. The cardiovascular system then gets congested like a traffic jam in the Holland Tunnel and the system fails. That's *congestive heart failure.*

If the blood vessels that supply the heart with blood and oxygen get clogged up with fatty deposits or a blood clot, the heart can't function. When the heart muscle cannot get enough oxygen, the muscle tissue affected dies off—that death is called an *infarct.* The word *myo*, means muscle. The world *cardio* means heart. Hence the term *myocardial infarction*, or heart attack.

When the heart muscle gets less oxygen than it needs, there's often a powerful warning alarm called *angina.* (It's Greek for "to strangle.") Angina is the crushing, squeezing pain that most—not all—heart attack victims experience. It's been described as "like an elephant sitting on my chest." The pressure is not always a sign of a heart attack in progress though, because stress, extreme emotions like fright or anger, exercise, or rapid temperature changes can also cause that symptom. Hopefully, you'll create a healthy heart for yourself and never feel it. But if you do experience chest pain of any kind, get medical help. It could be a pain in your left arm or feel like indigestion. I know dental hygienists who have identified pain in

> **The Major Risk Factors for Heart Disease**
> • High Blood Cholesterol
> • High Homocysteine Levels
> • High Blood Pressure
> • Cigarette Smoking

the jaw that was angina and helped save a life. Either way, know that sharp pain in the chest or arms or jaw could be a warning sign of angina and should never be ignored.

WHY HIGH CHOLESTEROL IS BAD FOR YOU

Cholesterol is a fatty substance that the body uses for many wonderful purposes. It is found in nerve tissues of the brain and spinal cord, the liver, the kidneys, and the adrenal glands. It's made by the liver and is a normal constituent of bile. It's also a precursor for various hormones in the body like testosterone, estrogen, and DHEA. In fact, cholesterol is a part of every cell membrane in our bodies.

However, when the amount of cholesterol is beyond what the body needs to function, the result is a yellow, sticky, fatty, mushy substance that flows through your blood vessels and adheres to the blood vessel walls as plaque. This hardening of the arteries is called *atherosclerosis.*

Too much cholesterol has been fingered as a cause of heart disease for almost one hundred years. How do you get excessive amounts in the body? Most people simply eat too many foods that are high in cholesterol. Others have high cholesterol and other blood fats called triglycerides due to a hereditary condition known as *hyperlipidemia*. Your doctor can use diagnostic blood tests to determine if this is the case with you.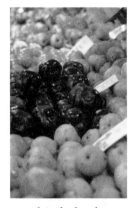

While cholesterol is strongly associated with heart disease, it is certainly not the only cause. A study done in Japan and Southern Europe demonstrated that even though these populations tended to have the same cholesterol levels as Americans, they had only one-third the heart attack rate. On the other hand, having lived in Switzerland many years ago, I can attest to the fact that it is a far more physically active culture than in America, with people walking or riding bicycles, for example, to go the grocery store or to work. Clearly, there are other lifestyle factors protecting the European and Japanese populations from the fatal effects of cholesterol.

WHAT'S A HIGH CHOLESTEROL READING?

Age	Moderate Risk	High Risk
20–29	over 200 mg/dl*	over 220 mg/dl
30–39	over 220 mg/dl	over 240 mg/dl
over 40	over 240 mg/dl	over 260 mg/dl

*deciliter

How do you decrease your cholesterol levels? Improve your diet. Decrease animal (saturated) fats like red meat, whole milk, cheese, doughnuts, bacon. Two more factors that contribute to high cholesterol are smoking and alcohol abuse. If you get control of these, you are also decreasing your risks for cancer, stroke, and heart attacks. If you can't do it yourself, contact the American Heart Association, the American Cancer Society, and Alcoholics Anonymous. The U.S. *heart disease death rate is dropping* and the average cholesterol level has gone from 220 in the 1960s to a current average of 205. We seem to be getting the message, but not all of us.

ISN'T THERE A "GOOD" CHOLESTEROL?

New studies question the traditional view that it is cholesterol itself that causes the destructive process arterial plaque. Kilmer McCully, M.D. a pathologist at the VA Medical Center Providence, Rhode Island, has spent thirty years gathering evidence that points to high homocysteine levels in the blood as the felon in heart disease. Homocysteine is an amino acid that can damage the walls of the arteries if it is allowed to reach high blood levels.

A safe range for premenopausal women is 6 to 10 micromoles per deciliter of blood, and 8 to 12 micromoles per deciliter for men and postmenopausal women.

Folic acid, vitamin B6, and vitamin B12 in adequate amounts control homocysteine levels. There's no need to megadose, as only a few milligrams per day of each will do the trick. Good sources are found in beans, green leafy vegetables, and whole grains.

Cholesterol comes in two types: either a high-density good guy (HDL) which helps prevent fats from sticking to arteries, or low-density bad guy (LDL) which clogs up blood vessels. The ratio between the two is used as an indicator of cardiovascular risk. Regular aerobic exercise raises the good cholesterol, but may not lower the bad cholesterol in everyone.

SOYBEANS VS. THE ANTICHOLESTEROL DRUGS

A new class of cholesterol lowering drugs called *statins* may prove to be a potent weapon in the battle against heart disease. But there are a lot of short-term side effects and the long-term effects of these drugs are still unknown. Current estimates, according to the *Wall Street Journal*, are that 4 to 6 million Americans now take statins. The drugs are also quite expensive—costing up to $2,000 to $3000 per year.

There may be a better alternative—tofu. Researchers from the University of Kentucky at Lexington reported recently in the *New England Journal of Medicine* that eating soy protein significantly reduces moderate to high concentrations of cholesterol in the blood. Those who averaged four grams of soy protein a day saw their cholesterol level drop about 10 percent. People with the highest levels of cholesterol benefitted the most, with an average reduction of about 24 percent. Most cholesterol-reducing drugs do about the same, but the soy products have no side effects.

WHY HIGH BLOOD PRESSURE SHOULD CONCERN YOU

An estimated 63 million Americans have hypertension, or high blood pressure. High blood pressure is symptomless, which is why doctors call hypertension the *silent killer*. Keep your blood pressure under control and you will live longer and feel better.

HOW TO LOWER YOUR BLOOD PRESSURE AND CHOLESTEROL

Go veggie. A Johns Hopkins University Study presented at the American Heart Association's scientific conference in 1996 reported that participants who consumed nine to ten servings of fruits and vegetables plus three servings of low-fat dairy products per day reduced blood pressure readings within two weeks to the level you would achieve with medication.

Go low fat. Just one high-fat meal may cause a release of the hormone *thromboxane*, which causes arteries to constrict and blood to clot faster. That's why so many heart patients get pains in their chest after a fatty meal and end up in the emergency room after a big holiday party. The good news is that making better, low-fat choices can improve blood flow to the heart in only a few weeks.

Stop smoking. Smoking adds to arterial plaque on the heart's blood vessels, the coronary arteries. Blood vessels narrowed by fatty plaque make the heart pump harder. Nicotine also causes blood to clot faster.

Lose weight. Reducing your body weight to normal may bring down even a high or moderately high blood pressure. As far as cardiovascular disease is concerned, we're literally eating ourselves to death.

Shake the salt habit. Do you add salt to your food before even tasting it? Try using herbs and spices like powdered garlic on your food instead. Sodium makes us retain water, which increases the volume of blood so that the heart has to work harder. A study in Britain found that cutting salt by about a teaspoon a day could prevent 25 percent of all strokes and 15 percent of all heart attacks. In America, 80 percent of our sodium intake is hidden in prepared foods.

Fill up on the fiber. Eating lots of fiber-rich fruits, vegetables, and whole grains helps speed food through the digestive tract and cuts down on the amount of cholesterol absorbed from food. There's also the added benefit of weight loss. Is this a real bargain, or what?

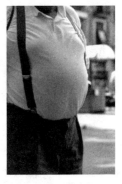

Move it and lose it. The American College of Sports Medicine says that regular huff and puff aerobic exercise can reduce systolic and diastolic blood pressure by as much as ten points. You don't have to start Olympic-style workouts to get these benefits. Walking at a brisk pace for half an hour five times a week can really give you a head start.

One study published in the *New England Journal of Medicine* compared 12,000 longshoremen between the ages of thirty-five and seventy-four who were vigorously active, moderately active, and inactive. The low activity group showed double the risk of sudden death from heart attack as the others. The American Heart Association says that lack of exercise is as significant a risk for heart disease as smoking.

Get some potassium. This important mineral can counteract the negative effects of too much sodium, and that helps keep blood pressure down. There's no need to take supplements for potassium (potassium overdose is dangerous). Instead eat potassium-rich foods such as beans, baked potatoes, peas, and bananas. Just four ounces of lima beans contains almost 500 milligrams of potassium, a baked potato gives 800 milligrams, and a banana gives you over 100 milligrams. And, of course, these all contribute fiber to your diet which helps reduce cholesterol, increase weight loss, and protect you from colon cancer.

Lighten up. Are you a *hot reactor*? Are you angry, tense, or full of negative emotions on a daily basis? You can learn to control your emotions and lower your blood pressure. Don't sweat the small stuff—try to solve your problems and make a conscious effort to relax. Exercise, biofeedback, meditation, a support group, or professionally taught relaxation techniques can help you live longer and enjoy life more.

You can have a drink, but only once in a while. Heavy drinking can do severe damage, but having a drink now and then can help raise your levels of HDLs (the good guys). Moderate drinkers are less likely to get heart disease than teetotalers or heavy drinkers. That translates to no more than three ounces of hard liquor, two five-ounces glasses of wine, or two twelve-ounce glasses of beer five days a week.

Menopause and your heart. In the Nurses Health Study of 48,000 healthy women, women who were taking estrogen after menopause had half as many heart attacks and cardiovascular deaths as women who had never used estrogen. Hormone replacement therapy (HRT) also decreases LDL (bad cholesterol) while raising HDL (good cholesterol) by approximately 15 percent each. There is a possibility that HRT may increase breast cancer, but a woman's chance of dying from heart disease is more than double that from any of the different kinds of cancer. That can be stated another way. The current risk of dying of breast cancer is one in nine. The current risk of dying of heart disease for a woman over fifty is one in two. For a more complete discussion of HRT, including natural therapies, please turn to Chapter 22.

Consider taking antioxidants like vitamin E. There is a vast amount of research saying that antioxidants prevent arterial plaque and the thick blood that build the clots that produce heart disease and strokes. For instance, the Cambridge Heart Antioxidant Study of 2,000 patients with clinical evidence of coronary atherosclerosis found a 77 percent decrease in nonfatal heart attacks after only 200 days of antioxidant supplements. Turn to Chapter 11 for a list of antioxidants.

Calcium guards against hypertension. If you eat lots of kale and broccoli, and drink calcium-fortified orange juice, you could reduce your risk of hypertension by 25 percent. Researchers who studied men and women between 1971 and 1984 found that one gram of calcium a day did the trick. Most Americans don't even get half the amount that's recommended. Turn to Chapter 13 to get more information on calcium-rich foods.

Don't forget the folic acid. Increased levels of homocysteine, a blood protein linked to arterial plaque, triples your risk of heart attacks. Folic acid, vitamins B6 and B12 all work together to help keep homocysteine under control. Foods high in folic acid are: spinach, collard greens, beet greens, legumes, and nuts. Good sources of B6 are whole grains, bananas, and seafood.

WHAT ABOUT TAKING SUPPLEMENTS TO PREVENT HEART DISEASE?

Vitamin E. Several decades ago, the Shute Brothers in Canada researched vitamin E, believing that this vitamin would increase oxygen uptake. They applied their findings to thoroughbred race horses. Northern Dancer, the first horse raised with the supplement, won many championship races.

Since then, thousands and thousands of studies have been done on vitamin E. The evidence on the benefits of the vitamin as a preventive and treatment for cardiovascular disease is staggering.

Vitamin E is an antioxidant. It prevents the LDL (bad cholesterol) from oxidizing so that this "bad cholesterol" cannot turn into artery-clogging plaque. In 1996, the *Lancet* medical journal reported on a study of 2,000 patients with coronary heart disease in which the participants who received 400 to 800 IU of vitamin E a day experienced a 75 percent reduction of heart attacks.

Omega-3 fatty acids. These essential fatty acids are found in oil of cold-water fish like

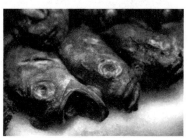

salmon or in flaxseed oil. In 1991, a study done on 25 men with high cholesterol found that supplementation with omega-3 fatty acids increased the good cholesterol HDLs and decreased triglycerides in just five weeks.

You can eat cold-water fish regularly or supplement with flax seed or omega-3 oils, which are available in any health food store. My at-risk patients take two tablespoons of flaxseed oil daily.

Coenzyme Q10. Often abbreviated as CoQ10, this antioxidant is a naturally occurring substance with a molecular structure similar to vitamin K. Found in humans, plants, and animals, it is also known as *ubiquinone* (from the word *ubiquitous*), because it is present in nearly every cell of our bodies. CoQ10 has an important role in heart health. Studies have shown it to be safe and effective in reducing angina spasms, increasing the efficiency of the heart muscle, and helping prevent major damage to the heart caused by heart attacks.

Vitamin C. Studies have demonstrated that vitamin C can lower cholesterol in animals. It is a powerful antioxidant that fights free radicals.

Niacin, or vitamin B3. This has been shown to lower LDL cholesterol and raise HDL cholesterol. The preferred form is *inositol hexanicotinate* or *hexaniacinate*, which can be bought in a health food store. Be sure to read labels, because regular niacin can cause some severe and unpleasant flushing reactions in the body.

Garlic. Considered a longevity food for thousands of years, we now know that the ancients were right. Clinical studies show that garlic lowers total cholesterol, increases HDL cholesterol, and lowers LDL cholesterol. Eat garlic bread tonight. Roast whole cloves and spread them on bread. Or go to the health food store and buy it in capsules. The important ingredient is *allicin,* so make sure you read the labels. Aged garlic extract, called *Kyolic,* has been proven to be a powerful antioxidant. It's popular with a lot of folks who want the garlic benefits without the garlic breath. You can get it at health food stores.

Gugulipid. It's a funny name for a plant extract that packs a serious threat to cholesterol. Gugulipid is an extract of an herb called *commiphora mukul,* which has been used in India for thousands of years. Studies show that it can lower cholesterol up to 27 percent and triglycerides by up to 30 percent. It's available in health food stores.

Folic Acid. New research published in the *Journal of the American Medical Association (JAMA)* indicates that many heart attacks might be averted if people consumed folic acid, a water-soluble vitamin-B complex. It functions as a coenzyme, working together with vitamins B12 and C. Folic acid performs an important role because it helps keep down the levels of homocysteine, as we discussed earlier. The *JAMA* article estimated that 35,000 deaths a year could be prevented in American men if folic acid intake was increased.

Folic acid is easily destroyed in food with high temperatures in cooking, by exposure to light, or even room temperatures. Oral contraceptives interfere with absorption, as do sulfa drugs. The best food sources of folic acid are green leafy vegetables, brewer's yeast, and liver.

Magnesium. Its been linked to heart health and prevention of heart disease for a while. The National Research Council recommends 350 mg. a day for adults. Dark green, leafy vegetables, nuts, seeds, and apricots are good food sources. Caution: High dosages over 1,000 mg. per day can cause diarrhea and could be toxic. If you have kidney disease, do not take magnesium supplements.

WHAT IS CHELATION THERAPY?

EDTA (ethylenediaminetetraacetatate) is a man-made protein that is used commercially as a preservative in canned crab meat to retard crystal formation and promote color retention. It is also used in salad dressings and carbonated beverages.

In cardiovascular medicine EDTA is used as a chelating agent, which means it binds to certain metal ions in the blood vessels and arteries. The metals are then excreted out of the body along with other waste products. One 1988 study of 3,000 patients with cardiovascular disease found that chelation therapy improved high blood pressure, leg pain from blocked arteries, and heart disease. EDTA chelation therapy has been controversial since its outset; it is not considered conventional medicine and the American Medical Association is against it. You decide. To find out more, read *Questions From The Heart*, by Terry Chappell, M.D., published by Phillips Publishing in Potomac, Maryland.

In short: Why wait until you get a heart attack or have a stroke to think about your health? There are many safe, natural ways to help yourself now. **Take charge and learn all you can about how to help yourself.** Put your heart into it—you're worth it. And if you want to learn more, check out *Dr. Dean Ornish's Program For Reversing Heart Disease*, published by Ballantine Books. Special discount rates for educational purposes are available; call 1-800-733-3000 for more information.

Also, Dr. Kilmer McCully's book, *The Homocysteine Revolution,* Keats Publishing, New Canaan, CT, is another winner; call 1-800-858-7014 for more information.

17

How to Prevent Cancer

Why pay for an ambulance to wait for you at the bottom of the cliff?
Isn't it saner to invest a little money to put some guard rails at the top?
—Gayle Olinekova

$\mathcal{E}$ach day we're bombarded with information about food and cancer, and it seems like each week there's a new miracle food that prevents cancer and yet another "bad guy" cancer-causing agent in some food you love. One friend responded to an announcement that steak causes cancer by saying, "Just leave my chocolate alone and nobody gets hurt!"

Yet it has only been in the last few decades that researchers have paid as much attention to preventing cancer as curing it. Ironically, the mid-nineteenth century health food "Naturalists," like Dr. John Harvey Kellog and Sylvester Abraham, once considered the lunatic fringe, pointed the way to cancer-free living. The Naturalist program of exercising, eating your veggies, fruits, and nuts, and achieving spiritual harmony is at the heart of most cancer prevention programs today. An incredible explosion of research in the last few decades has shown how effective these and other preventive measures truly are.

For instances, simply staying out of sun-tanning booths can cut your risk of melanoma and skin cancer by 90 percent. More than 700,000 men and women in America are diagnosed with skin cancer each year. Approximately 165,000 people a year in America die from tobacco-related cancers. Most of those deaths could be prevented. Abuse of alcohol accounts for another 17,000 deaths a year in America. Most of those could be prevented as well. In a study of 17,000 male Harvard alumni, there was a 25 to 50 percent lower incidence of colon cancer in those who exercised at moderate to high levels. And scientists now believe that 40 percent of men's cancer and 60 percent of women's cancers are food-related.

Because there are so many books available on cancer treatment, in the pages that follow I will restrict myself to an overview of some of the most common prevention techniques. Also, at the end of the chapter, I list some wonderful books you can use for research. If you have a resource that you have found particularly helpful, then please write to me so that I may share this valuable information with others in subsequent editions of this book.

WHAT IS CANCER?

There are an estimated one hundred different kinds of cancer. Cancer is the uncontrolled growth of cells derived from normal tissues. These abnormal cells may kill organs by spreading from the original site to other areas of the body. The word itself comes from the Greek word *karkinos*, meaning crab, presumably because a cancer adheres to the affected part so tenaciously. The study of cancer is named *oncology*, from the Greek word for tumor.

Cancer begins when the highly ordered genetic structure of the cells is changed or mutated. When the genetic material is altered, usually by something like cigarette smoke, X-rays, or other chemicals, and then stimulated by certain other *promoting elements*, then cell growth and division go haywire. For instance, alcohol contains compounds that are known to combine with tobacco by-products to increase the rate of mouth and throat cancers. Our bodies have powerful immune defense systems to eliminate and destroy cancer cells that may be wandering around in our bodies. And there are also other defense mechanisms within our immune systems that search out and destroy cells that are beginning to change so that tumors do not develop. These cells act like the Pac men of the eponymous video game and go around gobbling up the invaders. It's a complex system, but normal human cells have protein markers that stick out of them like a flag on the main mast. When the Pac men cells see what amounts to the skull and crossbones of a foreign invader cell, a cascade of reactions occur so that *natural killer cells, suppressor T cells, helper T cells*, and the Pac men (*macrophages*) can all work together to wipe out the unwanted pirate cells.

Risk Factors and Prevention

After mutated cells develop, it still can take decades for the cancer to cause symptoms. That's why it's important to get check-ups and catch it in the early and most curable stages. Cancer is rated in chronological stages from zero to four, with stage zero being the earliest and most curable. A stage two colon cancer, for instance, is 75 percent curable.

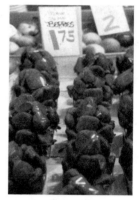

Our immune systems are powerful, intricate organizations that have over 2 million years of DNA replication behind them. That's a lot of time to get it right. However, too much dietary fat, unattenuated stress and depression, radiation, drugs, tobacco use, and lack of exercise are factors that exceed the design specs of our genetic inheritance. Additionally, some genetic markers that a person may be born with may also predispose him or her to developing cancer.

In the arena of cancer and disease prevention in general, knowing your risk factors may motivate you to change your health habits and reduce your risk. The Serenity Prayer written by St. Francis of Assisi hundreds of years ago takes on new meaning even in our high-tech era of applied nuclear physics and gene splicing: "God grant me the serenity to accept the things I cannot change, courage to change the things I can, and wisdom to know the difference." Some risks, like toxins in the workplace you were exposed to years ago or genetic markers that have been part of your DNA inheritance for many generations are examples of risk factors that you cannot control now. But knowing that there are risk factors that are unique to you may help you to watch out for symptoms or be very conscientious about getting regular check-ups that can lead to early detection. There are no guarantees that early detection automatically leads to a cure, but in many cases that's just what happens.

Knowing that you have a lifestyle that includes risk factors for cancer may motivate you to change. Giving up smoking, for instance, can rapidly improve the health even of people who have smoked *for fifty years or more*. Giving up your membership in the Couch Potato club can significantly increase your life span and quality of life. And learning how to be cheerful and seek the joyful experiences in life will undoubtedly not only improve your life, but the lives and safety of others around you, especially while you're driving on the freeway.

It's not as tough as it sounds. All the cards are in your hands. What better choices can you make today in order to invest in yourself and your future? What risk factors must you accept? And what do you need to know to tell the difference? Someone once told me that a healthy, harmonious lifestyle has to be what your heart and head can stand on a daily basis. Nobody has all the answers. But you can take responsibility for your own health one better choice at a time. And then you will be giving your own immune system what it needs to fight the good fight.

George Burns smoked cigars for years and outlived enough of his contemporaries to dedicate his book *How to Live to Be a Hundred or More* "To the widows of my last six doctors." He undoubtedly had genetic blessings that we can only envy. How do you know if you can smoke cigars and carry on like that and still have longevity? You don't. An interesting side note is that because of a slowing metabolism, cancer cells generally do not proliferate fast enough to kill you after about the age of eighty-five. Hearing that news prompted me to decide that even though I know that coffee is linked to various reproductive cancers and that high intake of dietary fat is certainly contraindicated for generalized good health, if I ever get to be a hundred years old, I'm going to eat croissants and brie for breakfast and wash it all down with a pint of cappucino and a chocolate eclair.

Getting back to reality, the following pages provide a number of suggestions for things you can start to do today to reduce your risk of cancer. As with any goal, health or otherwise, it seems that once you know the *what*, it's only a matter of the *how*. Your mission, if you decide to accept it, is to find ways to phase these better choices into your lifestyle on a daily basis. My advice is to make just one better choice for yourself the first day. Each time you do that, it becomes easier and easier to make better choices for yourself on subsequent occasions. Now let's get to it.

CANCER PREVENTION 101

If you do all of the things on this list, will it totally protect you from getting cancer? Even the legions of experts in this field won't give you that kind of guarantee. However, eliminating the known factors that cause cancer will minimize your risk. It's better than living in fear. Making better choices is a way for you to care for yourself and the ones that you care for and who love you. Here then, are some of the ways.

Quit smoking or using tobacco products. Tobacco contains forty-three known car-cinogens. One in five American fatalities is blamed on smoke-related illnesses—almost half a million deaths per year. Scientists now know that smoking also augments the risk of other cancers from toxic exposures like alcohol, industrial toxins, and the like. Staying away from smoky places like bars is also a good idea, because secondhand smoke is more toxic than what the smoker inhales and is estimated to account for 8,000 deaths per year.

Quit using marijuana. Marijuana produces five times as much carbon monoxide in the bloodstream as cigarettes. The lava lamp generation thought otherwise, but mar-ijuana has also been linked to lung cancer, just like cigarettes. Additionally, it is known to reduce immune system functioning. The immune system is our only defense against infection, so it makes sense not to mess with it. If you can quit on your own, great. If you need help, get it.

Avoid toxins from home, hobbies, and your workplace. That means working in well ventilated rooms, wearing protective clothing like gloves and goggles, and following safety guidelines for your occupation or hobbies. Avoid fabric dyes, sawdust, paint, glue, chemicals, and the like. Test your house for radon, the number-two cause of lung cancer in America. It is a by-product of naturally occurring uranium in soil and rocks. Testing kits are available. Refer to your yellow pages for a professional. Con-tact the American Lung Association for a list of common asbestos products in your home, including the "cottage cheese" that may be on your ceiling, floor tiles, and gaskets. Lawn chemicals, including pesticides, are another common source of cancer-producing substances in the home. Solvents like those used for stripping paint and electric blankets are other among other suspects that you may want to think about avoiding.

Stay out of the sun and don't go to tanning salons. The experts all agree on this one: More than 90 percent of all aging of the skin and skin cancer could be prevented by avoiding exposure to ultraviolet light. Wear a hat, long sleeves, and use a sunblock of at least 15 SPF (sun protection factor). Skin cancer is one of the most commonly known cancers, affecting more than 700,000 people in the U.S. *every year.*

Avoid the barbie. Not the doll, the barbecue. Grilling food over charcoal produces *nitrosamines*, some of the most potent carcinogens discovered, as well as several other cancer-causing chemicals.

Keep fit. The American Academy of Sports Medicine and the Centers For Disease Control recommend thirty minutes of moderate exercise at least five times a week.

Not exercising is as great a risk factor for cancer as smoking. Exercising rewards participants with protection against cancer for many reasons:

- Immune system function in general is increased, which stimulates the body's natural defense mechanisms against cancer. It's like grabbing for the brass ring on a merry-go-round. Exercisers have higher amounts of natural killer cells and, additionally, the other cells that fight infection have more chances to grab at the invaders because an active person's blood supply circulates more than a couch potato's does.
- Exercise may prevent colorectal cancer by up to 80 percent because it increases bowel contraction, so that waste can zoom on through at a faster rate, thereby limiting toxic contact with the lining of the bowel.
- Breast, uterine, ovarian, and prostate cancer are all reduced because exercise balances the body's production of testosterone and estrogen hormones.
- Exercise controls obesity and obesity is linked with increased cancer risk. Obesity is defined as being more than 40 percent over your ideal weight. The statistics on this are really quite astonishing: Obese men are 35 percent more likely to die of cancer. Obese women are 160 percent more likely to die of cancer than those who are within healthy weight limits.

Avoid eating meat. Numerous studies point to the fact that vegetarians have only a fraction of the cancers found among the meat-eating population. Red meat, in particular, is high in fat, and excess fat in the diet is known to be linked to suppression of the body's natural defense systems. High fat can also act as a tumor promoter. Some studies have linked the excessive amounts of bile acids and fatty acids as promoters in colon cancer because these substances increase the proliferation of cells in the colon. Increased cell proliferation is considered a risk factor for colon cancer. Additionally, an overabundance of protein and fat in the typical American diet seems to increase carcinogenesis, while a low protein intake seems to reduce the overall risk. However, soy products high in vegetable protein have been shown to significantly lower the risk of reproductive cancers in women.

Eat lots of fiber. The National Cancer Institute recommends at least twenty to thirty grams of fiber per day. That's easy to accomplish by eating five servings of fruits and vegetables per day. Turn to Chapter 11 for a list of high-fiber foods. Fiber prevents cancer by promoting healthy, regular bowel movements and speeding food along it's way in the digestive tract. This minimizes the length of time a potential carcinogen could have contact with the intestinal lining.

Get more antioxidants. Antioxidants are micronutrients that act as biotech "freedom fighters." They intercept highly reactive and cell-wrecking molecules called free radicals before they can do their dirty work in the body. For a list of antioxidant foods, turn to Chapter 11.

Eat less fat in your diet. High-fat diets are linked not only to higher incidence of cancer, but to increased risk of cardiovascular disease. Try stir-frying, baking, and steaming instead of regular frying; fat-free salad dressings; and smaller meat portions and larger veggie portions in each meal.

Avoid eating smoked, pickled, or salt-cured foods. Benzopyrines in smoked foods and nitrites used to preserve pickled foods are known carcinogens.

Consider supplements. Capriciously popping some vitamin pills whenever you feel guilty about a junk food binge does not get you out of the responsibility of honoring your body on a daily basis. That's the danger of relying on supplements. However, with no other dietary modifications, there are studies that show that melatonin, selenium, and the antioxidants vitamins A, C, and E offer both cancer and heart disease protection.

Chart your family tree. Knowledge is power. If you know blood relatives—direct lineage aunts and uncles, grandparents, parents, and siblings—have cancer, then you should be alert to symptoms, get early check-ups, and possibly prevent it. Cancer that develops fifteen or twenty years earlier than normal, cancer that spans more than one generation, or that affects more than one close relative is all very important information to know about. Remember, early surveillance is the key to stopping the progress of cancer in its curable stages.

Practice safe sex. Genital warts (human papilloma virus, or HPV) may be prevented by condom use. HPV increases the risk of genital cancers, particularly cervical cancer in women. Also for women: Don't douche too often. Women who douche more than four times a month are at greater risk for cervical cancer, presumably because douching upsets the natural defense immunological systems of the tissues involved.

Heal your life. Much has been written about the mind and cancer since the landmark book *Peace, Love, and Healing* by oncologist Bernie Seigel, M.D. However, the ancient Greeks and Chinese noted certain basic trends in personality type and cancers of all kinds. At this time, more research is clearly needed but, as with research into herbs, funding is not as easily forthcoming because there are not millions to be made in telling people to get rid of their toxic emotions and deal with the angering, depressing, and frustrating lives they may be living in quiet desperation. Author Henry David Thoreau talked about living our lives in quiet desperation, but were he alive today, I think he would be surprised at how noisy our desperation has become.

Get regular check-ups and screening tests. Cancer normally takes twenty to thirty years to develop, so time is really on your side. Most cancers are curable when they are detected in the early stages.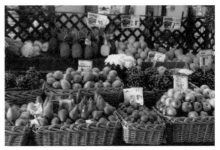

Drink lots of pure water. Are you drinking at least eight to ten glasses of pure water every day? Drinking water encourages frequent and regular bowel movements, nourishes the thyroid gland which regulates metabolism, and helps reduce body stress from dehydration.

Drink less alcohol. Moderation is the goal when it comes to diet, exercise, and drinking alcoholic beverages. Avoid binge drinking, which can promote tumor growth. While heart disease experts may say go ahead and drink up, cancer specialists remind us of the limit of four drinks per week, especially for those at risk for breast cancer. Guess what? The experts don't agree. Balance is the key, moderation is the age-old method, and as usual, it's up to you to make the best decision. Nothing new here!

Get in a Few Laughs Along the Way

There's enough fear, shame, and guilt in the world without adding cancer to the list. There are plenty of teetotalling, committed, exercising folks who never smoked a cigarette in their life and got cancer anyway. You can avoid industrial pollutants by never leaving your house, but some studies have shown that stay-at-home housewives are exposed to a tremendous number of carcinogens from common household cleaning products and pesticides, and they have above average rates of cancer.

This is the kind of information that can really drive you crazy. The best case scenario is to try to institute as many of the prevention lifestyle measures described on these pages as your heart and head and wallet can stand. To be able to have more energy and to be able to share life and enjoy it more as a result of a lifestyle that nourishes you is a wonderful thing. You are not helpless and alone against the threat of cancer. The power is in the knowledge that you use to help yourself.

MUST-READS

Cancer Free, The Comprehensive Cancer Prevention Program, Sidney J. Winawer M.D. et al, physicians at Sloan Kettering Cancer Center.

Peace, Love, and Healing, Bernie Siegel, M.D.

18

TAKING THE BITE OUT OF DENTAL PROBLEMS

I am escaped with the skin of my teeth.

—Book of Job 19:20

*E*ven if it's *only* a teeth cleaning appointment, I still think of that scene from the movie *Marathon Man* when Dustin Hoffman was being tortured by the sadistic dentist. It makes for a very white-knuckled visit. But compared to medieval times when candle wax, raven's dung, and stale bread were used for fillings, Hoffman didn't do so bad. I've never had a cavity in my life, but the fear of the dentist is well ingrained from going as moral support with family and friends, and it doesn't seem to matter how soothing the piped-in music is.

If you rate going to the dentist up there on your list of favorites right next to getting audited by the IRS, you're not alone. Fear of dentistry still prevents a lot of people from going to the dentist and committing to that all important basic: the twice a year cleaning. But get over it—modern dentistry has improved a lot since those bad dental memories when you were a kid, and it can save you from becoming toothless.

New advancements in the field of dentistry and new technology and equipment have allowed dentists to perform dental procedures without the discomfort, drilling, noise, and injections of yesteryear. The pay-off in terms of time spent in the dental chair is better too. To get a cavity filled twenty years ago, you could expect to sit there for at least an hour. Today, the same cavity takes about fifteen minutes from start to finish. There is even a type of chewing gum being developed that may heal small cavities that have started to form. Fluoride in toothpaste may also help remineralize soft spots on your teeth, preventing future cavities before they even become cavities.

That's happy news, because though we are keeping our teeth longer than our parents' generation, statistically speaking, when it comes to aging, the teeth are near the front of the line for warranties that wear out. And no amount of dental enthusiasm, even for the champion flossers and brushers among us, is singlehandedly enough to keep our teeth around forever unless we are willing to learn new techniques for home tooth care and prevention.

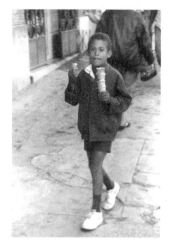

So hang on to your dental floss, and we'll take a whirlwind tour of some of the highlights of dental care that can have you flashing those pearly whites at your one hundredth birthday party.

BUT FIRST, A WORD FROM THE GUM LINE

Although the spotlight always seems to be on the teeth, be aware that gum disease accounts for more tooth loss than cavities. *Gingivitis* is the first stage of inflammation that occurs when gums become irritated from plaque. Plaque is the end product of food, bacteria, and saliva that stick to the spaces between our teeth and gums. When it is not cleaned by proper brushing, flossing, and dental hygiene visits, the gums become irritated and infected. If this goes on too long, the gums form pockets, the infection increases, and then another tooth is lost due to periodontal disease. Symptoms of this? Red, swollen, bleeding gums, bad breath, a bad taste in your mouth, and loose teeth. An estimated three out of four Americans will suffer from gum disease at some time. See a dentist before it gets to the loose tooth stage (pyorrhea), because then your choices are limited. Regular teeth cleaning, at least every six months, helps keep your gums in the pink and helps to prevent the gum problems that can lead to teeth problems.

SMILE SAVERS FROM THE PROS

Do you really know how to brush? If you were on a game show with a $100,000 prize and you had an hour to demonstrate the correct way to brush your teeth in order to win, would you go ahead and brush your teeth the same old way you do every day, or would you make a few telephone calls, talk to an expert or two, and *then* answer the question? Are you $100,000 worth of sure that you brush your teeth correctly? I pick that dollar amount, because the lifetime dental work to keep you from becoming toothless could very well add up to that amount, given all the cavities, root canals, bridges, gum surgery, partials, and eventual dental implants that you might have to endure.

Brushing your teeth can be one of your greatest weapons against tooth decay and loss—or one of your biggest enemies. Scrubbing your teeth several times a day with a highly abrasive toothpaste and a hard bristled toothbrush can eventually wear down the enamel and expose the soft dentin, which is more prone to decay. Additionally, scrubbing may wear away the gums around the roots. This can lead to cavities near the gum baseline.

The correct way to brush is to hold your toothbrush in a palms-up grip, similar to the way golfers hold a golf club. Your thumb should be extended. Now, hold the brush against your teeth at a 45-degree angle, and try to vibrate the bristles next to the teeth in a squiggly motion, so that they can reach under the all-important gum line. This should be done gently, over only a few teeth at a time. Flick your wrist up and down a few times while you're at it—this helps the bristles brush away food particles and bacteria that may be lining up on the sides of your teeth. It should take about three minutes to do a good job.

The best thing to do is have your dentist check out your technique on your next visit. After all, if you wanted to keep your tennis game in maximum shape, wouldn't you want a pro to check out your serve every once in a while? Ask your dentist for a demo. It's a sure bet to keep your smile at its brightest.

Treat yourself to some new tools. Most people seem to buy shoes more often than they spring for a new toothbrush. Get rid of that frayed, hard-tufted, bacteria-ridden thing you stick in your mouth every morning. Replace it with a soft-bristled beauty every four to six weeks.

A dentist friend once recommended buying a child-size toothbrush as an alternate brush, to use every other day. It really is easier to negotiate all the nooks and crannies of your mouth with the smaller toothbrush. And the kid-size brushes have a much better selection: You can get sparkle dust, favorite cartoon characters, and even a handle that changes color when you've brushed long enough. Think of it as the cheapest form of retail therapy.

While you're at it, buy one of those tooth gizmos you see next to the toothbrushes with the little rubber tip on the end. It's called a dental stimulator in case you're ever in a trivia challenge. Holding the tip at the right angles to the gums, gently work it in between your teeth, as if it were a delicate toothpick. It helps bring circulation into the all important gum margin as well as moving dislodging bacteria that may be trying to set up shop on your enamel.

Electric toothbrushes, sonic cleaners, and dental irrigators are all new tools that can help you keep your smile.

Paste, powder, or nothing at all? In the year 100 A.D., the Chinese brushed their teeth with a tooth powder made of soap beans. The Romans realized the value of oral hygiene, and the emery used in the early Italian tooth powder made teeth clean and shiny, but wore away the enamel until the pulp was exposed. Two thousand years later, the American Dental Association has developed a rating program with a seal of approval given to products that are low in abrasion. Most dentists recommend a fluoride-based product. Fluoride has had it's share of controversy over the years, but research has supported the fact that fluoride remineralizes the teeth. This means that teeth become stronger, less cavity prone, and less sensitive at the roots.

Some people don't use any toothpaste at all, but because of championship brushing and flossing techniques, they're still protected. Most of us prefer the psychological boost from toothpaste and the like, but you may want to choose a product that's free of saccharine (a known carcinogen). A note if you are using homeopathic formulas: The use of mint or peppermint is discouraged because it is believed to interfere with the homeopathic process.

You don't have to floss all of your teeth every day—just the ones you want to keep. This little sign has been fastened to the ceiling in my dentist's office for years. If you have difficulty negotiating the tiny spaces in your mouth, or if your hands are not as agile as they used to be, consider flossing helpers. Your dentist can help you with these small plastic wands that help get you between the teeth in the most effective way. While you're at it, ask for a free flossing demonstration from the hygienist while you're there. They're glad to do it, because it saves them from scraping off all the extra plaque that builds up if you don't floss or if you floss incorrectly. Flossing is the all-time greatest prevention tactic for gum disease, so commit yourself to this humble task at least once a day, and you'll definitely have something to smile about in the years to come.

What if you can't brush after every meal? Try carrying a small travel toothbrush or child-size toothbrush with you. Otherwise, swish out your mouth vigorously with water to loosen food particles and dilute the acids formed by sugary foods.

Beware of the "cling-ons." These are the sticky foods that cling to your teeth the most tenaciously and cause the most enamel damage. Raisins, crackers, bread, and sugary snacks are at the top of the list. Acids formed from sugar-fed bacteria park themselves on the tooth enamel and very slowly leech the calcium ions out of the enamel. When these tiny holes dissolve the enamel and work their way to the soft inner dentin of the tooth, a cavity is born. So either be prepared to brush right after eating or try to avoid sticky snacks in the first place. This strategy may do wonders for your tooth enamel *and* your waistline.

Feed your teeth and gums. Strong bones and teeth depend upon an adequate calcium and other mineral intake. Caffeine, the phosphorous in soda drinks, and a high-protein diet containing lots of red meat will all help to leach calcium out of your system. Turn to Chapter 13 for a list of some high calcium foods and the most absorbable forms of supplements for strong bones and teeth. Magnesium and zinc are two other mineral standouts for dental health: Zinc because it helps the body fight the inflammation of gum disease and magnesium because it is a component of bones.

Vitamin C and bioflavinoids help boost the body's immune system in the prevention of gingivitis and pyorrhea, or end-stage gum disease. Remember the scurvy-ridden sailors who finally made it to the shores of North America? To cure this vitamin C deficiency disease, the experienced Native American people made them a medicine from pine trees, high in vitamin C. Incidentally, *pycnogenol,* the latest in a series of powerful antioxidants, is extracted from pine trees, so what's old becomes new again.

This doesn't meant that you have to save your Christmas tree this year and start gnawing on the bark while you're watching television, but do eat your grains, fresh fruits, and veggies. Chewing on the fresh foods provides valuable stimulation for the teeth and gums and adds vitamins C and A, minerals, and bioflavinoids to your diet—all important for your dental well-being.

Don't smoke. Aside from turning your teeth yellow and causing beastly bad breath, smoking suppresses the immune system and creates twice the risk of gum disease.

For a Really Bright Smile

If you've noticed that your teeth aren't as white as they used to be, you're probably right. Over the years, teeth absorb minerals from food and water and as a result, lose their pristine white color. The good news is that the mineralization process helps teeth become stronger. Teeth can also yellow over the decades due to stains from coffee, tea, wine, tobacco, and some food additives. Minute cracks in the enamel allow the various dyes from food and drink to be absorbed. Have you ever observed the effect of red wine on a white porcelain kitchen sink? If the sink has been scratched up by abrasive cleaners, that stain will be hard to remove. The same goes for your teeth if they have been scrubbed up by abrasive dental products.

An emerging branch of dentistry is cosmetic dentistry. Dentists now have bleaching agents that can be applied either at home or in the dentist's office. The at home version involves wearing a custom mold of your teeth filled with a bleaching gel. You wear this for a few hours a day or overnight for a couple of weeks. The in-office procedure takes up to ten minutes and the dentist may use a strong peroxide that is activated by high-intensity ultra violet or laser light.

If you are thinking about bleaching your teeth, be careful of the drugstore products. They can be very abrasive. You need your teeth to last for the rest of your life, so leave it to the professionals.

"The Name Is Bond . . . "

No, not James Bond, 007, porcelain bonds. This is truly dental improvement for sissies. Ultrathin porcelain veneers can usually be applied without anesthetic. The bonding is achieved by way of a resin and high-intensity light that fuses the porcelain and resin to the tooth. Because of the variety of shades and the skillful contouring of the veneer, a bonded tooth can be indistinguishable from a natural one. Bonding can cover bad stains, cracks, chips, and even teeth with uneven spacing. They can last ten years to a lifetime.

PERMANENT DENTURES

Losing enough teeth so that dentures are required extracts a physical and emotional toll. Something as simple as smiling can be upsetting when dentures slip and eating, though still necessary, is no longer enjoyed. In the 1950s, before dental advancements, dentures were the only alternative for those who could not afford extensive dental work. It was simply cheaper to remove all the teeth and submit the patient to a life of taking his or her teeth out at night to soak in a glass of cleaning solution until the morning.

"When I lost my upper teeth, I was still in my thirties," Liz told me. "I instantly felt like my grandmother at night, and the emotional pain of losing your teeth is every bit as bad as the physical pain of having them pulled out. I stopped smiling for years, or covered my mouth with my hand when I was speaking. I never felt attractive after that. I stopped wearing lipstick because I didn't want to draw attention to my mouth."

Today, however, people like Liz have options. The dental implant process begins when tiny metal posts are surgically placed into the jaw where teeth once grew. It's done under local anesthesia. Then, after a period of time (about six months) bone actually grows around the titanium posts and they become part of the jaw. When the posts are solidly in place, a new artificial tooth is built over it. Then it's good-bye dentures.

A team of professionals may be involved with a patient's dental implants. Technically, they are named root-form implants and the skills of an oral or maxillary surgeon, a prosthodontist, a general dentist, and a team of dental laboratory technicians may all work together to produce the maximum result for the patient. Implants were first done in Sweden, almost forty years ago, but are newer to American patients.

"This has changed my life," said Liz, after the implants freed her from the false teeth she'd had since she was a young woman. "My confidence is way up—I enjoy things that make me feel young again, like kissing my husband, or laughing, or eating a piece of fruit without having to cut it up into little pieces."

It's expensive—each post usually costs around $1,000, but they last twenty years or more and, for many, they are a blessing of much greater value.

HOW OLD IS TOO OLD FOR BRACES?

Braces used to be strictly for kids, but now a lot of folks are opting to finally get their teeth straightened. Maybe your family simply couldn't afford them when you were a teenager, or perhaps you didn't want the "tinsel mouth" look.

Newer methods of straightening the teeth involve gentle, tiny braces instead of the big steel straps you may remember from your childhood. You can even have clear, ceramic braces and color coordinated elastics instead of the traditional wires. The colors can be mixed and matched to appease even the most strident fashion drives.

Correction for crooked teeth, spaces, and overbite can also be achieved through removable retainers worn at night. This is called braceless orthodontics, and is very popular in Europe.

And how old is too old for braces? Some dentists have reported treating patients in their eighties.

THE POWER SMILE

The power smile can be yours for the rest of your life if you follow the basics of brushing, flossing, and regular dental hygiene visits. Avoiding the blood sports of kick boxing, competitive karate, nail biting, and teeth gnashing are other obvious ways to hold on to your smile and keep your teeth from wearing out.

In a few years, xylitol chewing gum may be widely available in America to help prevent tooth decay. It's available in Europe now. As you read this, scientists are staying up late in the lab to perfect the cloning of tooth enamel. A similar technique is already being used to clone cartilage and then repair damaged knees and shoulders. And researchers are getting closer to inventing a "smart bomb" for cavity-causing bacteria that will stop cavities before they can even start.

In the meantime, keep smiling.

RESOURCE

The American Society for Dental Aesthetics is a peer-reviewed association that will provide a list of recommended dentists for cosmetic dentistry. Their address is 635 Madison Avenue, New York, N.Y. 10022.

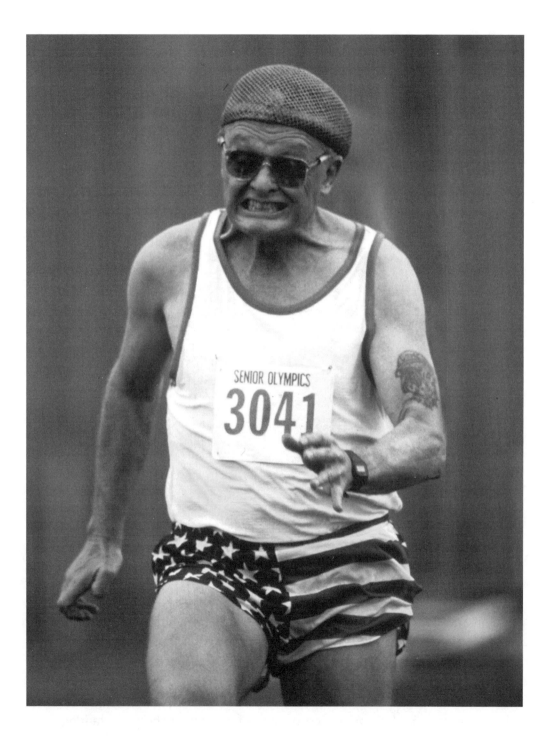

19

ASSORTED PARTS:
KEEPING YOUR VITALS VITAL

Have you ever heard of the Sugarplum Tree
'Tis a marvel of great renown!
It blooms on the shore of the Lollipop Sea
In the garden of Shuteye Town.

—Eugene Field (1850–1895), "The Sugarplum Tree"

For that elephant ate all night,
And that elephant ate all day;
Do what he could to furnish him food,
The cry was still for more hay.

—John Cheever Goodwin (1850–1912),
Wang: The Man with an Elephant on His Hands

GALL BLADDER

I have a number of patients who have had gall bladder surgery but when I go through their health history they forget that they've had any surgeries at all. When I point out the unmistakable broad scar or possible puncture wounds on the abdomen, it results in an, "Oh yes, that's right, I *did* have my gall bladder removed a few years ago." The next question always shakes me up a little, "Hey Doc, what's your gall bladder for anyway, was that something I really needed, or what?"

It shakes me up because it seems hard to believe that you could go through the pain and expense of a surgery without asking why the part in question is going to be permanently removed. So let's briefly go over the function of the gall bladder, and then how you could make better choices to avoid surgery. Because you know that bumper sticker *"Just one surgery could ruin your whole day"* actually has a lot to it.

What Is Your Gall Bladder For?

The gall bladder is a pear-shaped sac underneath the right side of the liver. Its whole purpose and meaning in life is to hold and store acid-rich bile that is made in the liver. Every day, about 500 to 600 milliliters of bile is secreted via ducts into the small intestine, where it helps to digest fats.

The most frequent gall bladder problem is an inflammation and swelling that results from bile backing up from gallstones. Most gallstones are of crystallized cholesterol, with bile acids and bilirubin—all products manufactured in the liver. Gallstones may form and stay in the gall bladder, causing no symptoms unless one of the stones slips into the common bile duct.

Risk Factors for Gallstones

There's a mnemonic that is often recited in lectures regarding likely candidates for gall bladder stones: fat, female, forty, and flatulent. However, other important risk factors for cholesterol stones are gaining or losing weight rapidly, ethnicity (Pima Indians and Scandinavian peoples seem especially susceptible), certain prescription drugs such as clofibrate (a blood pressure medication), estrogens, anticholesterol drugs, and some diseases of the gastrointestinal tract. Additionally, there are pigmented gallstones that contain calcium salts and risk factors for these are low body weight, Far Eastern ethnicity, a diet insufficient in fat or protein, liver cirrhosis, sickle cell anemia, and infections.

A nonsurgical treatment is increasingly available for both cholesterol and the unpigmented gallstones. Extracorporeal shock-wave biliary lithotripsy (ESBT) is the $50 word for a treatment that involves beaming ultrasound waves at the large stones to fragment them. Oral drug treatments area also used to dissolve the stones. Interestingly enough, lecithin, which is actually a component of bile, is also used to dissolve gallstones.

How to Avoid Gallstones

Everyone needs a hobby, but if growing gallstones is one you'd like to avoid, here's how.

Fill up on fiber, not fat. That means eating more veggies, grain, and fruit and less animal-origin foods. Populations that eat the undesirable high-fat, low-fiber diets are penalized with the highest rates of gall bladder disease.

Go lightly. A study in the *New England Journal of Medicine* that followed 89,000 women for four years found that every surgery for gall bladder removal was on a woman who was overweight.

Eat early and eat often. This is not an endorsement for making the whole day into one big mealtime. However, according to a report in the *American Journal of Public Health*, those who wait sixteen hours or more between meals increased the amounts of cholesterol (and the risk factor for disease) in the gall bladder up to twelve times more. Eat small, frequent meals of plant origin (vegetables, fruits, and whole grains) throughout the day and don't skip meals.

Avoid coffee. My first patient of the day one Monday morning came early, finished off an extra large espresso in the waiting room, and the next thing we knew, he was doubled over on the floor writhing in pain, clutching his stomach. He'd had the extra strong coffee to wash down the caffe latte he'd had earlier for breakfast. It was a classic gall bladder attack, triggered by coffee. Needless to say, the patient swore off coffee after that. Most folks who have gallstones have no symptoms. The pain experienced by my patient occurred when a stone blocked one of the bile ducts.

Feed your gall bladder, starve the stones. Lecithin helps reduce cholesterol levels and is found in the food sources of wheat germ and brewer's yeast. The B-complex of vitamins work with the body to help it produce lecithin on its own as well as stimulating the gall bladder to void. Phosphatidlycholine, the dietary form of lecithin, is also used sometimes to help the body prevent gallstones. Some researchers believe that vitamins A, the B-complex, and E may help dissolve stones. Because choline (of phosphatidylcholine) is synthesized in the body by an interaction of folic acid, cobalamine (vitamin B12), and the amino acid methionine, the B vitamins are commonly taken together in a complex form. Some researchers estimate that the average diet supplies about 400 to 900 milligrams of choline per day. Therapeutic dosages range from half a gram to several grams. *Note*: Consult a doctor experienced in nutrition to adjust the amounts for your age, size, weight, height, physical condition, and need.

HOW DO YOU LIVE WITHOUT A GALL BLADDER?

HOW DO YOU LIVE WITHOUT A GALL BLADDER?

This is a frequently asked question. Without a gall bladder, bile produced by the liver is stored in the large common duct that connects the liver and the small intestine. The body is curiously and wonderfully adaptive in this scenario, because the tube stretches to perform its new job and ends up functioning like the gall bladder that was surgically removed!!

However, avoiding the pain and expense of surgery seems like a better scenario, don't you think?

KEEPING YOUR PANCREAS HEALTHY

The Islets of Langherans: This sounds like an idyllic vacation spot somewhere in the British Isles. Actually, these hormone-producing tissues in the pancreas are home to 1 million microscopic beta cells, which are responsible for making insulin. Although beta cells weigh in at only about one to one and a half grams, when they malfunction, the result can be diabetes mellitus. Diabetes, among the top ten causes of death in Western nations, is a devastating disease that affects over 13 million Americans.

Every system of the body is affected. Diabetes doubles the chance of stroke; increases the odds of kidney failure; causes impotence, blindness, and nerve sensation loss in the arms and legs; and is responsible for more than 54,000 feet or leg amputations each year, according to the American Diabetes Association. Ten percent of diabetics develop kidney disease and between 15,000 and 39,000 people with diabetes become blind every year. And yet, diabetes and its after effects are partly preventable.

SYMPTOMS OF DIABETES

On a regular basis, have you experienced:
- Excessive thirst?
- Frequent urination?
- Extreme fatigue?
- Unexplained loss of sensation in arms and legs?
- Blurry vision?

Diabetes Can Be Avoided

Glucose, a fuel for our cells, is extracted by the body from the food we eat. The glucose is then moved from the food into the cells thanks to the magic of insulin. When we don't have insulin, glucose can't enter the cells, so it backs up into the bloodstream. Damage results.

Diabetes is actually the plural name for two different scenarios involving insulin problems in the body. Ten percent of diabetics are Type I, which usually develops during childhood. The beta cells produce no insulin and so the young diabetic must get injections every day. There is no known way to prevent this more serious form of diabetes.

The more common kind of diabetes is called Type II. This form, which accounts for over 90 percent of all diabetics, is often called adult-onset diabetes because it often occurs after the age of forty. Two major insulin defects are responsible: (1) a failure of the body to produce sufficient insulin relative to the glucose load, and (2) an inability of the body cells to respond to insulin and thereby allow glucose to enter them. This is called *insulin resistance*. In either scenario, the result is the same: Glucose backs up into the blood stream. Biomolecular havoc ensues.

In Type II diabetes, the symptoms can sneak up slowly. Genetics, overeating, and obesity play important roles, and increasing age is known to be correlated to increasing frequency of the disease.

The bright side of this equation is that much **diabetes can be prevented. Even after it has been diagnosed, diet and exercise can mostly overcome it.**

RISK FACTORS FOR TYPE II DIABETES:

- Over age thirty (risk increases with age)
- More than 20 percent over your ideal weight
- Being female, with more than one baby weighing over nine pounds at birth
- Native American, Hispanic, or African American descent (all groups have high rates of diabetes)
- Having a parent or sibling with diabetes (it tends to run in families)

Note: If you have any combination of symptoms and risk factors, see your doctor immediately.

HOW TO PREVENT DIABETES

Eat plenty of fiber in the form of fruits and vegetables, whole grains, and potatoes. Eat three healthy meals a day and two or three snacks of pears, apples, berries, beans, and whole-grains and slow-cooking oatmeal. Lose weight by exercising more. Eat less fat and lift weights.

Nothing new here. It's the ideal eating and exercising plan that everyone can thrive on. Nathan Pritikin proved this at his famous Longevity Center in Santa Monica, California, where thousands of people have overcome the need for insulin by combining a very low-fat, high-fiber diet and plenty of exercise. Fifty percent of those on insulin when they get to the center no longer need injections by the time they leave.

PREVENTING DIABETES

Cut the sugar, eat some fiber. In a study by the Harvard Medical School of 65,000 nurses ages forty to sixty years, women who ate the most sugar and the least fiber were two and a half times more likely to develop diabetes than those on a healthy diet. *Cut the fat.* For every extra forty grams of fat you eat every day, you increase your risk of contracting Type II diabetes three times.

Chromium. A daily 200 micrograms of chromium, a trace mineral, has been demonstrated to prevent mild glucose intolerance from becoming Type II diabetes. Most Americans get an estimated thirty micrograms of this nutrient each day.

Be nutty, go bananas, be a bean-counter, and take a veggie to lunch. Nuts, whole grains, legumes, and green vegetables are all high in magnesium. The *American Journal of Clinical Nutrition* reports that extra magnesium helps regulate blood chemistry and glucose processing in the body.

Ask your doctor about vanadyl sulfate. Preliminary research on this trace mineral has been very encouraging. Ask your doctor for an update. You can also check out new studies published on the Internet, if you are connected to Medline.

Get in some heavy breathing. For every 500 calories you burn in a given week, you cut your risk of Type II diabetes by 6 percent. So says researcher Dr. Susan P. Helmrich, University of California, Berkeley, who came to this conclusion after following 5,990 men for fourteen years. Five hundred calories' worth of exercise is one hour and a half of brisk walking, over an hour bicycling, an hour of swimming, and just over fifty minutes of jogging. (To find out more about food and the amount of exercise it takes to work it off, turn to Chapter 10's Exercise Chart for Cheaters.)

Pump those muscles up. The bigger your muscles, the more your body uses up the glucose in your bloodstream. This equation reminds me of those phony ads for weight loss: "Lose weight while you sleep." But it happens to be true when it comes to your muscles. Resistance weight training speeds up your metabolism, so you really do burn more calories, even when you sleep.

THE DIGESTIVE SYSTEM

Heartburn, gas, bloating, and the ill-behaved "rumblies in the tummy." I once heard a great explanation of why all of the above happens from a six-year-old patient. The theory was that certain foods like radishes, raw onions, and the like may look perfectly innocent when they are just laying there on your plate. But these foods are afraid of the dark. As soon as you swallow them they will do whatever is necessary to make their fear known, and until they can get out, they will let you know about it. They'll send you reaching for your favorite heartburn remedy in an instant.

For some strange reason, I have never been able to substantiate that point of view with a research paper on the special psychiatric leanings of any food in general, let alone the examples mentioned. However, the world of research is coming up with new theories, even as you read these words, so who is to say that this particular six-year-old was wrong?

All kidding aside though, because indigestion can mimic many serious health problems, like cancer of the stomach or colon, inflammatory bowel disease, ulcerative colitis, and a host of others, **you need to see your doctor about persistent digestive difficulties.** Bleeding with a bowel movement; black, tarry stools; abdominal cramping and pain; fever with any of the above; unexplained weight loss; or rectal itching or bleeding are all symptoms that need to be taken seriously.

The following are some tips for healthy living for your consideration, *after* you get your check-up:

Prevent constipation and deal with diverticular disease. Diverticulosis is a disease of civilization that can be avoided. Decades of low fiber and junk food can weaken the thin tissue walls of the colon and cause weakened pouches to develop. Food can get stuck in those pouches and cause a lot of pain. Most people diagnosed with this disease are over forty—decades of straining to pass hard, dried-up stools from a low-fiber diet have weakened the colon walls. Major gas and cramps, and even alternating constipation or diarrhea can result. It doesn't have to happen. Here are three important ways to prevent constipation:

1. Drink plenty of water. This doesn't mean tea, coffee, or cola drinks, all of which act as diuretics and can actually dehydrate you. Eight to ten big glasses per day of pure water is the minimum. Water helps maintain regularity by keeping stools soft, which speeds the time it takes for food to go through your system.

2. Eat lots of fiber. Roughage helps speed transit time. Most Americans barely get half of the recommended twenty-five grams per day. At least five servings per day of fresh fruits and vegetables is the ideal.

3. Huff and puff a little. Exercise also helps speed transit time of food in the intestinal tract. It improves blood supply to the intestines, helps tone and contract the abdominal muscles, and may activate intestinal hormones that also speed food along its way.

Eat less. You'll not only trim some fat from your tummy, but you will reduce the overload on your stomach. Overeating at any one meal causes the stomach to produce a lot of acid in order to digest the load. Instead, eat smaller portions, and eat more frequently throughout the day.

Don't eat a big meal right before bedtime. Remember the rule about swimming right after you ate? Same rule applies about eating before bedtime, but for a different reason. If you eat a big meal and then lie down flat in bed, you may be encouraging heartburn. Instead, limit your food intake at least two hours before bedtime, which will help prevent reflux of stomach acids back up into the esophagus.

Not milk? An estimated 70 percent of the people in the world are lactose intolerant. Their bodies do not produce the enzyme lactase, which helps us digest lactose, a sugar in milk. Milk sugar passes through their digestive tracts undigested, acting like a free lunch for bacteria. The resulting fermentation process causes gas, bloating, and pain. Additionally, some folks also experience colon spasms.

What to do? Don't drink milk. However, you may be able to eat yogurt, because the friendly bacteria in yogurt, labeled "active cultures" on the package, go into the intestine and break down the milk sugar. That's pretty cheap labor, by any standards. There are also lactose-free dairy products in supermarkets—check the labels.

If you're still determined to drink milk there are also lactase tablets on the market that you can buy at supermarkets and drugstores without a prescription.

Can the coffee. Tea and cola drinks have caffeine in them too. Caffeine is known to speed up the pace of food in the digestive tract, but may also cause abdominal cramping.

Forget the fat. Ice cream, cheesecake, french fries, and many meats are high in fat. Fat can really take a long time to digest, so it stays around in your stomach a long time, and gas and bloating can result. Ask yourself this: Would you eat a steak that was left out on the sidewalk for twelve hours on a hot summer's day with temperatures in the high nineties? Red meat can take up to forty-eight hours to digest, and your body temperature is 98.6 degrees Fahrenheit. That's a lot of fermentation. What would steak left out in a summer heat wave smell like after a couple days at that temperature? You've got the picture.

Don't smoke. Smoking adds nicotine to the body, which restricts blood supply. Abdominal cramps can be the result. Yet another reason to quit.

Ulcers. Up until very recently, the patient was simply put on a bland diet. It is now known that most ulcers are caused by a pesky bacteria called *Helicobacter pylori.* A brief course of antibiotics results in a permanent cure.

KIDNEY AND BLADDER HEALTH PRIMER

Even though movie stars tout adult protective undergarments on prime time television, incontinence is still one of the best kept secrets around. Regardless of how upbeat those advertisements are, nobody looks forward to wearing adult diapers for the rest of their life. Incontinence is associated with aging and becoming dependent, and fear and pride may keep people from seeking help for a problem that is controllable the majority of the time.

Often incontinence can be caused by prescription or over-the-counter medications. Dietary factors are common, including alcohol and overindulging on food to the point of being overweight. And, yes, for those who "negotiate" the times when they will actually take time to empty their bowels or bladders, incontinence can be the unwanted result of delaying trips to the bathroom by damaging the bladder muscles. Childbirth and fluctuations in hormone production can also affect the bladder muscles.

Of the many kinds of incontinence, however, the two most common are *urge incontinence,* an inability to control when you urinate, caused by infections or inflammation of the bladder muscles, and *stress incontinence,* in which urine "leaks" when you cough or sneeze, most often caused by weak pelvic floor muscles.

HOW TO AVOID VOIDING PROBLEMS

The word *void* comes from the old French word *voider*, which means to empty. If you have any problems regarding this, or any other health problem, you must see your doctor. Incontinence may be a sign of serious urinary tract problems such as infection or diabetes, so it's important to get it checked out. Spinal cord injuries, multiple sclerosis, and other immune disorders may also cause incontinence. After you rule out anything else, the following are some simple ways to prevent and deal with incontinence.

When you have to go, then go! Isn't it better to momentarily excuse yourself from a situation rather than embarrass yourself later on? Mother Nature knows what she's doing when she gives you that first nature call. Listen. Most people can hold their urine in for three to four hours. Longer than that, and you're probably stretching your bladder beyond its limit. Continued practices of withholding could lead to long-term problems.

Curb constipation. A full bowel can exert pressure on the bladder. Ditto for straining to eliminate dry, hard stools. Drink eight to ten glasses of pure water per day and eat at least five servings of fruits and vegetables to ensure that you get enough fiber in your diet.

Is it a prescription for your good health? There are many drugs, both over-the-counter and prescriptive, that could set the stage for incontinence. Your doctor is a good source of information here. Additionally, I find that most pharmacists are very helpful in explaining drug interactions and possible side effects. If you are the self-sufficient sleuth, delve into that drug insert—you know, the one written on tissue paper that is usually the first thing you put in the "round file" when you get home from the drugstore. Antihistamines, cold medicines, diuretics, seasickness medications, sedatives, and parasympathetic nervous system drugs called anticholinergic are all suspects.

Have a drink of water. Chronic alcohol abuse can lead to overflow and stress incontinence. Likewise many of the other diuretic and stimulatory beverages such as coffee, tea, and sodas. Some patients have told me that simply cutting out their bedtime cocoa is helpful. When you're thirsty have some water. It has no calories, and you save money too. A new way to get thin and rich.

Relieve some of the pressure. Extra weight around the abdomen can add pressure to the bladder. If you've ever squeezed into your "thin" blue jeans and then gone out to dinner, you know what we're talking about here. That extra five pounds (which is usually about eight or nine pounds to be very honest) is enough to really put some pressure on. Try trimming a little from your exterior architecture, and you may be helping yourself out in the plumbing department.

Quit smoking. This one seems to come up during the discussion of every body system. In this case, some experts believe that the excessive coughing that smokers experience may weaken the pelvic muscles and lead to stress incontinence.

Muscle in on the problem. Kegel exercises to the rescue. Not only do these exercises strengthen the muscles of the pelvic floor, many Kegel exercise enthusiasts say that they improve their sex lives. To do the Kegels, try to stop the flow of urine when you are urinating. Squeeze the muscles and hold for a count of five and then relax and let the urine flow for a count of five. That's the sensation you're after. When you've got the hang of that, you will be able to control the start and stop of urination.

It's hard to tell at first, but you'll quickly get better and better at the exercises. You can hold for five seconds at first, then build up to twenty or thirty seconds of holding. As you get better, also try tightening the rectal muscles, as if you are trying not to pass gas. Most people urinate at least five or six times a day, so that will give you plenty of practice to start. Once you can identify the muscles, then you can practice at any time: while waiting for traffic lights, while you're in line at the supermarket, or any time you're put on hold while on the telephone.

The best thing to do is practice early and practice often. Kegel exercises have better than a 60 percent cure rate with incontinence. Ask your doctor for more information.

When Cystitis Strikes

I have had patients come into the office because they have lower back pain, complaining "I think I threw something out over the weekend." But the accompanying fever, abdominal pain, and urinary symptoms help clinch the diagnosis: cystitis. Few patients who have cystitis ever forget the symptoms—there's burning and pain on urination and the feeling that they have to go all the time even when there's nothing there but a trickle. Some people notice blood in the urine or a strong odor.

Women tend to get cystitis, a bacterial infection of the bladder and urinary tract, more often than men. This is because the female urethra that carries urine out of the bladder is only about two inches long. That makes it an easy trip for bacteria from the vagina and rectum to the bladder. Once the microorganisms get to the bladder, antibiotics can be prescribed, but the best way to treat cystitis is to avoid it. Don't delay getting treatment if you have any of the symptoms listed above, because a urinary tract infection (UTI) can travel all the way up to the kidneys and cause some nasty problems.

Drink early and drink often. Water helps to keep urine plentiful and dilute nutrients, foiling the bacteria who love to thrive on scanty, concentrated urine.

Consider cranberry. Cranberry juice is an age-old cure with modern research to back it up. At Harvard Medical School, scientists found that those who drank cranberry juice regularly had a 42 percent lower incidence of UTIs than those who didn't. Ten ounces a day was the amount of juice consumed. However, read your labels carefully. Many popular cranberry drinks have a tremendous amount of sugar in them. Bacteria love sugar. Fresh cranberry sauce prepared with a minimum of sweeteners, and even cranberry powder or capsules may be alternatives to sweetened beverages.

Wipe from the front to the back. Most experts agree on this bathroom technique. The reason? It helps keep E. coli bacteria from the rectum away from the vagina and urethra. Washing the rectum after bowel movements may not only help prevent UTIs, but might decrease the incidence of colon cancer.

Urinate after sex. This helps flush out bacteria that may be pushed up into the urethra during intercourse. Some patients have reported to me that urinating immediately after using the hot tub or swimming pool has reduced the rate of infections as well.

Ask your doctor about alternative contraception. Diaphragms and barrier contraceptives with spermicide are linked to proliferations of the E. coli bacteria that cause UTIs.

20 BREATHING EASY

A thing of beauty is a joy forever:
Its loveliness increases; it will never
Pass into nothingness; but still will keep
A bower of quiet for us, and a sleep
Full of sweet dreams, and health, and quiet breathing.

—John Keats, 1795–1821

*O*ne of the special privileges of sailing off the coast of Southern California under the power of a strong northwest wind is that you are breathing sea air that has not touched land for thousands of miles. That's fresh. When I inhale that oxygen-rich air deep into my lungs, I think of it nourishing every cell in my body. It is sweet medicine. I picture how wonderful it is to stand on the bow and experience the ocean breeze whenever I'm stuck on the freeway and the famous Los Angeles smog is burning my eyes.

Your lungs were built to last a lifetime. They weigh about twelve to fourteen ounces each, with the left lung slightly smaller than the right because of the placement of the heart on the left side. For years, exercise physiologists agreed that diminishing lung capacity with aging was a given, and concentrated their efforts on measuring the amount of decline with each passing decade.

However, new research has many of the same scientists scratching their heads. Guess what? It seems that regular cardiovascular exercise throughout a lifetime can keep the lungs vital, strong, and functioning with minimal loss of capacity. This should have exercise enthusiasts breathing a lot easier. For those who have never been accused of athletic overachievement, starting today, if you do some cardiovascular exercise, you could still increase your lung power.

Normal lung tissue is pink and elastic and stretched out. Pollution, smoke, bacteria, viruses, and other impurities in the air all give the lungs a beating and cause lung tissue to contract. Sadly, in this day and age of cigarette smoking and polluted cities, chronic bronchitis and emphysema are becoming rampant, affecting large segments of our population.

HOW TO KEEP BREATHING EASY

Don't smoke and avoid the smoke of others. Smoking is the number-one avoidable cause of death in our times. Lung cancer is now the number-one cancer killer of both men and women. And secondhand smoke contains fifty times more ammonia, five times more carbon monoxide, and twice as much tar as what the smoker inhales.

Nicotine is physiologically addictive to the body, whether it is smoked or chewed. Whatever it takes to quit, why not make this the year you do it? The American Can-

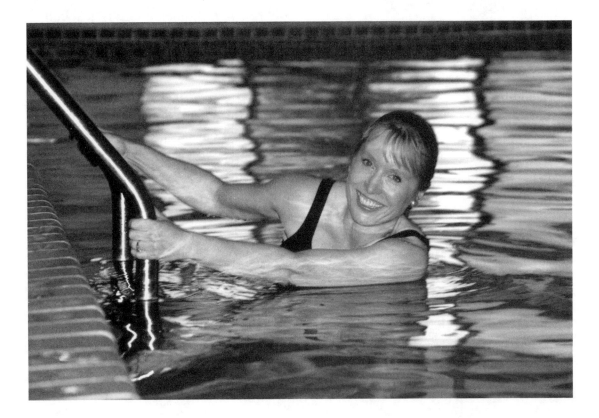

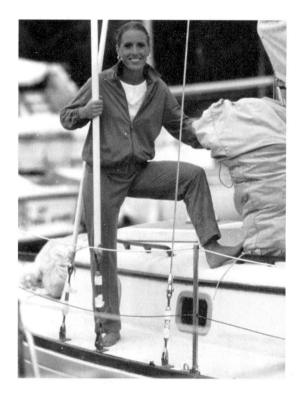

cer Society and the American Lung Association both have nonsmoking information with tips and support groups you can join.

Food will taste better, you will feel better about yourself, and you will be healthier and live longer. Smoking affects every system of your body, from the discs that absorb shock in your vertebrae to the tiny capillaries that nourish your skin. Most of all, you will have pride in yourself for overcoming something that has a negative effect on almost every cell in your body.

Practice deep breathing to de-stress. The old time strong men and physical culturists throughout history practiced deep breathing exercises as a source of youthful energy.

1. Lie comfortably on your back on the floor, knees bent, with a small towel rolled up under your neck. Imagine yourself to be in a warm, safe, relaxing place, anywhere you would like to be—perhaps it's by the ocean, floating in a tiny pond in little wooden boat, or on a cloud. Wherever it is, make it a favorite, cozy place that feels inviting and relaxing to you.
2. Clasp your hands loosely over your abdomen.
3. Inhale slowly and effortlessly, pushing your abdomen out as you inhale. Feel the air feeling up your lungs, filling up your whole body like a breath of life.
4. Hold your breath for a slow count of three.
5. Exhale slowly through your nose.
6. Repeat the whole sequence again three times.

Monitor your breathing throughout the day. I have noticed people in a variety of professions who do work that requires so much concentration *that they actually forget to breathe.* It may sound incredible, but it is true. Surgeons, dentists, computer workers, writers, crafts people—they often are so engrossed in their work that they hold their breath. I have had several patients complain to me of shortness of breath. On close questioning, and on observation of them at work, I have seen them actually breathe in a more and more shallow fashion until they go without taking in another breath for up to thirty seconds at a time. Presumably, the body carbon dioxide sensors kick in about that time, which can have them gasping for a new breath and noticing heart arrhythmias along with the whole process.

Monitor yourself. Be aware of how you are breathing. To relax and de-stress, simply try to focus on your breathing for several minutes while you are comfortably seated. Repeat whenever you feel the need for a "mini-vacation" at your desk. One of the reasons smoking is relaxing for people is that a smoker takes a deep breath while inhaling. Read over the deep breathing exercises above—perhaps you could try them instead of reaching for a cigarette.

Do some huff and puff exercise. There are muscles that operate the rib cage, and if you don't use them, they weaken, lose flexibility, and stiffen up. The key to keeping elasticity in the rib cage is to keep using it. That means huff and puff exercise that will expand the rib cage and lungs and allow the muscles in between the ribs to contract. Have you ever seen how thick the meat is on a spare rib? That is the same muscle that is in between your ribs. In my experience with patients, those who have exercised vigorously throughout their lives have wide-spread rib cages that are resilient and expandable. Those who have led sedentary lives have ribs that are narrowly spaced and rigid. These folks also have a thorax that is capable of expanding very little, even when the biggest breath is inhaled.

The minimum for a healthy lung oxygen workout is thirty minutes of an activity, such as brisk walking, five times a week. Turn to Chapter 10 to get the skinny on how to keep your lungs operating at maximum capacity. Be sure to check with your doctor first for health clearance to start an exercise program.

Humidify to defy the bugs. The lungs can boast of over 600 square feet of surface area. That's because of all their spongy surfaces. Cilia are the bronchial fine hairs that move like fields of grain to help keep bacteria, dust, dirt, viruses, smoke, and other irritants out of the lungs. Mucous, nasal hairs, and specialized lymph cells called macrophages and dust cells do the rest of the work.

During winter months when central heating dries out the air, a humidifier can do wonders to help keep your lungs and all their helpers in top fighting form.

When you have a drink, your cilia can get drunk. Those tiny bronchial hairs that help sweep out your respiratory tree can be impaired workers under the influence after two drinks. It's a little known piece of anatomical trivia, but they just don't seem to be able to stand up and do the job under the influence of alcohol. That can give "the bad guys" of dirt, dust, pollution, bacteria, viruses, and other irritants a foot in the door and give your lungs an unwelcome disadvantage.

Get tested for TB. Tuberculosis (TB) had been declining for decades, but it's back with a vengeance. The reason? AIDS victims, the homeless, and newcomers to America from other countries are all causes of the rapid increase in tuberculosis. Additionally, new drug-resistant strains of the disease have surfaced because many patients in low-income areas start on medication with good intentions, then fall out of the system or stop the drugs once they start feeling better. The drugs are generally taken two or three times a day with meals. However, homeless or low-income individuals may only eat one meal a day, so the therapeutic dose is not maintained and the bacteria become resistant to it.

TB is spread by simple breathing. The bacteria are transferred from person to person through inhalation into the lungs. If you think that you have been exposed to TB, then contact your doctor. Many people who are carriers of the disease do not have the classic TB cough or weight loss and exhaustion that characterized the disease in the 1940s. A chest X-ray or a quick skin test can determine if you have TB.

Foil the dust mites. The excrement produced by these microscopic critters who love to live in your mattresses, pillows, comforters, and teddy bears can cause waking headaches from allergic reactions, as well as chronically stuffy sinuses. For pillows and teddy bears and comforters, try putting them in the dryer for thirty to forty minutes on a high setting. You can buy mattress covers that prevent them from escaping and HEPA filters for your vacuum cleaner to roust them from the carpet without blowing them all around the house.

21

HOW OLD IS TOO OLD TO HAVE A BABY?

While with an eye made quiet by the power
Of harmony, and the deep power of joy,
We see into the life of things.

—William Wordsworth (1770–1850)

$\mathcal{F}$or Tiffany, it seemed to happen imperceptibly. While she was taking a business flight from L.A. to New York for her ad agency, an infant started screaming two aisles up. Barely missing a beat, she winced and cast a frowning glance toward the harassed mother, reached into her briefcase, pulled out a pair of earplugs, and continued pounding out her report on the laptop. The next day, before meeting her clients for lunch at the Russian Tea Room, she was negotiating her way through a gaggle of four-year-olds when one of the rambunctious little brats snagged her pantyhose with his backpack.

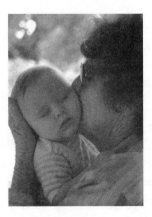

She was ready to fume, but when the child turned toward her with those big wide eyes, the tiny brow knit in remorse, and the tearful "I'm sorry" squeaked out so sorrowfully, Tiffany felt all her executive armor melt and crash to the ground. After all, she always carried an extra pair of stockings anyway. The funny thing was, she wasn't upset in the least— just mortified at having snapped at the poor kid. And then it hit her like a five ton megabomb. It was one of those "Eureka" moments, as they said at the agency when a big idea was about to hit: she wished that child was hers. She wanted that baby; she wanted to hold it and comfort it and wipe the tears from

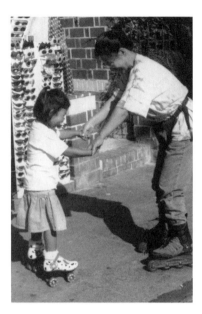

those chubby cheeks. She stood there until the doorman broke the spell: "Are you all right, Miss?"

She felt like she was in a daze for the rest of the day. In a gesture completely uncharacteristic of her usual professional persona, when a client mentioned the birth of his latest grandchild, she pressed him for photographs and *ooh*ed and *ahh*ed over them with the fervor of a religious convert. "You must have some little ones at home yourself!" chuckled the proud grandfather. "Why no—I mean, not yet," she stammered. Tiffany had a sinking elevator feeling in her stomach that made her ill at ease.

From then on, she felt the baby craving more and more. She was a successful nineties woman and, at forty years old, fulfilled and full of confidence and business savvy. Except when she strode through the airport and saw a child crying, except when she hailed a cab and caught the eye of a smiling infant in a stroller. "It's a craving that's hard to explain. When you see a baby, you wish that baby was yours. You see pregnant women walking in a mall or at the hairdresser, and you envy her. You walk by a toy store and *ooh* over all the cute little toys in the window. The bottom line is that you feel that craving and you can't explain it in a rational way—it's just there, and it tugs at you in that quiet, powerful way."

At this writing, Tiffany and her husband are deciding whether or not he will have his vasectomy reversed.

THE BIOLOGICAL CLOCK

It's a reminder that seems to get louder every year. "You're not getting any younger, you know," intone aunts, neighbors, your mother. For many women, the ticking of their biological clock is almost loud enough to drown out the well-meaning advice of relatives. But how old is too old to have a baby? These days, the answer is—much later than you think.

Not so long ago, Mother Nature held all the cards and was in complete control of who had a baby and when. A woman got pregnant, went to the hospital nine months later, and went home with a baby. If a couple couldn't conceive, and really wanted a family, they adopted. There were few other options available.

These days, there are many options. Revolutionary techniques are making headlines all over the world. Women are giving birth at age fifty, sixty, and even older. At sixty-one years old, an Italian woman gave birth in 1992. That was topped by a sixty-three-year-old American woman who recently gave birth. Grandmothers are bearing their own grandchildren via implantation and assisted hatching procedures. The first test tube baby was born in 1981 and people around the world reacted with a mixture of fear and surprise. Less than two decades later, children conceived in laboratory test tubes and petri dishes are born every day and nobody gives it a second thought. Yet when a sheep was cloned, the world reeled with fear and wonderment once again. The president of the United States held a nationwide press conference asking for a moratorium on human cloning experiments. As the old saying goes—the only surprise is that you can still be surprised.

OLDER MOMS AND DADS

A friend of mine, a retired professional tennis champion, married at age thirty-eight, had her first child just before she turned forty. "I used to take such a dim view of clients who were late for their lessons with yet another excuse about their kids, or the babysitter, or the carpool. Now that I've got a baby, I think it's amazing that they got there at all. It takes so long to get organized just to get out the door. It feels like two hours of preparation even to go to the supermarket, by the time you pack in the stroller, the diaper bag, the car seat, and all the rest of the paraphernalia. I have total sympathy for any parent who manages to get anything in their day that's not kid-related. My house is no longer spotless, there are teething biscuits all over the carpet, and I'm so totally exhausted that I don't even care. When I got tired of trying to fit the car seat in my sports car, I got rid of it and bought a truck. And I wouldn't trade any of it in for the whole world."

Parenthood can mellow even the most driven people. But what's the real scoop on older moms and dads? Are they better or worse as parents? Critics of older parents are quick to point out that bringing a child into the world when you are in your fifties is selfish when you consider that you may not be around to see the child into adulthood. Yet older parents who are more established in their careers may be able to give the child a more privileged life of better preschool, tutors, educational experiences of travel and college without the burden of student loans—even if the child ultimately graduates college without their parents at the ceremony.

Most older parents don't have children by accident, and after full lives of diverse business and personal experiences and the intense emotional and financial energy that they put into being parents in the first place, they may be less likely to complain that their lives are being put on hold because of parenthood.

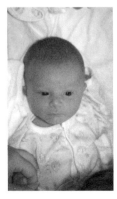 The prospect of having a baby can be a daunting one at any age, but psychologists studying older parents are finding them to be patient, caring, and devoted—simply older. From the bold new world of high-tech baby making, a recent report by a British team of psychologists states that the quality of parenting in families with a child conceived through in vitro fertilization (IVF) or donor insemination (DI) exceeds that observed in well-functioning families with a naturally conceived child. Furthermore, adoptive parents also show higher quality skills, on a level with those parents who have medical technological assistance in conceiving, according to an article in *Child Development*. Researchers concluded, "The findings suggest that genetic ties are less important for family functioning than a strong desire for parenthood."

Down syndrome. This is one of the most common causes of mental retardation. It is a combination of physical deformities and mental retardation as a result of a genetic defect in chromosome pair 21. Hence it is also known as Trisomy 21. You and your partner can be *karyotyped* (chromosome analysis) to help predict your chances of having a healthy baby. According to the National Institute of Child Health and Human Development under the auspices of the U.S. Department of Health, the relationship of Down Syndrome to maternal age is as follows:

Mother's age	Incidence of Down syndrome
Under 30	less than 1 in 1,000
age 35	1 in 400
age 40	1 in 105
age 42	1 in 60
age 44	1 in 35
age 46	1 in 20
age 48	1 in 12

The risk of having a child with Down syndrome increase with maternal age.

How to Stay Healthy when You're not Quite Ready to Be a Parent . . .

Even if you want to scream when hear about that biological clock, chances are it still may be earlier than you think. Most experts agree that fertility peaks in your early twenties. After age thirty-five, eggs do get older and the outer coating, or shell, does get a little tougher, making it less penetrable by sperm cells. However, there is still a strong chance of getting pregnant in your forties.

To preserve your fertility, the following suggestions may be helpful.

Don't smoke. Or, for that matter, inhale the secondhand smoke of others. On average smokers go through menopause two years earlier than nonsmokers. Obviously, that's two years off your reproductive time. Would-be fathers who smoke may reduce their sperm count and motility. Children of fathers who smoke are also more likely to suffer from childhood cancers.

Keep yourself fit. Yo-yo dieting with severe weight fluctuations plays havoc with your hormones and your reproductive system. Very overweight couples may experience difficulty conceiving simply because of the physical restraints that result in shallow penetration, if they are successful at all. Additionally, overweight women may also have difficulty conceiving because of excessive estrogen levels, which can affect the uterine lining.

Exercise has the added benefit of keeping your muscles and cardiovascular system in good shape, and the overall healthiness of your body is a plus when trying to conceive.

But don't get too skinny. Most doctors agree that a woman must have at least 10 percent body fat to sustain ovulation. Bulemics, anorexics, or highly competitive athletes with lower than the 10 percent often have ovulatory and menstrual irregularities, but usually regain their reproductive equilibrium when their normal body fat returns.

Eat a well-balanced diet. No big surprise here. Lack of vitamin C and some amino acids has been linked to decreased sperm counts and poor sperm motility as well. Mineral deficiencies in women have also been associated with fertility problems, as well as protein-poor diets. Orange juice anyone?

Turn down the heat. If you are a man, that is. Exposing the testicles to the heat of the hot tub, the bath tub, tight jeans, or lycra bicycle shorts can drastically cut down on sperm production. Is this why Victoria's Secret now sells men's boxer shorts in the Christmas catalogue?

Don't ignore pain or fevers. Abdominal pain and fever could be a symptom of pelvic inflammatory disease (PID). See a doctor. After only one untreated episode of PID, 35 percent of the 8 million women who suffer from it have become infertile. Three

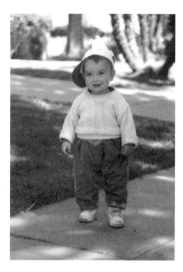

untreated episodes can cause infertility in 75 percent of the women. Since PID may have no symptoms ask your doctor to check for it at your regular exam.

Find out why your periods are painful. Endometriosis is a painful condition in which the lining of the uterus grows outside the organ in the abdominal cavity. For 20 percent of infertile women, endometriosis is the cause. Heavy menstrual cramping is one sign, so have it checked out.

Avoid environmental toxins. This probably sounds too obvious to even list here, but radiation, exposure to pesticides, heavy metals, high gauss electromagnetic fields and a host of other pollutants from the job site may prevent conception when either partner is exposed. Evaluate your workplace. Ask if other people in your job environment are having trouble conceiving. This information might help you solve the problem.

Become an expert. The more you know about your body, the more power you will have understanding conception, fertility, and a healthy life in general. Join a support group or gain advice from others who have been there and done that. Outline your

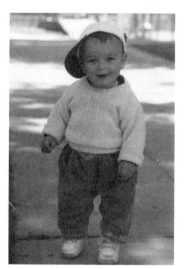

limits to baby-making: financially, physically, emotionally, and even time-wise. If all else fails, will you consider adoption? There are resources listed for you in the reference section at the end of this chapter.

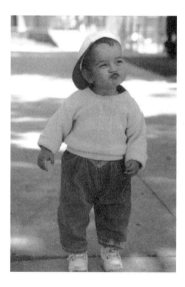

Do your Kegel exercises. More than half a century ago, Dr. Arnold Kegel demonstrated that strengthening the pubococcygeal muscles not only improves bladder control and helps prevent incontinence, but also adds to sexual satisfaction and an easier childbirth experience. To initially identify these muscles, try to stop the flow of urine or tighten the rectal muscles as if you are trying to prevent the passing of gas. Then lie down, breathe normally, and try to draw up these same muscles for a count of five. Relax for a few seconds and try again. Work up to a count of ten and repeat ten times. When you can hold the contraction for a count of ten, then try several short, strong contractions in a row. Repeat. How often should you do these exercises? Every day, many times. During TV commercials, while stopped at traffic lights, while you're waiting on hold on the telephone, find the time to work these exercises in. How many repetitions? Work up to at least two minutes of Kegel exercises, which averages out to be about 200 repetitions.

No jelly. Jellies and lubricants are believed to impair a sperm's motility, so don't use them if you are trying to get pregnant.

Avoid a lot of alcohol. Alcohol can play havoc with regular ovulation schedules, making it difficult to predict peak availability of eggs.

TURNING BACK THE CLOCK

There are more options in the baby arena than ever before in history. From egg donors, test tube babies, and assisted hatching, baby-making is a big industry, as the baby-boomers are finding out. However, nothing is 100 percent sure as many frustrated couples will tell you. The following glossary of terms is by no means all inclusive. With new techniques constantly appearing on the front pages of newspapers these days, here is a simple overview of some of the options available for stretching time on the baby clock.

Adoption. It can be exhausting, challenging, and ultimately incredibly fulfilling. Friends have warned me of the unspoken bias against parents over the age of forty. However, there are many adoptable children of color in America and also from Third World and war ravaged countries, so if the desire to be a parent is the issue, rather than being the biological parent, adoption is clearly a wonderful choice to override the biological clock.

Alphafetoprotein from maternal serum (MSAFP). The mother's serum is analyzed in this technique to determine women who may be at risk for producing babies with abnormalities such as Down syndrome, spina bifida, and some heart conditions. This test is preformed within the same window as amniocentesis, sometimes from as early as the fifteenth week of pregnancy. It is not a guarantee of the baby's health because it is basically a screening test, and the results could be very skewed indeed if there were twins, or the calculation of conception was incorrect. MSAFP has a 40 percent accuracy rate in predicting Down syndrome. An *enhanced MSAFP* screen technique generally has a 60 to 65 percent prediction rate.

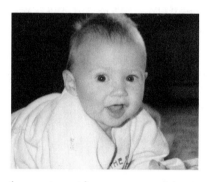

Amniocentesis. This is most often used to test for Down syndrome, as well as other chromosomal, biochemical, and metabolic disorders. However, it is not a guarantee of a baby's health. Between the sixteenth and eighteenth weeks of pregnancy, a small amount of fluid is removed from the amniotic sac surrounding the fetus. The fluid sample is then sent to a lab for analysis. It can be done as an office procedure, and results may take up to two weeks—a nerve-rackingly long time if you are waiting to see if there is a health problem with the baby. Risks: Possible complications include a 0.5 risk of miscarriage, infection, fluid leakage, vaginal bleeding, or fetal injury.

Assisted hatching. As we age, our eggs age too, with the covering of the egg, the zona pellucida, hardening. This makes it difficult for the embryo to "hatch" and break open the shell when it reaches the cell division of about 100 cells. To counteract this problem, specially trained scientists use a tiny amount of acid on the outside surface of the embryo, creating a minuscule hole, weakening the shell enough for the embryo to break loose and expand. The hatched embryo is then put back inside the mother's uterus, where the chances of successful implantation and a continuation of the pregnancy are increased by up to 53 percent.

Chorionic Villi Sampling (CVS). Yet another technique to try to determine chromosomal or other genetic disabilities. It can be performed earlier than amniocentesis, at ten to twelve weeks. Its popularity is waning, however, because miscarriage can be as high as more than 1 percent with this technique and the test itself may cause other fetal abnormalities.

Cloning. Monkeys were near-cloned at the beginning of 1997 by a technique called nuclear transfer. The genes from unfertilized monkey eggs were stripped, then scientists added new genetic material by fusing the eggs to a monkey embryo that had grown to an eight-cell size. The monkeys were not true clones because two different embryos were used as sources. Will human clones be next? If you ever wished to live in interesting times, you got your wish.

Donor insemination (heterologous insemination). An option to consider when the husband's sperm is not viable, this process involves introduction of viable donor sperm into the vagina, cervical canal, or uterus by artificial means. The semen is obtained from a donor other than the husband.

Egg donation. In this technique, the eggs of a fertile woman are harvested. The donor may be known or anonymous. Sperm from the partner of the infertile female are then mixed with the egg. Once the egg is penetrated by the sperm, the embryo is then implanted into the uterus of the infertile woman.

Fertility drugs. A hormone drug is given to the woman so that she will produce multiple eggs all at once. This is often done so that the eggs may be harvested for in vitro fertilization.

In vitro fertilization. In vitro comes from a Latin phrase meaning "in glass." Eggs are harvested from the mother and then the father's sperm is added. When one sperm cell swims inside the egg—voila! The fertilized egg is then transplanted back into the uterus of the mother. The egg, the sperm, or both, may be donated.

Intracytoplasmic sperm injection. In 40 percent of all infertile couples, the man has the fertility problem. With this technique, the woman is given a fertility drug and produces about a dozen eggs to be harvested and taken to the laboratory. Then, a very tiny pinprick is made in the egg membrane with a small needle and a single sperm cell is

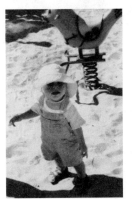

injected into the egg. This is a big help when sperm are not really fast swimmers. Early clinical pregnancy rates have been recorded at up to 62 percent with this method, which proves that you don't have to be an Olympic champion to win the prize.

Surrogate moms. These days, it could even be a surrogate grandmother. A fertilized egg from one couple is transplanted to the uterus of another woman, who carries the pregnancy to term, delivers the baby, and returns the child to its biological parents.

Ultrasound imaging. This technique can be done either abdominally or vaginally. It is an imaging test that is done to determine the location, position, and structural and organic architecture of the fetus. Twins or triplets are also visualized with this technique.

Vasectomy reversal. This procedure now has 50 percent chance of success.

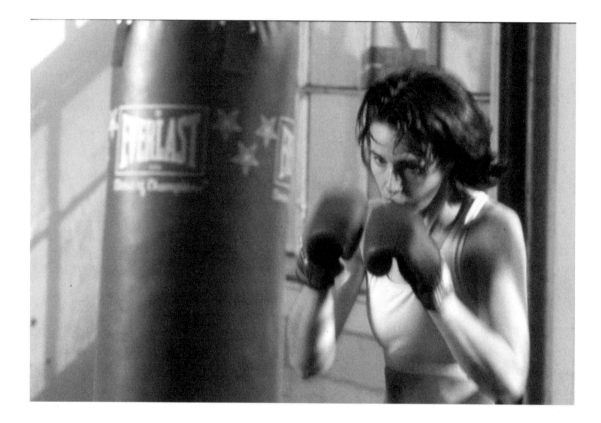

THE FUTURE RIGHT NOW

Frozen eggs for later use—researchers are concentrating on this one right now. The immature eggs of a woman would be harvested and frozen for future use. This is similar to current strategies of saving frozen sperm as a hedge against aging, illness, or medical treatment that may alter sperm such as chemotherapy.

RESOURCES

The American Society for Reproductive Medicine
1209 Montgomery Highway
Birmingham, AL 35216-2809

Can provide success rates for various procedures and general information. There is a charge for their various publications.

National Adoption Center
1500 Walnut Street, Suite 701
Philadelphia, PA 19102
1-800-TO-ADOPT

Packets of general information are available for a small charge (under $10).

Resolve
1310 Broadway
Sumerville, MA 02144-1731

Write to this support group for infertile couples at the above address.

22 HOT FLASH: MENOPAUSE

Everything in life that we really accept undergoes a change.
This is the thing that in the greatest is a shining light,
a pure white fire; and in the humblest is a constant radiance,
a quiet perpetual gleam. When we stop running away,
when we really accept, that is when even tragedy succumbs to beauty.

—Katherine Mansfield (1888–1923)

"*D*uring an annual industry gathering, the regional manager of a communications giant began to feel warm. The air conditioner must be on the blink, she thought. But then she realized that everyone else in the room—all men in suits—seemed comfortable with the temperature. Suddenly the heat surging through her body became as intense as that of a big-block V-8 idling in New York City's gridlock traffic. 'The hair on the back of my neck was soaking wet,' the woman, then 43 recalls. She frantically searched her briefcase for a wad of tissues to dab the perspiration and then made a discreet exit to the powder room, where she splashed cold water on her face. As she later learned, this was her first encounter with menopause."

Less than 10 percent of women find hot flashes or any menopausal symptoms to be disruptive to their lives, but I remember reading this story in *Fortune* magazine with the dull fascination of trying not to look at a freeway accident cleared to the side of the road. I had the same kind of mentality, thankful I wasn't in that wreck: "Menopause—thank goodness I don't have to start thinking about *that* yet! I'm too *young*." Denial is a big reason that we allow ourselves to build up fear about menopause.

WANTING TO KNOW AND AFRAID TO KNOW

For many of us, we want to know about menopause, but we avoid the topic—as if knowing about it will somehow detonate the bomb sooner and we will be hapless victims of our own curiosity. "Knowledge is power," says one side of our brain. The other side screams, "What you don't know right now, won't hurt you—and besides, you're too young anyway."

Even the medical community has essentially neglected the topic. "The majority of practicing doctors in the U.S. have never been taught anything about menopause." says Dr. Wulf Utian, director of obstetrics and gynecology at University Hospitals in Cleveland in a recent *Fortune* magazine interview. In the same article, Dr. Robert Barbieri, a professor of obstetrics and gynecology at Harvard Medical school acknowledged, "Many people who finished training before 1980 did not have much exposure to menopause." However he stated that Harvard and other medical schools have now developed courses on the topic.

These new doctors will be putting that information to good use. Although the average age for menopause—or more accurately, cessation of menstruation—is fifty-one years old, hormonal shifts can begin in the mid thirties to late forties. It's estimated that by the year 2000, the number of baby-boomers going through menopause will grow at the rate of 2 million a year.

And who wants to talk about it anyway? "Am I going to lose my looks, my sex drive, and dry up like a prune now?" asked my forty-nine-year-old patient who had her first hot flash at age forty-eight, virtually in tears at the prospect. "Because that's what happened to my mother—and then she got one of those humps in her back."

To be very candid, this woman's mother "lost" her sex drive twenty years before menopause because of an unhappy marriage. Her looks had actually begun to vanish when she was unable to shed the eighty extra pounds gained during her pregnancy. Furthermore, the "hump" on her back was from obesity and a lifetime of incredibly poor posture with her shoulders and head hunched over. It had nothing to do with menopause or osteoporosis.

We must first conquer the anxiety factor of the unknown so that we can deal with this life event in an effective way. After all, menopause is not a disease! In many cultures around the world, menopause is seen as a positive event. We are effective when we learn as much as possible so that we can then make informed choices that can take us out of the victim role into the power role. Talk to other women who have been through menopause and you may be surprised to learn that it's not the big deal you might think.

There are many books written about menopause, but the must-read I recommend for every woman is: *What Your Doctor May Not Tell You About Menopause: The Breakthrough Book on Natural Progesterone* by John R. Lee, M.D. It is literally a blockbuster because it debunks some very long-standing and widely held beliefs about traditional synthetic hormone replacement therapy based on replacing estrogen, and offers a natural hormone treatment regime using a progesterone cream that can be applied to the skin. After reading stacks of contradictory research articles on hormone replacement therapy (HRT), this book made so much sense I started sending out copies to everyone I could think of.

Do you remember hearing the horror stories about menstruation? Were you convinced that you would be wearing white tennis shorts the day it happened? Of course, we all learned to cope just fine. The menopause hype in the press reminds me of a classic description by Clarissa Pinkola Estes, Ph.D., in her wonderful book *Women Who Run With the Wolves*. She is referring to descriptions by anthropologists of the temporary forced exile of menstruating women by tribal societies. Supposedly the women were banished because they were considered to be "unclean."

"All women know that even if there were such a forced ritual exile, every single woman, to a woman, would, when her time came, leave the village hanging her head mournfully, at least till she was out of sight, and then suddenly break into a jig down the path, cackling all the way."

Most women stride right through menopause without a break in their daily lives. Some feel so good they may be tempted to break into the kind of jig that Estes describes. However, you'd never know it from all the conflicting claims and negative reports in the media. So let's backtrack a little and get to the facts on exactly what menopause is and what are the options.

THE HORMONE SHOW

The word *hormone* is derived from the Greek root meaning "I arouse to activity." These chemicals are released by specialized glands into the blood stream and either circulate to a target organ or another gland triggering chains of chemical reactions. There are a few key hormones in the reproductive cycle of a woman. To understand what happens when reproduction slows down and ceases during menopause, we're going to look at the major players in this show.

Ovarian hormones. The two types of sex hormones primarily produced in the ovaries are the *estrogens* and the *progesterone.*

The word estrogen has an interesting history in itself. It comes from the Greek word *oistros*, which means "mad desire" and from the word *gennan* which means "to produce."

While estrogens and progesterone are the dominant female hormones produced by the ovaries, some small quantities of testosterone, the dominant male hormone, are also produced. The adrenal glands also make a small contribution of estrogen and progesterone. All of this production, and indeed most hormonal production in the body, is regulated by the pituitary gland which is located in the brain.

There are three main types of estrogen: estrone (E1), estradiol (E2), and estriol (E3). The principal of these is estradiol and it is twelve times more potent than estrone and eight times more potent than estriol. You will recognize these types on your lab report.

During childhood, estrogens and progesterone are secreted only in minute quantities, but beginning with puberty, twenty times that amount is secreted by the ovaries. In response to the increase in these and other hormones, the female sex organs change into adult size, with the uterus alone increasing two to three times in size. Estrogens stimulate the development of the female sex organs, breasts, and secondary sexual characteristics. Progesterone stimulates the mucous production of the uterus and also helps promote the development of milk secreting glands in the breasts. The key point is that estrogen and progesterone are antagonistic to each other, meaning that they balance each other out.

For instance, while estrogen increases blood clotting, increases body fat and promotes salt and fluid retention, and decreases sex drive, progesterone decreases blood clotting, helps the body use up fat for energy, increases sex drive, and acts as a natural diuretic.

Estrogen also causes women's blood vessels to become more elastic, especially during pregnancy when the mother's blood volume expands. If her blood vessels were as inflexible as a man's, then the increase in blood pressure during pregnancy could kill the mother and the baby by the fifth month.

Ever wonder why your husband or boyfriend seems to be able to eat just about anything and never gain weight and yet you have to watch every bite? The dominant male sex hormone, testosterone, can increase a man's metabolic rate by 10 to 15 percent more than a woman's metabolic rate. Additionally, estrogen dominance causes increased fat to be deposited primarily in the thighs and derrière. That's why the figures of women are different than those of men—the fat distribution overall and the protein to fat ratio in male versus female bodies are not the same.

The more potent metabolic effect of testosterone in men is why a man and woman of the same height and weight could eat exactly the same diet, but the woman could gain weight and the man could lose weight—a fact that has dismayed many women over the years! However, a woman's more efficient metabolism is designed to help store fat as an emergency reserve in case of pregnancy—a small consolation if you don't happen to be in the middle of a famine while you're having a baby, but important information if you're ever placing bets on a man and woman in an ultra long distance running event. Given a male and female athlete of roughly the same abilities, put your money on the woman in a 100-mile-plus event. Female runners tend to do very well at very long distances and, if you consider life to be an endurance event, women *do* live longer than men.

Finally, the balance of estrogen and progesterone helps promote and maintain bone density and health as well as affecting such varied functions as memory, fluid retention in our skin, blood fat levels, blood sugar levels, and immune function of the vaginal and urinary tracts. You may have guessed that estrogen and progesterone balancing acts are very major players in a woman's body—they're found in over three hundred different tissues in varying amounts.

Progesterone, estrogen, and menstruation. Progesterone is secreted by the ovaries and it has the important function of causing changes in the uterus after ovulation (release of an egg from an ovary) each month just in case the egg is fertilized and needs to be implanted. Estrogen builds up the endometrial lining of the uterus. Progesterone nourishes the lining, but stops it from building up too much. If the egg is not fertilized, the uterine lining is routinely shed once a month as a menstrual period and the whole cycle of hormone secretion, ebb and flow, build-up, and shedding begins all over again to prepare for the next occurrence of ovulation.

Other Hormones

Androstenedione. This is the hormone that is secreted by the adrenal glands and then converted by the body's fat, muscle, and skin cells into estrone, the main type of estrogen that still continues to be produced after menopause. Some doctors of natural medicine hypothesize that women who have had a lifetime of heavy caffeine and diet pill consumption seem to have a harder time at menopause because they have exhausted the adrenal glands with decades of stimulant abuse and then the adrenals are less capable of producing estrone.

Testosterone. The ovaries and the adrenal glands produce this hormone in women, with the adrenal glands taking over after menopause. Both men and women produce testosterone, and while it is the dominant male sex hormone, produced in the male testes, it is often called "the libido hormone" for either gender.

Pregnenolone. This is the precursor of all steroid hormones.

DHEA (dehydroepiandrosterone). The most abundant hormone in the body, it's made primarily in the adrenal glands and is a precursor to estrogens and testosterone.

WHAT HAPPENS AT MENOPAUSE

The cause of menopause is generally a relaxation of duty by the ovaries. Menstrual cycles gradually become irregular and the production of progesterone and estrogen gradually decreases. When a complete hysterectomy has been performed and the ovaries and the uterus are surgically removed, then this is a sudden and immediate halt of most estrogen production and a different, immediate menopause results.

At the time when estrogen production decreases to a certain level, the pituitary gland in the brain, which controls most hormone production, senses the change. The pituitary then goes into overdrive and increases its production of stimulating hormones to fire up the ovaries.

These stimulating hormones are called FSH (follicle stimulating hormone) and LH (luteinizing hormone). Blood tests can determine exactly how much of these stimulating hormones are being sent out to fire up the ovaries, and when the levels are above 40 MIU per milliliter of blood, this is considered to be diagnostic of menopause.

Here is where Dr. John R. Lee challenges the widely held medical belief that estrogen decline is the main cause of postmenopausal symptoms. He points out that, during menopause, progesterone may decrease to zero while estrogen drops by only one-third or one-half of premenopausal levels. Therefore, Western women suffer a decade and a half of estrogen *dominant* symptoms, he emphasizes. The opposite, older belief of estrogen deficiency has many doctors prescribing even more estrogen in synthetic form. "This is a kind of backwards science," he states in his book. "It leads to ridiculous ideas—like calling a headache an aspirin deficiency disease." Instead, Dr. Lee has researched the important role of natural hormone replacement cream and administers it with the admonishment, "Since progesterone has so many positive benefits and no known side effects, there is no reason to discontinue it. I tell women to continue until age 96 and then we'll reevaluate."

At the time of menopause, a woman is adjusting her body's physiology from one that has been stimulated by estrogen and progesterone production, to one with less of these hormones. Finally, the medical community, led by people like Dr. Lee, is echoing the advice of earlier naturalistic health care providers: that adherence to a healthy, mostly vegetarian diet free of fatty foods, sugar, and stimulants, and a lifestyle of exercise and effective stress management seems to have most women in other cultures sailing through menopause and enjoying life.

WHAT IS MENOPAUSE?

Menopause is a gradual, natural process usually defined as the cessation of menstruation for at least six months. The average age of menopause is fifty-one. In most cases, periods start to be irregular at about the age of forty-five and by age fifty-five there are no periods at all.

This is important to know because many people think of menopause as a line you suddenly cross over when it's actually a slow series of changes spread over a period of some ten years. Menopause is a unique experience for each woman and it's important to know that the change of cycle is not a big deal for most. The Massachusetts Women's Health Study detailed the menopause of 2,500 women ages forty-five to fifty-five for a full ten years. An interesting finding was that a majority of women have neutral or negative feelings before menopause, but that these feelings became more positive as they actually experienced menopause.

The first concern many women have about menopause is hot flashes and 60 to 70 percent of menopausal women may experience them. This is a feeling and sensation that heat is coming up to the upper body and head and there may be sweating associated with it. Many women learn the value of dressing in layers and then the flashes are not a problem. Statistics vary, but most data confirms that menopausal symptoms are disruptive to only about 10 percent of women. For 85 percent of women, the symptoms stop within one year after their last period.

The second concern of women in menopause is vaginal dryness. Women who are sexually active, take hormone replacement therapy (either the natural progesterone cream or "traditional" oral HRT), or use lubricants do not find vaginal dryness to be a problem. It can be uncomfortable, but it can be easily treated and does not mean that you are "turning into a prune." Vaginal dryness does *not* mean that your sexuality is drying up. It *does* meant that you and your partner can experiment with more foreplay, a change in sexual positions (woman on top works very well here, according to some), lubricants (some are even flavored), and a return to petting and sexual play. For certain couples, this means a positive change, as men at a similar age often take longer to attain an erection and ejaculate. Couples often relate an associated good change in not only their sexual relationship but their whole method of relating to each other because the "change of life" has forced them to communicate.

There have been some reports of a decrease of libido, while others are beginning new relationships and experiencing the excitement of "postmenopausal zest."

In *The Complete Book of Menopause*, Drs. Landau, Cyr, and Moulton sum up many feelings related to me by my patients and friends: "One way to not only enjoy menopausal years but to rejoice in them is to read other women's stories. If we do, we will learn that each of us is unique and that menopause may well be easier than other stages of life! Women who fear menopause and have negative beliefs about it may do worse than women who have an optimistic attitude. So it is our attitude and our outlook toward midlife and not our hormones that can lead us to sadness, depression, and preoccupation with physical symptoms."

HISTORY OF HORMONE REPLACEMENT

The Chinese have been extracting sex and pituitary gland hormones from urine since the second century A.D. A textbook dating back to 1025 details the necessary processing steps of what was called "autumn mineral" crystals used to treat various and wide-ranging problems from impotence to hermaphroditism. It wasn't until 1927 that Western scientists were able to isolate estrogen and progesterone in the laboratory. In the 1960s estrogen replacement gathered momentum until 1975, when the first bad news about estrogen supplementation emerged. But the stutter-step in the progress of synthetic hormone use was a short one, as researchers blamed only "unopposed" estrogen as the culprit. When paired with progesterone, either synthetic or natural, the process was renamed hormone replacement therapy instead of simply estrogen replacement therapy and the forward march continued.

Today, Premarin, the synthetic estrogen derived from and named for the urine of pregnant mares, is the most commonly prescribed drug in the United States, with sales estimated at $700 million. More than 8 million women take Premarin every day, and more than 30 billion tablets have been sold to date.

THE HRT DECISION VS. NATURAL PROGESTERONE CREAM

The question of whether hormone replacement therapy (HRT) is right for you is an important decision that requires you to be informed so that you can make better choices. You're not alone—the number of women facing this decision is growing dramatically. According to *American Demographics*, 35 million American women are currently menopausal. That number is expected to grow to 61 million by the year 2010.

HRT aims to replace hormones at a premenopausal level. If the woman still has an intact uterus, then both estrogen and progesterone are replaced. If the woman has had a hysterectomy with the ovaries also removed, then commonly only estrogen is given. Before you submit to oral HRT therapy, consider reading Dr. John R. Lee's book *What Your Doctor May Not Tell You About Menopause* and give a copy of the book to your doctor to read while you're at it. The effectiveness of natural progesterone cream that can be applied easily to the skin in order to be absorbed certainly spares your liver from having to process the oral medication, and it may be far more effective and much safer than HRT.

BENEFITS OF HRT

- Effective in treating hot flashes
- Reverses vaginal dryness
- Helps prevent osteoporosis
- Prevents heart disease
- Prevents colon cancer
- Helps preserve skin elasticity
- Improves longevity
- Helps vaginal and urinary tract immune system
- Improves skin and muscle tone
- Reduces mood swings, fatigue, depression, and insomnia

Possible Side Effects of HRT

Not all women experience these symptoms and side effects. Proponents for natural progesterone creams hypothesize that some of the common HRT symptoms might be from an imbalanced estrogen/progesterone ratio. In fact, when the patient complains of any or all of these symptoms, often *more* estrogen is prescribed and the balance could be tipped even further.

- Fluid retention and bloating
- Headaches
- Abnormal spotting or bleeding
- Nausea
- Vaginal discharge
- PMS-like symptoms of irritability and moodiness

Health Problems That Need to Be Ruled Out Before HRT

- Cancer of the uterus
- Estrogen-dependent breast cancer
- Diabetes
- Hypertension
- Blood clotting disorders
- Benign Uterine Fibroids
- Endometriosis
- Gall bladder and Liver Disease

Do the Benefits Outweigh the Side Effects?

It's no wonder that women considering HRT are confused. On June 15, 1995, the *New England Journal of Medicine* reported that long-term use of HRT increases the risk of developing breast cancer, regardless of the type of formulation. Just thirty days later, the *Journal of the American Medical Association* reported that women who took the estrogen-plus-progestin formulation did not face any increased risk of breast cancer.

"The fact of the matter is that it is surprising how little taking hormones increases the risk for breast cancer," said Barbara Hulka of the University of North Carolina at

Chapel Hill School of Public Health in an interview with *Science News* in August 1995. "While not all studies show increased breast cancer from either oral contraceptives or HRT, the ones that do typically gauge the risk as 1.3 to 1.7 times the normal chance—a number that pales in comparison to the risks seen with [being born with] the BRCA1 and BRAC2 genes" (which carry a genetic risk of breast cancer).

"HRT benefits outweigh the risks in terms of basic deaths from any disease," said Louise Brinton of the National Cancer Institute in Bethesda, Maryland, in the same article.

Another key issue: Why do up to half of all women who opt for HRT quit within a year? "The point is, when it comes to HRT, one size doesn't fit all," cautions Dr. Brian Walsh, director of the menopause clinic at Brigham and Women's Hospitals in Boston. He was quoted in a *Prevention* magazine article discussing how regimes need to be tailored to each woman's needs.

Luckily, there are patches, pills, creams, implants, suppositories, lots of different brands and combinations available to you and your doctor. Which of the dozens of combinations you choose depends on the severity of your symptoms, if you have a family history of osteoporosis or heart disease, and whether or not you've had a hysterectomy.

"I just felt draggy and depressed after my hysterectomy," says Molly, an athletic thirty-four-year-old professional woman with two children. "I have a wonderful husband but I simply had no desire for him until I switched to a combination that included a tiny bit of testosterone. I had to switch doctors to find someone who didn't just say, 'There, there, maybe you're just feeling a little overtired.' But now I feel super—really back to my old self, and my husband and I just went to Las Vegas for a mini romantic vacation to celebrate."

Susan, a painter, age forty-eight, remembers, "I was actually scared at the beginning because my family has a history of cancer and heart attacks, but I talked it over with my doctor and he said we could try the lowest dose necessary to help my hot flashes and insomnia. But I get even better results with the natural progesterone cream and now I'm not worried about the cancer risk."

Some women are sensitive to the dose, others to the duration of the medication. For many more, there is basically a problem with even the idea of turning a natural event into a health problem that results in years of medication.

"I had one hot flash only and I just said to heck with it all when my doctor started talking about all the creams and pills and everything else." says Beth, now eighty-two.

"It's not like I had a disease or anything. I honestly didn't feel much of a difference—I just went on about my usual business."

In the final analysis, there's more than one way to go. The decision about HRT is highly personal and individual. The most a woman can do is educate herself about the risks, the benefits, and face the real honest truth that scientists are still arguing about the data. Then make a choice. The results of all the new research studies will be in by the turn of the century. Hopefully there will be more answers as a new generation of women approaches menopause. Perhaps the most important thing a woman can do when she walks into her doctor's office is to simply ask: "What's new?"

THE NATURAL ALTERNATIVES

For preventing osteoporosis. Get regular weight-bearing exercise like walking and lifting weights. (See Chapter 13: Keeping your Beautiful Bones.) Supplement with calcium or calcium-rich foods.

For preventing heart disease. Don't smoke. Smokers also reach menopause two years earlier on average than nonsmokers. Get regular huff and puff cardiovascular exercise. Eat a low-fat diet. Build a low-fat body. (See Chapter 10.)

For hot flashes. Mexican yams and other soybean foods like tofu and soy milk contain weak plant estrogens called *phytoestrogen*. The actual amount of estrogen activity that they can supply is speculative at this point, but some experts hypothesize that Asian women have few, if any, menopausal symptoms due to frequent soy consumption. Tofu, tempeh, soy hot dogs, tofu cheese, and soy milk are available at health food stores and some supermarkets. Paavo Airola, Ph.D., perhaps the most classic American naturalist, advocates up to 1,200 units of vitamin E per day as well as vitamins C, B6, PABA, and pantothenic acid in his book *How to Get Well.* Oil of evening primrose, don quai, or angelica, licorice root, fenugreek, sarsaparilla (smilax), and elder are herbs that are used by herbalists to treat menopausal symptoms. Caution: Be prudent when taking herbs. If you don't have the time or inclination to educate yourself about them, consult an expert.

For better skin. Become a "shady lady" and avoid the sun. Use sunscreen. Exfoliate and moisturize. (See Chapter 8: Skin Deep.)

For yeast infections. 8 oz. of yogurt per day was just what the doctor ordered at Long Island Jewish Medical Center, where it was found that it led to fewer yeast infections.

This is of particular note to menopausal women because the vaginal dryness that may occur with a drop in estrogen can increase the risk of yeast infection.

Ginseng. It's been used in Asia for thousands of years as an anti-aging plant. In keeping with traditional, preventive Chinese medical practices, it is used as a tonic to gain health each day and not just when there's a crisis. Because it has estrogen mimicking qualities to it, ginseng is sometimes used to treat some side effects of menopause like hot flashes and can be taken as a tea.

For memory, loss of concentration, and headaches. The herb ginkgo biloba was reviewed strongly in the *British Journal of Clinical Pharmacology* in 1992 for alleviating these symptoms. It's the number one prescription drug in Germany and is also sold over the counter in Europe and North America. Check out Chapter 7 if you'd like more information on how to forget about losing your memory.

For sexual well-being. The best way to keep your machinery humming is an active sex life, which stimulates pelvic circulation and burns calories. It's the use it or lose it rule once again. For vaginal dryness, there are nonprescription lubricants like Astroglide, Gyne-Moistrin, and Replens. Check out Chapter 4 for more strategies.

DHEA. Traditional oral HRT lowers DHEA levels, while natural progesterone cream can elevate DHEA. This is one of the new kids on the block with a great deal of promise. It is the most abundantly produced hormone from the adrenal glands in the body. It is important for production of estrogen, progesterone, testosterone, and corticosterone, and levels fall off rapidly in the body after about age forty-five to fifty. It is available from health food stores. Rather than self-dosing, I recommend that you get your DHEA levels checked by a simple blood test from your health care practitioner. Find out where you are on this one. Optimal levels are considered to be: 750 ng/dL or above in men, 550ng/dL or above in women. Read up on DHEA, and then remember, that if you decide to take it, it is a commitment to your endocrine system, and should not be taken capriciously, but every day. Find a health care provider who is up on DHEA and dosages. Then you can monitor DHEA levels and be respectful of what your body needs. If you have cancer of the female reproductive organs or any medical condition, you should only take DHEA or any supplement under the care of your physician.

For weight gain. The average American woman watches more than thirty hours of television a week or more than four hours a day, according to a report from the Nielson Media Research. According to the *American Dietetic Association*, the prevalence of obesity is 19.2 percent for those who are watching the tube for four or more hours per day. Unless you're participating in all those dance aerobics programs on TV, your couch potato habits are going to sneak up on you—most likely around your waist! According to Dr. John R. Lee, natural progesterone cream help post-menopausal women maintain healthy weight by balancing the estrogen/progesterone ratios.

For emotional well-being. The ebb of hormones may coincide with many life events such as children leaving home, a husband who has become impotent or is going through mid-life crisis, a spouse having an affair/leaving you for a younger woman, parents who become your children and a myriad of other scenarios. "The more a woman feels valued in her life, the less likely she is to have emotional symptoms at menopause. Working women tend to do better than women who stay home," said Dr. Stotland of the University of Chicago in a feature article in *Newsweek* magazine.

23 MENOPAUSE: NOT FOR WOMEN ONLY

> For without belittling the courage with which men have died, we
> should not forget those acts of courage with which men . . . have lived.
> The courage of life is often a less dramatic spectacle than the courage
> of a final moment; but no less a magnificent mixture of triumph and
> tragedy. A man does what he must—in spite of obstacles and dangers
> and pressures—and that is the basis of all human morality.
>
> —John Fitzgerald Kennedy (1917–1963), *Profiles in Courage*

Surrounded by gleaming chrome and a swarm of fit bodies in lycra, Mel clenches his teeth and psyches himself for one more rep in his bench press. It feels heavy, but he pushes himself and gets the bar straight up above his chest. "One more for the Gipper," he grunts to himself and this time strains to hoist the bar. It wobbles slightly. "Here, let me spot you on that," says a leggy blonde, supplying the extra guidance to get the heavy barbell up into the safety rests.

He used to bench press 250 pounds, four sets of ten repetitions, no problem, he remembers. At fifty-two, Mel has always kept in shape. He's six foot two, with a full head of hair graying slightly at the temples. Okay, so it's not quite a full head of hair anymore. He stares up at the blonde's body while he is still horizontal on the bench. Definitely a ten. Thank God I'm not wearing Spandex, he thinks and smiles to himself, feeling the stirrings of an erection. At least there's something to feel good about in *that* department. He's been comfortable with making love to his new thirty-five-year-old girlfriend whenever he can fit a getaway into his busy executive schedule of traveling and deal making. Last weekend, he had trouble getting an erection. Too much wine at dinner? Yeah, that was all.

Yet, the effects of Mel's far-from-healthy lifestyle were becoming more apparent to his friends. Mel confides to no one about the vodka and tonic at lunch as the regular routine these days, nor the increase in his smoking, from half a pack since he "quit" last year, to over a pack a day now. He'd put on a few pounds, just temporarily, until the divorce was finalized, he told himself.

Basically, Mel is stressed out and feeling it. He has been through some major life events and it's affecting him in some unhealthful ways. What kind of self-talk do you think is going on in Mel's head? If you were Mel's friend, would you say anything? If you were his girlfriend? What if you were his doctor?

MALE MENOPAUSE

The above scenario is very surely not the norm. It's actually a compilation of what many male patients have told me about their lives, and it does raise the interesting question: Is there such a thing as male menopause? It may become the new buzz phrase for the nineties as the postwar baby boomers reach their late forties and fifties. But the term is clearly confusing and misleading. "The phrase 'male menopause' does not make sense," states Alvin M. Matsumoto, M.D., professor of gerontology at the Veteran's Affairs Medical Center, Seattle. "The word *menopause* means the cessation of a woman's menstrual period, so applying that word to a male is not a useful thing to talk about. It's something you'd expect to see as a headline on a TV talk show."

But, he adds: "There are changes in testosterone, human growth hormone, insulin growth factor number one, and other male hormones. I think we need to understand these changes more and then evaluate them in some individuals if they are having symptoms. Also, this is not a male functional problem that only affects men. Because anything that affects a man will have an effect on female health—the spouse and significant others who are in a man's life."

IF THERE IS SUCH A THING, WHAT ARE THE SYMPTOMS?

There is very little written at this time about a male climeractic or male menopause. A few journal articles, some popular magazine features, but not an abundance of hard-core, detailed data in which a large group of men have been studied. "There are not enough studies right now," states Dr. Matsumoto. "I feel very strongly about the need for research in this important area."

One of the few studies available, the Massachusetts Male Aging Study of over 1,500 men between the ages of forty and seventy found that half of the men suffered from persistent erection problems at least half of the time. However, the self-esteem and other emotional issues that can result from those problems were not studied.

So what's the difference between male menopause and midlife crisis? "I've gone through at least one big-time crisis every five or ten years of my life," said one age forty-eight patient. "Because I'm having one now, it's labeled *mid-life* crisis." David Ryback, Ph.D., author of *Look 10 Years Younger, Live 10 Years Longer*, addresses the difference in his book: "Whereas midlife crises can be a passing phase based on a single-issue challenge, male menopause is a psychological/medical syndrome which is experienced as a passage of the spirit from one way of being to an entirely different, more thoughtful way of life."

In my experience with patients, I have noticed that certain trends may be a signal for some of the midlife hormonal changes that are often chronicled by events large and small, both physical and psychological. Some individuals experience nothing at all, and it's business as usual without even a missed step or a mixed feeling. Others may experience the whole list of symptoms, others only a few, but those few may be felt very intensely.

A depressionlike anxiety. There are limitless reasons for this in any of us at any time however, in male patients in their late forties and fifties, I have noted some trends. These are a selected review of symptoms reported by my patients:

- occasional episodes of impotence
- an injury that takes longer to heal than any other injury—whether it's a sprained back, an ankle injury, a shoulder strain, or the like
- a change in the employment arena, whether it's being cut in a corporate downsizing, a move to another department, a self-induced change, or suddenly finding the job intolerable
- the sudden necessity of reading glasses
- the awareness that physical fitness is slipping—the waistband that is too tight, hair loss that is accelerating, blood pressure that is rising, libido that is dropping
- divorce or separation
- unexplained chills or hot flashes that are unrelated to disease
- a sudden increase in the use of alcohol, caffeine, and tobacco
- difficulty falling asleep or staying asleep at night
- all or any combination of the above

Denial of changes. Spouses or family members may be quite mindful of the changes and report them in the initial consultation, yet the patient may deny that there are any. The denial of physical symptoms may tend to increase anxiety, stress, negative emotions, anger, depression, or generalized fatigue. And so the vicious cycle escalates.

WHAT IF YOU HAVE SOME OF THESE SYMPTOMS?

When a patient relates these changes, after a physical examination I will check for testosterone or DHEA levels and other hormones in addition to the usual complete blood count and tests of insulin, cholesterol levels, and the like. Naturally, it's wise to rule out any underlying disease process. Based on this information, we discuss the next step, whether it's a referral to an endocrinologist, a counselor, an opthamologist, a personal trainer, or a stress/relaxation specialist.

Do all men experience these symptoms? Just as with women and menopause, many men experience no symptoms whatsoever. However, others may experience a few of the symptoms quite intensely. What are the percentages? At this point, no one knows for sure and any guesses of how many men out there are going through an intense process are just that—guesses. "There needs to be more research," states Dr. Matsumoto.

However, author and psychologist Dr. David Ryback offers another interesting perspective in his book *Look 10 Years Younger, Live 10 Years Longer*: "If we could accept it [male menopause] as a common experience among middle-aged men, there would be less loneliness and pain among such men and their partners." He also says that "loss requires grieving and grieve he must if the menopausal male is to move on to a healthy acceptance of his new role, with sufficient support from spouse and/or close friends and receptivity to professional counseling when necessary."

THE NEXT FEW STEPS

Get some sleep and take a vacation. Depression is anger turned inwards, and depression loves to ride in on the heels of fatigue. Anxiety, depression, frustration, anger, low self-esteem—psychologists recognize that these emotions are often painted with the same brush. In the headlong rush toward paying off the big mortgage, getting the kids through college, evaluating whether this is where you really want to be right now, or simply sur-viving corporate downsizing, taking a break, even for a day, may be worth its weight in gold. It can give you the needed opportunity to reflect on your goals, where you are now, and what kind of changes might be necessary to cope with it all in an effective way.

Ego integrity versus despair. Psychoanalyst Erik H. Erikson proposed that as we age, we go through eight distinct stages of development from birth to death. He believed that each stage was the result of a crisis that evolved from the combined forces of bio-logical drives and cultural, economic, and societal demands.

In the sixth stage according to Erikson, no matter how successful you are in your work, you have not completed yourself until you are capable of intimacy. In the seventh stage, he proposed that once you know who you are, and have achieved intimacy, you enter the crisis of *generativity versus stagnation*, which many people resolve by becom-ing parents or becoming creative and nurturing through their work and relationships.

The eighth and final crisis identified by Erikson was named *ego integrity versus despair*. The ultimate goals of spirituality, balance, wisdom, and acceptance of one's life and role in the world are the striving of this important stage.

Perhaps these challenges are part of male and female menopause in ways that we will understand with more research. Does any of this sound like something you may recognize in yourself or in others in midlife?

Facing reality by taking stock in your life and deciding what needs to be rearranged in order for you to meet your highest personal and spiritual values is an important step toward reshaping your actions. It's a valuable coping mechanism. Ask what you really want out of your life and figure out how you can get it. That act alone may ban-ish the most virulent forms of male menopausal anxiety.

CHANGING WITH THE TIMES AND YOUR BODY: TWO CASE STUDIES

"The emotional changes of male menopause were real for me," a sixty-two-year-old physicist told me. "It accounts for the dissolution of job and personal relation-ships. There is not much we can do about it under our present rules. They call it 'the change' and the solution seems to be *to change*.

"I read lots of books on how to satisfy women and learned new ways of being close and we tried a lot of them," he continued, referring to his newfound romance. "Bet-ter than staying home and only wishing I had made changes. I'm a better lover now than when I was as a kid at eighteen or twenty. All in all, male menopause was good for me."

"The love, understanding, and support of a good woman are the keys to understanding some of my medical problems that started at about age fifty," stated Bob, another patient, a Vietnam vet who experienced a diminished sexual drive and "a feeling of no self-worth."

A physical exam and blood tests revealed low testosterone levels. After a few months of testosterone supplementation, the patient's symptoms were relieved. "I also learned during that time once again to love myself, taking pride in myself and all that I do," he says.

Bob is an exceptional patient who has healed his life from some serious war injuries that left him with a debilitating and progressive back condition, heart disease, and a rare form of skin cancer. "Learn to be happy in your world. Life goes by too rapidly. Guard your precious relationships fervently! Show love and compassion to anyone who needs it. Be aware of your body and mind changes and seek help from professionals whenever you feel you need help. Eat healthy and try to grow older with grace and understanding that changes happen. Feel young, act young with dignity—stay healthy and happy as long as the higher power allows you to."

Bob and his fiancée, Anne, plan to be married next spring.

MEN'S HEALTH PROBLEMS

IMPOTENCE

Impotence is defined as the consistent inability to maintain an erection with enough rigidity to allow for sexual intercourse. *All* men have had temporary experiences with erection problems in their lives, for diverse reasons. Stress, finances, the flu, tiredness, certain drugs, and even a fight in the marriage or relationship can all temporarily defeat erections. William Shakespeare noted of alcohol, "It provokes the desire, but it takes away the performance."

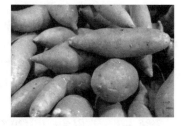

Approximately 10 million men are thought to be affected by impotence, and, in contrast to the belief a few decades ago, most cases are due to physical, nonpsychological factors. And, also unlike twenty or thirty years ago, men are not told "It's all in your head." Good treatment is available. Treatments range from mineral and herbal supplementation to external devices, drugs, implants, and hormone therapy. There is not the space here to review every treatment, but ask your urologist to inform you of your options.

A simple zinc deficiency, for instance, can be corrected by supplementation and a blood test can make the diagnosis. Many medications, including those for high blood pressure, can cause impotence. Ask your doctor or pharmacist to tell you about possible side effects.

To discover whether or not your impotence is permanent or not, there is a simple test available that you can do yourself. All men who are physically intact will achieve erections during their sleep. Wrap a strip of postage stamps around the penis at bedtime. (Not the self-adhesive kind.) If the roll of stamps is still intact the next morning for an entire week, then you're not experiencing nocturnal erections. Get a thorough medical examination from a urologist.

Sexual intercourse is an important part of our expression of emotional well-being and life enjoyment. Impotence can cause a lot of unhappiness and loss of self-esteem that is unnecessary, because effective treatment is available. Seeking treatment is a way to care for yourself and enjoy life, so for the sake of yourself and your partner, find out the cause and use the wealth of information available to you.

In Chapter 4, we discuss sexuality in the second half of life. Satisfying, even breathtaking sex is possible at age sixty, seventy, eighty, and beyond. If you feel like skipping to that now, turn to page 29. In the meantime, what follows is a thumbnail sketch of some of the reasons for erection failures and some of the methods that are now being used to deal with it in an effective way. Even as this is being written, current methodologies are being developed that may make this list obsolete.

REASONS FOR ERECTION DIFFICULTIES AND SOME TREATMENTS

Drugs that cause impotence. The dozens of possibilities include alcohol and marijuana, as well as prescription drugs such as antidepressants, tranquilizers, high blood pressure medication, and even over-the-counter antihistamines used for colds, sinus conjestion, and allergies. There are high blood pressure drugs that do not cause impotence, *so ask your doctor to switch you.*

Drugs that treat impotence. Bromocriptine, isoxsuprine, pentoxifylline, papaverine, and phentolamine are a few in usage.

Yohimbine. This Chinese herb to treat impotence is gaining popularity.

Acupuncture. Based on the ancient Eastern principle of balancing the body's hormones and stimulating body systems, acupuncture has been used as a treatment for impotence by the Chinese for thousands of years. Faced with drugs or surgery, many have found this nondrug system of healing very effective.

Atherosclerosis (hardening of the arteries). The penis requires a good supply of blood for all healthful functioning, just like every other part of the body. In Chapter 16, prevention strategies for atherosclerosis are discussed.

Nerve disorders. Chronic alcoholics tend to be impotent because long-term abuse of alcohol causes nerve damage. Long-term diabetes that is not managed effectively may also result in nerve damage. The key to managing diabetes is to practice the guidelines for controlling insulin levels on a daily basis: maintaining a healthy weight, exercising, following dietary restrictions, using insulin as instructed.

Hormone deficiency. Testosterone could be the key here. However, thyroid and pituitary gland functioning should also be investigated. A simple blood test can provide information in these cases.

Stress. Fatigue, depression, anxiety, stress—how easy is it to seek the joy of intimacy when it feels like the entire planet is crushing you down? Impotence is itself very stressful, even when it is an occasional event. It is important to rule out physical causes of depression, and then seek psychological medical intervention.

External devices. Condomlike devices that work via vacuum pressure to draw blood into the penis are successful. A ring around the base of the penis helps the erection last. When the ring is removed, the penis returns to normal. The devices can be either hand pumped or electronic. Many couples use the devices as part of foreplay, just as would be done with applying condoms.

Surgical implants. These have been around for almost thirty years. The three types in common usage are: semirigid, intermediate rigidity, and completely inflatable devices. Some of the implants can be inserted using only a local anesthetic. Ask your urologist to discuss the advantages of each.

ACUTE EPIDIDYMITIS

The epididymis is the first part of the duct that conducts sperm from the testicles to the vas deferens. In people under age forty, inflammation is usually the result of a sexually transmitted disease like gonorrhea or chlamydia. (Can you hear Dr. Ruth intoning you to practice safe sex right about now?)

Non-STD forms of epididymitis may be associated with prostatitis and urinary tract infections. Pain commonly occurs in the scrotum and may radiate to the side or flank of the abdomen. Fever, pain, and difficulty urinating along with swelling of the epididymis are other symptoms. Often men will delay treatment because the pain may occur after lifting weights or a sports-related trauma.

Prompt treatment usually results in a favorable prognosis, but promptness is the key here, as delay could result in infertility from scarring.

Benign Prostatic Hyperplasia (Enlarged Prostate)

The prostate is a part muscular, part glandular structure located below the bladder. A job description for the prostate is to secrete a thin, slightly alkaline fluid that neutralizes vas deferens and vaginal fluids in order to enhance sperm motility. It surrounds the neck of the bladder and the outlet of the bladder (the urethra) like a doughnut. This is a seeming design flaw that no one has been able to explain satisfactorily. It's tiny in boys four to six, smaller than a marble, but it increases to the size of a golf ball at sexual maturity.

In some men, the prostate can reach the size of a large orange by the age of seventy. If it didn't surround the urethra, but merely made its contributions via a side-lying duct, like those of the nearby seminal vesicles, there would be no problem. But swelling constricts the urethra and spells trouble. This is the architectural and engineering layout that has all the experts scratching their heads in disbelief.

Getting up a few times at night to urinate? Urinating with less force? Hesitancy before voiding is another key symptom of an enlarged prostate. However, these symptoms also mimic urethral strictures, bladder stones, prostatitis, and cancers of the prostate and bladder.

Benign prostatic hypertrophy (BPH) is age related, with about 20 percent of men experiencing it from age forty-one to fifty. Over 80 percent of men eighty years and older may have BPH, with about 50 percent complaining of a decrease of force and caliber of their urinary stream by age seventy-five. The cause is not completely understood. A digital rectal exam will explain whether the enlargement is in one area or more generalized.

The big question is, why does the prostate swell up? Experts theorize that hormonal changes are the cause. Testosterone is converted in increasing amounts to a slight variation called 5-alpha dihydrotestosterone (5-alpha DHT) after age forty. Male pattern baldness, male acne, and extra hair growth as well as prostatic hypertrophy and prostate cancer are all linked to specific types of 5-alpha DHT. Inhibitor drugs that block the enzyme (5-alpha-reductase) that is responsible for the conversion of regular testosterone to 5-alpha DHT have been tested and can shrink an enlarged prostate by about 30 percent. Finasteride (Proscar) is the first of a new class of 5-alpha-reductase inhibitors that targets unwanted androgenic hormone activity of 5-alpha DHT, producing significant relief of BPH. It works slowly, requiring about three to four weeks to shrink the prostate by just under 30 percent. Ninety percent of users experience significant improvement in urine flow, but only as long as they take the drug, and it's expensive. Experimental usage for prostate cancer and male pattern baldness offers new and exciting possibilities for this class of compounds. As a side note, in Chapter 9, you may read about topically applied DHT blockers that are being used to help reduce the effects of male pattern baldness.

Additionally, certain unsaturated fatty acids, such as gamma-linolenic acid (found in soybean and canola oil), are potent 5-alpha reductase inhibitors. Knowledge of 5-alpha-reductase is expanding rapidly at this point and further research will likely herald both biological and clinical roles that will help millions of men who suffer from BPH.

Treatment

At the moment, treatments for enlarged prostates include drugs such as alpha blockers, hormones, surgery, and dietary modifications (avoid irritants like spicy foods, too much alcohol, and anything that makes symptoms worse). Laser treatments and microwave hyperthermia, used experimentally until recently, may gain further ground. Balloon dilatation has been popular, but the results seem to be temporary. Removal of obstructing prostatic tissue by transurethral resection surgery (TURP) is the second most common surgery for men over the age of sixty-five.

As a dietary supplement, some men find saw palmetto berries and an extract from an African plant, pygeum, reduce symptoms. Peer-review research is scanty on this, because drug companies can't make money researching and marketing something that can be bought right now at any health food store.

The *British Journal of Pharmacology* published a 1984 study of 110 men with enlarged prostate glands. Patients on the saw palmetto extract experienced improved urine flow and 45 percent fewer nighttime urinations, to name only two symptoms. Those given a placebo had no improvement.

In my own experience with patients reporting their symptoms to me, I have noted their success with these dietary herbal supplements. Naturally, there is no indication that everyone will have the same results. Also, please understand that while this is a self-help book, I am *not* advocating that you diagnose and give treatment to yourself. The symptoms of BPH can mimic many other serious diseases, so get it checked out if you have any symptoms.

PROSTATITIS

Lower back pain, perineal pain around the anus, fever, chills, and irritative symptoms while urinating are the unforgettable and uncomfortable symptoms of acute prostatitis, inflammation of the prostate gland. These symptoms could be related to a bacterial infection or a localized inflammatory reaction with no infection present. It's important to get medical attention on this one right away. Not all of these symptoms may be present at the same time because not all prostates read from the same textbooks.

I have had patients come in with a complaint of lower back pain and "a feeling like I'm getting the flu or something." And it turns out to be acute prostatitis. This malady responds well to medical treatment if it is the bacterial kind of prostatitis. Otherwise, sitz baths (a big, plastic square basin large enough to sit in filled with hot water and epsom salts) can be effective.

However, *don't* try to diagnose this yourself, because if it's bacterial and you try the sitz bath routine, you could make matters worse for yourself. Leave it to the experts.

PROSTATE CANCER

"When you're a general, the doctors don't tend to do a thorough digital rectal exam," said the leader of the Gulf War forces in a *Los Angeles Times* headline story. A result, Gen. Norman Schwarzkopf's prostate cancer almost went undetected. Even though he had no symptoms, the general had been reading up on prostate cancer, so, during a routine hospital visit, he asked the doctor to do a more thorough exam. A lump was found, the biopsy confirmed prostate cancer, and he had a successful surgery. "Everything is absolutely, totally back to normal," he enthused after the surgery. "I feel like a million bucks," said the sixty-year-old general, who was spared incontinence and impotence because of a new nerve-saving surgical technique.

After the age of forty, men should get a yearly digital rectal examination by their doctor. However, many don't, and as a result, their cancers go undetected and untreated because the exam seems embarrassing or undignified. Perhaps it would be helpful to consider that undignified physical examinations are par for the course for women and, as a result, cancers of the genitalia are detected much sooner.

One in nine men will develop prostate cancer and 38,000 men die from it every year in America. Yet, if it is detected early, it can be cured. It would be great if there was a prostate screening test as good for male genitals as the Pap smear is for women, but for now, digital rectal examination and a blood test for prostatic specific antigen (PSA) are all there is. The problem with the PSA test is that elevated levels may indicate cancer, but 20 percent of men with prostate cancer have a normal PSA, and there is a 30 to 50 percent increase in men who have the common benign prostatic hypertrophy. A rectal exam *and* a PSA test are necessary, because a rectal exam alone could miss 32 percent of cancers present and an elevated PSA may be present in up to 50 percent of men who have no cancer.

PEYRONIE'S DISEASE

Abnormal curvature of the penis occurs in this condition, which affects middle-aged men and those older. A fibrous, calcified plaque on one side of the penis causes painful erections that are bent to one side. It is usually a self-limiting condition that often resolves itself spontaneously with no medical intervention. However, treat all lumps, thickenings, or sores that bleed or that do not heal with a lot of respect—go to a doctor and have them checked out. Unfortunately, there no statistics on how many men have Peyronie's disease, because many men are too embarrassed to see a doctor and don't seek treatment.

URINARY INCONTINENCE

Urinary incontinence is most often a problem in the elderly. Total incontinence is usually a result of nerve damage from previous surgery or disease. Overflow incontinence, in which urine is released without any sensation that the bladder is full, is thought to stem from a chronically distended bladder. Stress incontinence is leakage during activities that increase abdominal pressure on the bladder, such as coughing, sneezing, or lifting weights. Laxity of the pelvic floor muscles is the culprit here. Arnold

Kegel, M.D., developed the Kegel exercises as a nonsurgical alternative for incontinence. A stronger pubococcygeal muscle, a muscle that stretches from the pubic bone in front to the tail bone in back, will result from the workout. This muscle supports all the internal pelvic organs in men and women, and it will atrophy if it is not used. (For a fuller description of the Kegel exercises, please turn to page 258.)

TESTICULAR, PENILE, AND BREAST CANCER IN MEN

Male breast cancer accounts for 1 percent of new breast cancers each year. Cancer of the penis occurs in every one of 250 male cancer malignancies in America. Testicular cancer is found primarily in white men, with black or Asian men 75 percent less at risk. In all of these, early detection is the key to early and highly effective treatment.

LEARN HOW TO EXAMINE YOURSELF AND BE PROTECTED

At the same time every month, when you pay your bills on the first, for instance, make an appointment with yourself to do your own physical exam of your genitals. Ask your urologist to instruct you.

In the shower usually works best, because the testes contract when exposed to cold temperatures. Start by rolling each testicle between your thumb and fingers, comparing each one for symmetrical shape and size. They should be firm and rubbery and about an inch to an inch and a half in overall diameter. You can feel the epididymis, like a piece of spaghetti, running up the back of the testes. You are checking for any masses or lumps. Only a small percentage of lumps or masses turns out to be cancer, but leave it to the professionals here and go to your doctor if you find anything unusual. Since there are several thousand cases of male breast cancer each year, also palpate your chest every month checking for firm nodules or lumps.

Treatment for testicular cancer is also highly effective and excellent—*if it is diagnosed early*. This is one way to care for yourself and stay healthy, one month at a time.

24 COPING WITH CRISIS: GRIEF AND LOSS

Love knows not its depth 'til the hour of separation.

—Kahlil Gibran (1883–1931)

$\mathcal{G}$rief is natural, emotional suffering caused by any loss, misfortune, or disaster. This dictionary-based definition, however, only begins to describe it. In the silent soliloquys of our heart, grieving is the terrible pain and despair that knows the face of crisis. We cannot be immune to the windstorms of life. No amount of money can protect you—and no one else can help you survive it. No one escapes, as it is intrinsic to being alive. The loss of a loved one, especially the loss of a spouse or child, is considered to be one of the most powerful stressors in anyone's life. In the twenty-four months after the event, the survivors are more susceptible to illness and other physical ailments and their mortality rate is higher than expected.

The Chinese have a written character for the word *crisis*. It is a pictogram that shows both danger and opportunity. The danger is that of the wrenching emotional pain, the spiritual panic that affects us. The opportunity comes in the way that the ability to feel mental anguish can define us as sentient beings.

The loss of a loved one, for instance, presents with it the possibility of closing off our hearts and facing the world with only bitterness so that we will never have to open our hearts again. Even the loss of a loved one without death—a broken relationship, for instance—has caused many to withdraw into a shell so that they will never be wounded by their concept of love in the future. Of course, if we do that, we also block our chance to experience the ecstasy of love another time, perhaps in an even greater dimension.

Yet even in the midst of the most tremendous upheaval, there is the ability to cultivate our finest qualities as human beings—those of forgiveness, love and hope; the opportunity to face reality with acceptance and serenity; the chance to reach into ourselves and find the gentleness to create something new and beautiful out of a tragedy. These are the radiant possibilities that crisis can bring. The deep well springs of courage are something that you may never know until crisis demands their existence. In this way, the ancient Chinese symbol of opportunity in crisis is that of growth.

Parents so often try to shield their children from crisis. Yet how will they learn to cope with the windstorms of life if they are never exposed to them? Are we protecting them, or protecting ourselves from watching our children grow through the necessary pain of living? One study stated that a person who had faced childhood adversity and bounced back might even fare *better* in life than someone whose childhood was relatively easy. The same researcher followed up on the "new strain of resilient kids" at age forty and found that they tended to marry later, had fewer signs of emotional turmoil, were more likely to report that they were happy, and were 70 percent less likely to report mental health problems.

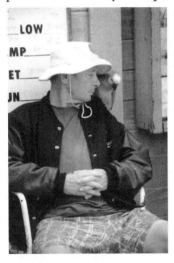

An example of this phenomenon is the best-selling author Dr. Ruth Westheimer, the sex therapist who fled the Nazis at age ten. Her parents died in the Holocaust and she grew up in an orphanage. "The values my family instilled left me with the sense I must make something out of my life to justify my survival," she has said.

Famed psychoanalyst Erik H. Erikson defined eight stages of life, each one a result of our biological demands and societal drives. He described each stage as a series of crises that must be resolved. The eighth and final stage of life, he described as *ego integrity versus despair*. As we age, we strive to reach the ultimate goal—wisdom, spiritual tranquility, and acceptance of our life and role in the world.

In living through the death of someone very close, we may be reminded of our own mortality. "Just as a healthy child will not fear life," said Erikson, "the healthy adult will not fear death." A thirty-nine-year-old patient who has been HIV positive for seven years told me: "Living each day as fully as possible is the most important way to keep me from being fearful of death. After all, everyone dies—the only difference is that with me, I know the *how* ahead of time."

The old expression, "Nothing good comes easy" makes its truthfulness felt as we struggle to recover from tragedy. Remember the sea plankton of prehistoric times? The crushing weight of layers of rock on the ancient sea beds produced diamonds, the hardest natural substances on earth. Will we allow ourselves to be crushed by our crisis or will we become diamonds?

The following are steps that may be useful to you in the future times. They have been helpful to me as I have struggled through the loss of loved ones most near and dear.

HOW TO HELP YOURSELF

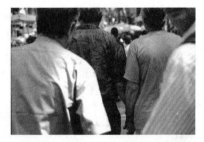

Take care today and build a strong body. The pure physical stamina that you cultivate can be an inextricable part of your ability to handle the pressure effectively. *Learn ways to manage the everyday stresses of living now.* The day-to-day management of stress establishes well-worn, comfortable pathways to power that will serve you in times of greater need.

Seek ways to express your painful feelings of despair. As a child, I found innate comfort in writing poems and lyrics. People with the established habit of keeping a journal or creating something with their hands and hearts know this tool. Another way to express your grief can sometimes be found in the action of helping others in a support group. Catharsis and cleansing comfort, as well as feeling that you are not alone in your grieving, are all part of the process. Hospice volunteers can be found in most hospitals.

When the grieving person feels the pressure of school or work and doesn't take the time necessary to fully mourn, a future loss may trigger an even more intense reaction. I remember that while I was in graduate school, several close friends died. Shortly after I graduated, yet another friend was lost, and I felt an exponentially intense period of mourning that shook me to the core. Finally I realized that I was mourning for all those who had died while I was too headlong into the rush of graduate school to take the time to grieve. You don't skip steps in your recovery from grief.

Don't expect a timetable. We are used to having a timetable for everything: nine months to have a baby, eight hours in a work day, seven days in a week, three minutes for a soft-boiled egg.

But grief does not follow a timetable or even a straight line. Instead, it's a crazy-quilt pattern of feeling that might be reasonably in control for a week or so followed by days on end being of disconsolate. This is when well-meaning, but misguided friends can do more harm than good with: "It's time to get on with your life!"; "What you need is to get out of the house"; "You'll get over it"; "You've been like this long enough." It's enough that you have to be patient with yourself without having to come up with an extra measure for others.

When my closest and dearest friend died at a young age, I remember how meaningful it was to receive a condolence card six months later. It was from a colleague I had really just met. Not surprisingly, we became very good friends over the years and I count that new friendship as one of the great blessings in my life. As a result, I now also send a note of condolence several months after a loss, when the other well wishers have moved on, but when the survivor is still grappling with the grief.

Become closer to the ones we will still have with us. Through the crushing pain and emptiness that we feel for the loss of a loved one, we can become closer to the ones we love now and realize that we should take every opportunity to express that love. Indeed part of the grief of loss is the guilt at never having expressed the love we felt as fully or as often as we would have liked. It is not too late now to tell the people who are close to you how much you love them, how much you care.

Develop and refine your spiritual beliefs. "Terminally ill patients who have some spiritual aspect to their life fare far better and suffer less than those who don't," says seasoned registered nurse Ellen Henehan, a practicing hospice nurse. "I don't care who the man is or what he's done," states chaplain Bill Glaser, of the Ventura County Jail. "If the worst criminal will just let God into his life, he can cope, feel God's love and forgiveness. He can survive the crisis of jail, the loss of freedom and family and with a spiritual commitment, he can become a man."

HOW TO HELP A GRIEVING FRIEND

Spend time with your friend and avoid platitudes. Don't bombard your friend with advice like "You'll snap out of it" or "It was really for the best" or "I know how you feel." Realize that no one knows how the grieving person feels except the grieving person him- or herself. Mourning is an important process and one that each individual must go through and not around.

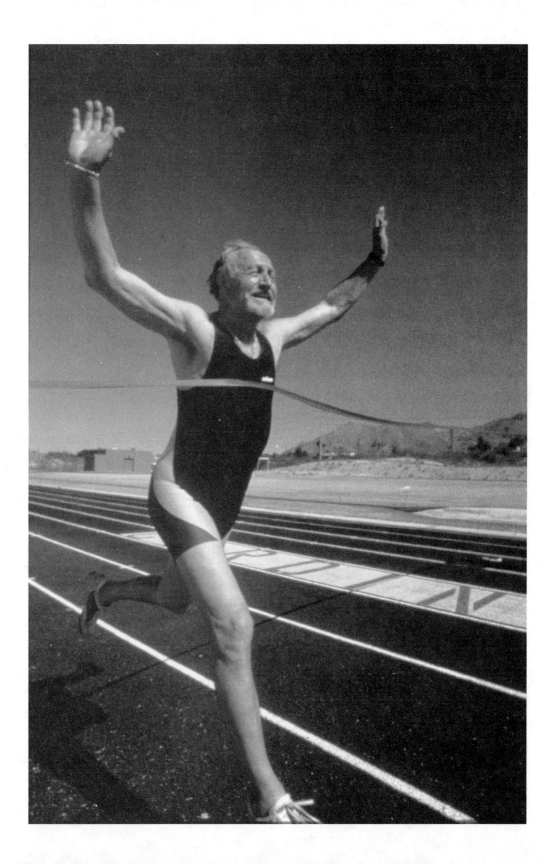

Don't say "If there's anything I can do to help." And then leave it at that. I appreciated the sentiment when I was grieving, but I derived the most comfort from a friend who noticed that my house was in a shambles and actually came over with her vacuum cleaner and started to help me clean up. "I'm going to the store—what can I pick up for you?" said another friend and the relief I felt at not having to face that chore myself was enormous at the time. So be specific in your offerings of assistance and you will be the most effective.

Let them talk—and listen. I had a loving friend who would simply listen as I told the stories of all the fun and adventures that I had experienced with my deceased friend. Talking about the wonderful times and having such an attentive listener was an important healing act. This can be especially true if your loss involved a younger person who died suddenly. When an older person dies after a lengthy illness, the mourning for the person often occurs while the person is still alive, but this is not to say that there are not still many emotions that need to be resolved.

If you can't visit, send cards and notes. You don't have to say much—simply that you care, that they are in your thoughts. There is comfort in any correspondence, even printed sympathy cards, just knowing that someone cares.

I asked my great-grandmother what is was like to live so long (she danced at her daughter's fiftieth wedding anniversary). I wanted to know if it was lonely to outlive all her friends, most of the people she loved. What do you do, I asked? How do you get through it? "You find new ones to love," she said. And then she gave me a chest-crushing bear hug.

Kahlil Gibran, the great Persian poet, wrote, "Your pain is the breaking of the shell that encloses your understanding." Of course, it's not only the great writers who know these truths. Each of us comes to know them, and at the times when this knowledge comes to you, I hope that you will be inspired to your highest healing powers.

25 EXTENDING THE HEALTH OF YOUR WEALTH INTO RETIREMENT

Skill'd to retire, and in retiring draw
Hearts after them tangled in amorous nets

—John Milton (1608–1674), *Paradise Regained*

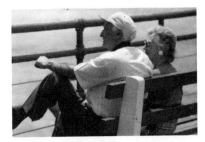

$\mathcal{B}$rides in the United States devote more than 180 hours and often up to $16,000 planning a wedding, while more than 70 percent of all American women have never determined how much money they will need to cover their retirement. And while women outlive men by five to seven years, they still earn nearly 30 percent less than men for doing the same jobs. That means that there's less money going into Social Security and pension plans.

Most people spend more time planning for their annual two-week vacation than they do planning their whole retirement. Job hopping, sabbaticals, corporate downsizing, switching careers, and entrepreneurial pursuits have left many of us with a checkered history of retirement savings vehicles, IRAs, and pension plans, if we have any at all.

Times have really changed since the early years after World War II when the postwar baby boom began. In 1948, for example, the median-income family in America paid 2 percent of its income to the Internal Revenue Service. In 1990, the same median-income family paid 24 percent of its income in federal income taxes and an additional 6 to 9 percent in state and local taxes.

Do you know why May 15 should be a national holiday? As of that date, you are earning money for yourself. All your paychecks prior to that date come to the amount you needed to pay your taxes.

Retirement, wills, and plans for how you want to spend the rest of your life are often topics that inspire people to a variety of emotions, from fear and anger to hope and enthusiasm. Did you know that less than 20 percent of attorneys have a will? I read that accountants have savings of less than 4 percent per year and that only 11 percent have made gifts or investments to minimize estate taxes. And these are the people we most commonly go to asking for financial advice.

RETIREMENT: WHAT DOES IT MEAN TO YOU?

There are no guarantees in life, but the percentages are greatly in your favor if you follow the health practices of staying young in this book. Chances are, you're not going to be sitting around in a rocking chair when you turn sixty-five, you're going to be out there roller-blading with your grandchildren. Indeed, if you are part of the late bloomers club, you could even be attending natural childbirth classes—for yourself!

With improved health practices, there is as much a growing trend toward early retirement as there is toward later retirement. There are more people celebrating their one-hundredth birthday in this country than ever before. Retirement used to mean you had ten years at most to defy the statistics and outlive the median age. Nowadays retirement at age sixty-five could mean that you have another forty years to reinvent yourself.

If you ask folks like my parents a question about retirement, they will talk excitedly about how these are the best years of their lives. "It's like a wonderful dream come true," they often exclaim. They're past the pressure of working at hard jobs, and they love the freedom to grow a big vegetable garden, travel, and enthusiastically pursue their fitness regimes.

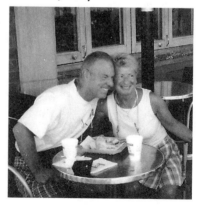

When one of my neighbors retired after a career he loved as an aerospace engineer, he called himself "a dinosaur." I'll never forget the night he and his wife returned from his retirement party and he was just standing in the driveway, hands in pockets, head down. His voice was cracking with emotion as he described to me his sense of loss. "How is a gold watch going to make me feel like getting out of bed tomorrow morning? What's the point of even waking up? I'm a has been."

Meanwhile, Maria retired from her job a month early. "It would have been twenty-five years today if I had just waited a little longer," she said, "but I figured, it's only a formality, I'm already sixty-five, so what's the big deal about getting a pen and pencil set if I wait another few weeks?"

You may identify with one or more of these attitudes about retirement. Or you may disagree with them based on your own experience when the time comes. Perhaps you will experience varying reactions at different points in time. One patient explained to me that even after almost forty years of marriage, living with her husband on a twenty-four-hour-a-day basis was a challenge and an adjustment that made her wonder how she was going to be able to stay married. All that togetherness was creating new conflicts that had to do with him wanting to tag along to every activity with her. "It drove me crazy until he took up golfing," she explained. Another couple spent more time together than ever, and it had another effect: "Our marriage is experiencing a wonderful renaissance. We're getting to know each other all over again and last night we went to a drive-in and fooled around like we were teenagers."

EARLY RETIREMENT FORMULA

"Save Plenty, Invest Aggressively, and Live Frugally." That was a headline from the *Wall Street Journal*, and it really sums up just about everything you need to know about retiring early. Naturally, there are other details, but devising a detailed financial program is not the focus of this book. Nonetheless, without claiming to have any financial answers, I have come up with many of the questions you should ask yourself, your accountant, tax advisor, or financial counselor to help you plan and provide for your retirement.

1. How can I plan for a successful retirement?
2. How can I develop my financial objectives and achieve my goals and aspirations?
3. How can I minimize my taxes?
4. How can I inflation-proof my income and savings?
5. How can I avoid unnecessary financial risk?
6. Where will we live?

7. How much money will we need for health-care, dental care, and prescriptions? What will the copayments, deductibles, and insurance payments be if one of us needs long-term care?
8. How much money do we want to leave behind for our families? Our favorite charities? To others who are important to us?
9. How can we achieve financial fitness in our young age and carry it over into our old age?
10. How much Social Security can I expect to receive?

Do You Really Want to Retire and Become a Couch Potato?

I'll never forget a couple who were friends of my parents when I was growing up. I remember hearing their voices in the living room when my sister and I were reading under the covers with flashlights and rolling our eyes at some of the things the adults were saying when they thought we were sleeping.

"We're not taking any vacations now and spending the money," the man boasted. "No sirree, the wife and I are saving up every penny until I retire, and then we're going to take a trip around the world. We've been planning for this trip for ten years already, and we're gonna get the money to go on that trip if it kills us."

So the couple worked. "Nose to the grindstone never hurt anyone," this man used to say to everyone. Well, do you know that after thirty years of working six and seven days a week on the railroad, this man finally retired. He died three months later and he never went on that trip. He was absolutely right when he said, "We're going to get the money to go on that trip *if it kills me*." Several years later, his widow finally was persuaded by the children to go by herself.

This story is so sad because we often treat happiness as if it were a destination. When we're young enough to enjoy it, we often defer those dreams of a special vacation together, a weekend getaway without the kids, an afternoon at the beach, because we'll do it *when . . . when* I get some time, *when* I get a better job, *when* the kids get older.

The problem is that when the kids get older, it's no longer cool for them to be seen with you; when you get a better job, there's more responsibility that goes with it often meaning that you have to take home work on the weekends; and when you get enough time, you'll be in your golden years and you may not want to or even be able to travel.

And it's not just about traveling. It's about how you want to experience today. Yes, I know—one must plan for the future. But certainly not at the price of enjoying the present. How many couples dream of taking a cruise "someday" and dancing under the stars? My parents went on a cruise to Alaska, and do you know that everyone was so on in years that the decks were practically deserted by nine o'clock because everybody had already gone to sleep?

Now is the time to take that cruise, while you know you can still enjoy it. Don't wait until you retire, like that couple who saved everything for a trip around the world and then could not make it together. So maybe you go on a shorter cruise for a long weekend or travel to a nearby bed and breakfast so that you can wake up late and eat crepes if you want them, without the kids creating a ruckus. *Now* is the time to do the things you want; shorten the way for yourself *in the present*.

Finally, let me share this with you: The people I interviewed for this book—in their seventies, eighties, even over a hundred years old—when I asked them if they had any regrets, they all said virtually the same thing, "It's not the things I did in my life that I regret—it's the things I *didn't do*."

A DREAM DEFERRED

Millions and millions of people dream of making more money, of getting rich quick. If they don't, then who is buying all those lottery tickets? What can we do about dreams deferred, plans that go awry? "I always thought I'd be retired by now,"

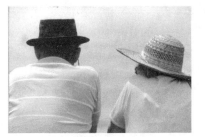

one man told me. "What happened? I have to face the reality that I can't afford to do that. I'm still helping the kids, running in the rat race more than ever."

I've heard that story many times, but perhaps the biggest problem we have, financially or otherwise, is thinking and expecting that there will be no problems. You show me a family, or a couple, or a person who has no problems in life, and we'll have to ask to see their membership card to the human race.

It's so hard to see tough times, especially tough financial times, as an opportunity, but in the long run, the incomparable opportunity to grow can make for the most excellent changed life.

Consider the following advertisement: "Wanted: Young, skinny, wiry fellows not over age eighteen. Must be expert riders, willing to risk death daily. Orphans preferred. Wages $25 per week."

If you fit the description from this 1800s help wanted ad, you'd have a job with the famous Pony Express. How would a want ad for your life read? Wanted: A workaholic with unlimited hours and a lot of local driving in exchange for room and board; must answer to the name *Mom*. Or, Wanted: Must love kids, dogs, and have an unlimited capacity to experience joy and beauty?

There is an endless list of financial scenarios that can make us feel that working that Pony Express job would be an improvement. A costly divorce, an untimely and expensive health problem, a grown child who still needs help, or a corporate downsizing are just some of the more common ones. A lot of people are thinking that it's hard enough getting through their youth, let alone planning for their old age.

Well, the line forms to the left. A lot of people are going through this. I know couples who will have to keep on working, regardless of the most well-thought-out plans for their golden years. Yet there are still possibilities. "When we realized that we were going to have to keep on working, at first, it was devastating and depressing," one woman wrote me. "But we're from North Dakota, and we decided that if this is our 'winter,' we'd figure out how to make the best of it." This couple reinvented themselves. She got extra training from a local college extension program and started her own medical transcribing business. He not only survived, but triumphed over a corporate downsizing by using his marketing and management skills to build a successful maid service company.

The tax code still gives small businesses big incentives to sock away money for retirement. As for the couple who reinvented themselves, they're making more money than they did before, but this time, they're investing in a diversified portfolio, not for a standard retirement, "because we're getting so much out of this, we want to do it for as long as it's interesting to us." Their savings are invested in an "in case we decide to chuck it all someday" fund.

NAME THAT TUNE . . .

What kind of life do you envision for yourself in the future? There are more options all the time and, in that spirit, here is a list of some of the more common choices.

There is an excellent book titled *Growing Older Together* from which I garnered a few golden nuggets of information for this list. Friends, patients, and my own experience were additional sources.

Not retiring. There are those of us who would prefer to die with our boots on. I absolutely love my work, and, God willing, I aspire to be the fittest chiropractor on the block when I'm ninety years old. I can't imagine not working and writing. The downside of this plan is that one could easily become a workaholic. Balance in life in the form of hobbies and relaxation pursuits with family and friends must be viewed as a necessity and not a luxury, because a disability derived from overwork could force retirement—just what you don't want.

Retiring into another job. About 25 percent of retirees continue to work, or go back to work as part-time or seasonal workers. Part-time income can supplement Social Security payments. The downside of this plan: Earnings above a certain level may prevent payment of full Social Security benefits until age seventy. Check with your local Social Security office to be sure.

Plan a second career. Reinventing yourself can be an exhilarating experience. Do you have a hobby like art, carpentry, or crafts-making? Betty turned her love of clothes and shopping into a wardrobe consultancy and personal shopper service. Ed, a retired architect, parlayed his long-standing devotion to the family garden into a freelance landscaping company. The downside of this plan is that the words "exciting new adventure" can be translated into "unwieldy burden" if you lack the entrepreneurial skills and training to handle your own business. Here's an idea: Transferring a long-standing love of sports may make you into a wonderful high-school basketball coach. Try volunteering for a season to see if it fits with your image of what it could be like. Then apply for a salaried position.

Become a health nut. My seventy-something mother regularly runs a few miles before breakfast every morning. Gypsy Boots, the ageless athlete, likes to build up an appetite for lunch by playing a few sets of aggressive single tennis. He's eighty-seven. Upside of this: Exercise will make you healthier and you may live a lot longer. Downside to this: You may, ironically, spend more time at the doctor's office. I often have a waiting room filled with enthusiastic weekends warriors with Monday morning sports injuries. Be sure to warm up thoroughly, and get good instruction on correct form when golfing, playing tennis, roller-blading, cross-country skiing, or whatever. Then go for it. And, of course, get a physical exam before starting an exercise program.

Go back to school. If you have a dream to be in a certain profession then go right ahead and start taking classes for it. You will be four years older whether you start college today or not. Why not get four years older and have the training you've always dreamed of? Downside to this plan: You will make new friends and think new ideas. Not for pessimistic, stick-in-the-mud types.

Volunteer to unretire. One friend spends every Wednesday volunteering at a local hospital. "We've made enough money to last us for the rest of our lives, so it doesn't make sense to get a job that pays me in dollars," she says. "When I was in the hospital, it was a volunteer who helped me feel at home in a painful and scary environment. Now that I am a volunteer, it feels wonderful to help make others a little more comfortable."

The Meals on Wheels program was the choice for a neighbor who wanted to put back something into the community. One man, a retired barber, volunteered to give shaves and haircuts to disabled patients at a local veteran's hospital. A lively patient has described her excitement at helping out as teacher's assistant at her granddaughter's elementary school. Her five-year-old granddaughter, thrilled at having her grandma as a teacher, said, "Grandma, when I grow up, I want to be retarded just like you!"

Would you like to help save the environment, mentor a new business owner, use your professional skill to help someone else get a leg up on life, work in a zoo? In 1987, there were twenty-three Peace Corps volunteers over the age of seventy.

Downside of this plan: You may have to structure you own involvement or define your own parameters of a job description if the organization you hook up with is unused to tapping the energies and talents of older volunteer workers.

Become a tightwad. Don't buy stuff you don't need, and take your lunch to work. The money saved from brown bagging could be $5 to $10 per day. Let's say it's $6 a day. That's about $1,200 a year. If you invested that money in a tax-deferred fixed annuity earning only 7 percent interest, you'd have over $10,000 in only seven years. For other savings tips, you can subscribe, for a measly one dollar a month, to the *Skinflint News* (P.O. Box 818, Palm Harbor, Florida 34682-0818).

On the one hand, all the experts say to live really frugally—some warn against ever eating out or going to a movie theater, better to stay home and eat popcorn with a video instead. Some books I've read have advised giving away your car and house *now* in order to save for the future. While these ideas may be too extreme for you, there's a lot to be said for simplifying your lifestyle. I was sent the following quotation about living life in the simple lane, and unfortunately I do not know the author, so I cannot give credit the person who wrote it: "One hundred years from now it will not matter what my bank account was, what sort of house I lived in, or what kind of car I drove; but the world may be a different place because I was important in the life of a child."

Downside of this: You may not always be in the mood to read about how to make wonderful papier-mâché objet d'arts out of dryer lint in lieu of buying holiday gifts.

Postpone your retirement another twelve to twenty-four months. If you defer retirement from age sixty-four to age sixty-six, you may increase your Social Security benefits by 13 percent for the rest of your life. Additionally, you will be adding to your retirement savings because, of course, you'll be dipping into them several years later. Downside of this: Stretching out your career may not be possible in the current corporate setting.

Retire early. There is often a lump sum available as an incentive toward helping employees make the decision to cut out early. If you were to find another job to pay the bills for say, two years longer, that lump sum could mushroom into a tidy little amount in a tax-deferred fixed annuity. Downside to this: It may be hard to find a job you like, and it might pay less than what you're used to.

ACHIEVING BALANCE

If you think that I'm sending out a mixed message here about retirement, you're right. You must walk the line between saving and investing in the future while squeezing the juice out of life right now.

About half of all workers age forty-five and older are concerned that they may outlive their savings, according to one survey by Merrill Lynch that I read about in a magazine whose name sums it up nicely: *Better Choices*. The bottom line is that retirement can be either wonderful or frightening, depending on how you look at it—either the greatest opportunity to reinvent yourself or not. The only thing that's guaranteed is: If you decide well, it won't be dull.

If you're not a financial wizard, exquisitely poised in matters of savings and investments, get some professional help from a financial advisor. I like the following view from *Better Choices* magazine: "Fortunately, it's not too late. If you're a typical fifty-something worker, you can still pull off some cunning financial moves that will transform your retirement outlook from gloomy to good—or downright glorious."

I'd say more about that, but I'm right in the middle of making a gigantic papier-mâché piggy bank out of the dryer lint I've been saving, and I gotta go . . .

Profiles in Living

No wise man ever wished to be younger.

—Jonathan Swift (1667–1745)

It's sad to grow old, but nice to ripen.

—Brigitte Bardot

*M*ost people are afraid of what time will do to them. Even children. An eight-year-old patient of mine was watching as I helped a ninety-seven-year-old woman to the door. "Does it hurt to get old?" she asked.

It was the most simple and most complex question that I've ever been asked. In that one microsecond, I thought of hundreds of answers—from the existential quandary of it all to the fidelity of misery, the emotional, spiritual, and even physical growth earned with the currency of pain. Before I replied, I recalled the pain of too much tenderness, the bittersweet anguish of parting from loved ones, the gripe of sore joints and backs, the ache of loneliness, of winning and losing, and even the throb of a heart bursting with joy.

"Not always," I answered. "Why do you think it might hurt?"

" 'Cause that old lady walks so slow it looks like it hurts."

"Well, she was in a car accident, but she's getting better."

"Oh. I wanted to ask you something else"

I waited, almost dreading the next question.

"Have you got any more of those peppermint candies?"

A temporary reprieve—I knew that it was only a matter of time until I'd be stumped by this eight-year-old again! But the point is that most people are afraid of what time is doing to them when it would be far better to think about what they are doing to their time.

This book was inspired many years ago when I saw the enthusiasm for living in my great-grandmother. The ceiling in her kitchen was painted fire engine red. She lived alone and grew her own garlic and danced the polka at my grandparents' fiftieth wedding anniversary with an energy that made me huff and puff. I was her partner in a vigorous troika with my grandmother in the middle of this classic three-person Ukrainian dance. I remember breaking into a sweat and glancing over at my great-grandmother in amazement as she picked up

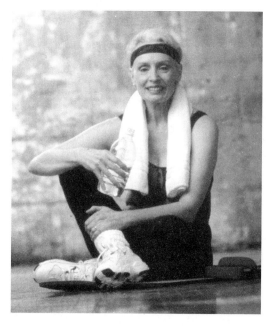

the pace and made a few more rounds on the dance floor—my grandmother was egging her on!

I was already a world-class athlete at the time, so this romp around the dance floor created an even greater impression. I remember thinking that Baba must have arteries the size of cannons! What makes some people ripen like that into fireballs of energy, while others are slumped on the sidelines, so tired they can barely shuffle through life? You'll meet some very inspirational people in this chapter who will share their learning with you.

MARVIN B. SMALL

At six-foot-two and three-quarters inches tall and 170 pounds, Marvin B. Small is anything but undersized. He's a commercial pilot in active retirement as a champion bicycle rider and an aspiring actor. Hometown: Gadsden, Alabama. Age: seventy-three. Father of four children, grandfather of four. A World War II pilot, he attended Vanderbilt University before the war. After the fighting was over, he graduated on a football scholarship from the University of Kansas as a member of the 1948 Orange Bowl team. He has won two gold medals in the 1985 Senior Olympics and has a winning attitude that is so infectious that after talking to him for five minutes, you want to drop to the floor and start doing push-ups.

"I've had a life filled with something I dearly loved—flying. Every day flying is like a play day. I used to say: You mean to tell me that they *pay* you to do this? I look forward to every day on the job."

"The outdoors is God's gift," says the energetic Southerner with contagious enthusiasm. "Bicycle riding puts you right up there in God's world—for me, up there in the mountains. People ought to get outside and do something. They spend so much time fixing up things around the house and just let their bodies go to pot."

I asked Marvin to prioritize the key values that have motivated him: "The most important thing in your life is *health*. The second most important thing is *family*. The third most important thing is *friends*. And the fourth most important thing is having enough money to enjoy the first three."

Marvin "walks his talk" as they say on the streets of Los Angeles. "I've always thought about the future—you have to live within your income on the frugal side." Same principle carries over into what you eat: Marvin drinks no coffee, tea, or soda and learned early in his career as a pilot that the jet-set lifestyle was not for him.

"A lot of martini drinking," he says.

The key to enjoying life? "I try not to worry about too much or take myself too seriously. You have to laugh at yourself. People ought to have goals, have hope, have faith. You only go down this road once—try to have a good time. It's a bright new world out there every single day."

EDITH BUTLER

Edith Butler did all the typing for my first three books. When I first met her, she opened the door and I saw a light surrounding her, as if her kindness was shining out from her. She looked like a guardian angel straight out of heaven. She was even wearing a long diaphanous dress that added to the effect. In the years that have intervened, I have come to know Edith and admire her courage and go-for-it attitudes about life. She was a "Rosie the Riveter" on the assembly line of a munitions factory during World War II.

When I met her, she was working part-time playing the organ for the shopping plaza across the street from her apartment in Coral Gables, Florida. Apartment-bound because of ongoing foot problems, she now manages a nursing referral service at night, which requires a constant vigil by the telephone to handle medical emergencies of every type. She is a twice-widowed mother of one son and grandmother to his two children. I asked for her recommendations on conquering loneliness and isolation.

"Frankly, it is a never-ending battle and some days one method will work better than another. Primarily, one should savor the obvious pleasures and privileges of solitude. Indulge yourself. According to your mood, prepare a quick snack to eat on a tray table in front of the TV, or place a few flowers in a pretty vase and lay a formal place setting of the best china on the dining table for a special time and effort gourmet meal.

"Go to bed as early or late as you want. If awakened in the night, read a good book or get up and make a cup of hot tea without fear of disturbing a companion. Play the type of music you prefer. Consider some type of pet for which you must be responsible, a living thing to greet you when you come in the door of your empty home.

"Develop a hobby that produces some sense of achievement, such as growing flowers to exhibit in shows, to sell or donate to a church or hospital. Flower seeds are inexpensive and dirt is free outside. Join a church or volunteer organization, study something that interests you, or take a job that will occupy your free time and keep your mind alert. They will hire seniors at fast food restaurants.

"Find comfort yourself by comforting someone else who has more recently suffered the same type of loss. Don't overwhelm the person with your well-meant good intentions and don't offer platitudes that may be resented, such as 'Time will heal,' 'It is God's will,' etc. Express your understanding and sympathy for their grief and despair based on your own personal experience. For instance, a person who was never a parent can't empathize with someone who has just lost a child in an accident.

"There are, of course, some people who are beyond help. They can't or won't lift themselves from a bog of self-pity and irritability that totally ignores their remaining blessings, and these people are to be avoided like the plague. They will bog you down in their negative output. We must learn to distinguish it from a truly courageous attempt to overcome adversity."

"Travel, if finances permit. In my case, I make do with an occasional trip to a big shopping mall in an adjoining town. I find that one of the hardships of living alone in a small apartment is that redecorating or large purchases for the home are reduced to a mere trickle. Therefore, when I feel at a low ebb, I try to take advantage of a sale to buy a few towels, a small flower arrangement, or even a new blouse.

"I spread my Christmas shopping over a couple of months, taking time and care in selecting something special rather than making a hasty decision. Engrossed in thoughts about someone else's happiness and returning home with a package in hand keeps the real world in focus.

"One does tend to feel isolated from the main stream and without purpose in life—if we don't search for one.

"Last, but not least, it's important to preserve one's femininity. There's nothing as rejuvenating as a warm, interested glance from a nice looking man. Unfortunately, we're greatly outnumbered as we get older, but for some of us, life can still be beautiful if we give it a chance."

Edith continued playing the piano and organ and got several jobs playing Christmas carols during the holidays each year. She was a regular contributor to the Letters to the Editor section in her local newspaper as well as a regular baby-sitter for her two grandchildren. I had the honor of being the last person to speak to her, and she told me of her desire to be with her husband, George Butler, who had died almost twenty years before. She went on to meet him while this manuscript was in preparation.

TONY URBAITIS

Tony Urbaitis, eighty-five, first introduced me to cayenne pepper by way of an old-country remedy from his homeland in Lithuania. *Nastoika* is made with a handful of pepper pods along with peony root, berries from ash, coriander, and cardamon. All this is added, naturally, to a bottle of vodka and then stored for a few months.

A one shot-glassful was given to me after I had finished a gruelling cross-country ski race, complete with frost bite and hypothermia (the opposite of heat stroke). After one swallow, my lips, mouth, and throat were aflame. Irreparable damage seemed imminent! After a few tense minutes though, the fire subsided and I felt positively glowing—and very warmed up.

Years later I learned of cayenne's styptic qualities when Tony sprinkled some cayenne pepper on a deep cut from a wood knife. The burning was incredible. I yelled at him, but he only laughed like crazy. But the bleeding stopped in seconds, a scab formed, and I didn't need stitches. There was no infection later, but *kids, don't try this at home!*

Besides harboring a wealth of herbal lore, Tony, a confirmed bachelor, has an eye for pretty women. "Just looking at them—they keep you from getting wrinkled," he says. He and his betrothed were separated on a train traveling to one of the many Gulag camps written about by Alexander Solzhenitsyn. He promised to wait for her, but he was never able bring her back. So he never married.

To what does he credit his youthful energy?

"Be kind, have charity for all the Lord's little ones. Anything that is living needs help—and some of the little creatures of the earth can't ask." There are bowls of cat food and saucers filled with grains and seeds for the birds and squirrels outside his door on the cold days of the Canadian winter. He cut a large window in the basement wall of the apartment where he lives in an old Gothic house in old Toronto. "This is the best TV in the world," he says, pointing to all the animals and birds feeding outside in the snow. In his lurching 1948 Chevy truck, he heads out in snow storms to distribute food to the homeless people he finds tucked into the nooks and crannies of High Park, the forested haven near the center of the city.

Tony is a wonderful cook, baker, and maker of everything from wooden shoes, candles, and herbal remedies to curtains that he makes on his vintage sewing machine. Fresh dark rye bread fermented for a day, raisin-honey wine, and the rust removing *Nastoika* are only some of his specialties.

"Give all the people who need it all they can eat. A poor man or a hungry family, human, animal, or bird—feed them all. Love means never having to say you're hungry."

CURLY KRIEGER

"A guy scaling a vertical wall doesn't say: 'What am I going to do?' he says: 'Where are the crevices?'

"Financially, most people don't win because they don't plan. Put something away for a rainy day, because it rains a lot later on in life."

Milton "Curly" Krieger, now eighty-four, is a muscular six-footer. But when his father died of a stroke at forty-four and his sister died of leukemia five months later, the teenage Milton "felt like I was a goner," he recalls.

He took up running twenty-five years ago after seeing a man jogging in the rain by the roadside when he was driving. He started running speed intervals at age seventy-three and finished ahead of 51 percent of the field at the classic Beverly Hills 10K footrace one year later. Swimming and tennis are two other activities in addition to his voracious reading.

"Getting the essence out of this one trip in life is vital," he says in his deliberate, thoughtful style of speaking. "Being the best I'm able to be. 'What's a heaven for?' is that old corny saying of Browning's. I like to benefit from the best of what people have poured into books and scholarship.

"When you're in there slugging, you can't help but worry, but I would have worried less in life. You win some here, you lose some there—so don't be afraid. Be positive. The fun's in the journey."

GYPSY BOOTS

"I've always tried to throw myself into everything I've done. Selling newspapers on street corners and marketing fruit on a highway won't impress most people if they see it included in a formal job resume. But the important thing is not what you do in life, but how you do it.

"I can't say that I've made much money, but I haven't had an unhappy day. That is more valuable than all the money in the world to me."

A zany naturalist with the wiry body strength of a teenager at eighty-six, this father of three and grandfather of five still does hard physical labor unloading hundreds of pounds of organic fruit each week from his health food delivery truck, "the Bootsmobile."

Gypsy is truly an ageless athlete. He runs and throws a football hard enough to knock the wind out of you—or sprain your wrist, which is why I won't play catch with him anymore. He was a guest on more than twenty-five episodes of the Steve Allen show. I met him one fine sunny afternoon almost twenty years ago when I opened the front door of my Venice Beach condominium to find the dirtiest pair of tanned feet I ever saw waving back and forth in front of my face. Gypsy, standing on his head and playing the tambourine was singing "I eat the nuts and fruits—my name is Gypsy Boots!" He then sprang to his feet and opened a big box of fresh Medjool dates and handed it to me saying "Make sure you tell all your friends about all the dates you had with Gypsy Boots!" That was some special delivery!

"I have walked until my feet were worn out," he says, although a glance at his bare tanned feet and muscular legs and you have to assume he is talking about a *lot* of walking.

"But I slept each night better than a king. Never have I taken a sleeping pill, like so many of the 'successful' and 'happy' people I know. Indeed, those successful and happy people come to me for help."

Gypsy's two books, *Barefeet and Good Things to Eat* and *How To Stay Young at Any Age*, are full of recipes, philosophies, and the humor that are part of his "nutrition ignition" program.

"My motto is this: Have a good time in life and take care of the body God gave you. Eat properly and laugh. Laugh your way to health. Wash all that down with plenty of Kyolic everyday and you've got it made!"

It's true. He acts like a crazy nut, but it is just his way of getting the message across in an entertaining way.

"The food you put in your heart and mind is more important than the good food you put in your stomach. If you feel lonely or sad, then fast for a day or two and you'll feel a lot better.

"We're living in a spoiled world. It's okay to have a car and a radio and all. But we came into this world with nothing but innocence and pureness and love and we leave

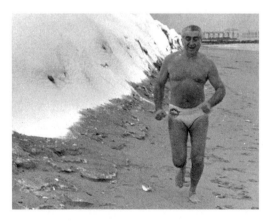

with nothing. The only way to space the bookends of life is to do one good and loving deed each day."

VIC BOFF

Some people love to warm themselves in a summer breeze, others love to walk in the crisp clean fall air. But when the weather turns cold and blustery, that's when Vic Boff puts on his bathing trunks and heads for the beach at Coney Island. You see, he's the founder of Brooklyn's world famous Iceberg Athletic Club.

"It's a tremendous stimulant. You're out in the air; your body's bombarded with cold; your blood is circulating; and when you come out of the icy water, you're a bright red. It's just a great, great feeling.

"There are days so dark and cold when we can't see another human being out there. Sure, I'm proud of this club. There isn't another outdoor club in the world that can boast of the day-in day-out attendance our club has shown in the last sixty-eight years.

"Fear of the cold is psychological. In order to appreciate it, you've got to try it. If you turn blue, it's not for you."

Vic Boff didn't miss a Sunday in over fifty years. On Sunday December 28, 1952, he spent a record twelve hours on the beach—9 A.M. to 9 P.M.—and swam in the icy ocean waters twelve times every hour on the hour, while the city of New York suffered through the coldest weather of the season: seven degreess below zero.

Now, at eighty-one, the man who aspired to learn physical culture as a boy in Red Lion, Pennsylvania, will always be respected by the countless people he has helped to a more natural way of living through his many health books and daily advice given from his Natural Foods store on 86th Street in Brooklyn. His mentors have been the Mighty Atom, Bernarr McFadden, Joe Bonomo, and John Grimek.

"If my induction into the Natural Hall of Fame does anything to eliminate kids taking drugs like steroids, then I'm happy," he says. He abhors the current bodybuilding superstars who have used drugs to achieve their success. "Many of today's athletic stars are setting dangerous examples for the youngsters who look up to them."

Now living in Boca Raton, Florida, he misses the colder climes in winter, but still takes ice baths regularly. Each year, he organizes the annual banquet for the Oldetime Barbell and Strongmen, an international organization dedicated to honoring physical culturists of this century. Vic is a man who's spent a lifetime staying close to Nature and his own ideals. Carry on, Vic!

People learn new skills and lose old ones throughout their lives. This book is dedicated to helping you acquire new talents and guide you toward examining some habits that may be getting in your way. I'll bet you already have some wonderful strategies of your own. May you take what you need and leave the rest. Let's ripen and improve into the most powerful people we can be. Here's to a lifetime of breathtaking intimacy, of unlimited brain power, of restful sleep, and joyful vitality and vigor. Let's make aging become the most interesting and powerful thing that we do.

Write to me and let me know how your journey is going. I'd love to hear how you are staying alive and well and we'll put you on our mailing list for future information. In the meantime, I hope you enjoyed reading this book as much as I've enjoyed writing it. I've tried to give you the most up-to-date information available, but please understand that knowledge is a dynamic quantity—even as you read these words, new data and discoveries are being announced somewhere in the world. My hope is that you will use the information, build your healthy future and have enough energy left over at the end of your day to share with the ones you love.

Yours in health,

Gayle Olinekova, D.C.

Selected References

ANTIOXIDANTS

Haran, D. "Free Radical Theory of Aging: The "Free Radical" Diseases. Age; 7:111-131.

Kushi, L.H., et al. "Dietary Antioxidant Vitamins and Death from Coronary Heart Disease in Post-menopausal Women," *New England Journal of Medicine*, 1996; 33:1156-1162.

Pandey, D.K., et al. "Dietary Vitamin C and Beta Carotene and Risk of Death in Middle-Aged Men." *American Journal of Epidemiology*, 1995. 142:1269-1278.

Raloff, Janet. "Novel antioxidants may slow aging." *Science News*, January 25, 1997. Vol.151;53.

Tappel, A. "Will Antioxidant Nutrients Slow Aging Processes?" *Geriatrics*, 1968;23:97-105.

Wu, Corinna. "How antioxidants defend cells." *Science News*, February 15, 1997. Vol 151;111.

ARTHRITIS

Adler, Tina. "Mending Joints." *Science News*, November 12, 1994; Vol.146:31-319.

Colt, George Howe. "The Magic of Touch." *Life*, August 1997.

Drovanti, A., et al. "Therapeutic activity of oral glucosamine sulfate in osteoarthritis: a placebo-controlled double-blind investigation." *Clinical Therapeutics*, 1980;3(4): 260-272.

Vas, A.L., et al. "Double Blind clinical evaluation of the relative efficacy of ibuprofen and glucosamine sulfate in the management of osteoarthritis of the knee in out-patients." *Current Medical Residence Opinion*, 1982;8: 145-149.

Whitaker, Julian, M.D., *Health & Healing*, August 1996;Vol.6 No. 8

BACK CARE

The U.S. Department of Health and Human Services Clinical Practice Guidelines from the Agency for Health Care Policy and Research Number 14 : "Acute Low Back Problems in Adults" is a most excellent resource, compiling 360 research articles. This one publication is written for doctors, but contains accessible information that a motivated reader could find useful.

Anderson, R., et al. "A meta-analysis of clinical trials of spinal manipulation." *Journal of Manipulative and Physiological Therapeutics*, March-April 1992;(15(3) : 181-94.

Haldeman, S., et al. "Guidelines for chiropractic quality assurance and practice parameters. Proceedings of the Mercy Center Consensus Conference," 1993. Gaithersberg, MD: Aspen Publishers, Inc.

Hadler, N.M., et al. "A benefit of spinal manipulation as adjunctive therapy for acute low-back pain: a stratified controlled trial." *Spine*, September, 1987;12(7): 703-6.

Jarvis, K.B., et al. "Cost per case comparison of back injury claims of chiropractic versus medical management for conditions with identical diagnostic codes." *Journal of Occupational Medicine*, August, 1991;33(8) : 847-52.

Manga, P., et al. "The effectiveness and cost effectiveness of chiropratic management of low back pain." University of Ottawa, Canada, 1993.

Mathews, J.A., "Back pain and sciatica: controlled trials of manipulation, traction, sclerosant and epidural injections." *British Journal of Rheumatology*, December, 1987;26(6) ; 16-23.

Nykvist F., et al. "Social factors and outcome in a five-year follow-up study of 276 patients with sciatica." *Scandanavian Journal of Rehabilitation Medicine*, 1991;23(1):19-26.

Spengler, D.M., et al. "Back injuries in industry: a retrospective study." *Spine*, April 1986;11(3):241-56.

Waddell, G. "A new clinical model for the treatment of low-back pain." *Spine*, September 1987;12(7): 632-44.

CANCER

Ames, B. University of California, Berkeley. "Understanding the Causes of Aging and Cancer"

Clark, L.C., et al. Effects of selenium supplementation for cancer prevention in patients with carcinoma of the skin." *Journal of the American Medical Association*, December 25, 1996;276(2): 1957-1985.

Maugh, Thomas H. II. "The Disease Men Try to Ignore." *Los Angeles Times*, January 2, 1995.

Raloff, J., "Aged Garlic could slow prostate cancer." *Science News*, April 19, 1997. Vol. 151;239.

From the United Nations and World Health Organization First Joint Conference on Healthy Aging, April 29-May 1, 1996, New York, NY.

Sternberg, S. "Can selenium ward off deadly cancers?" *Science News*, January 4, 1997. Vol.151;6.

EYES & EARS

Brownlee, Shannon, et al. "The Senses" *U.S.News & World Report*, January 13, 1997;50-59.

Dunlop, Marilyn. "Cell regeneration could reverse hearing loss." *The Toronto Star*, July 10, 1993.

Raloff, Janet. "Eyeing fetal cells to reverse blindness" *Science News*, November 3, 1996. Vol.

Sardi, Bill. "Eradicating Cataracts" *Townsend Letter for Doctors*, June, 1995; 50-59

Seachrist, Lisa. "Growing In and Out of Focus", *Science News*, November 11, 1995. Vol.148;318.

Seddon, J.M., et al. "The use of vitamin supplements and the risk of cataract among US male physicians." *American Journal of Public Health*, May 1994;84(5): 788-792.

Seddon, J.M., et al. "Dietary Carotenoids, vitamins A, C, and E, and advanced age-related macular degeneration." *JAMA*, November 9, 1994;272(18): 1413-1420.

Sternberg, S. "Smokers risk vision loss in twilight years." *Science News*, October 12, 1996. Vol.150;213.

The University of California at Berkeley Wellness Letter, June 1995. "Wellness Made Easy" (re: halogen lamps)

Uhlmann, R.F., et al. "Relationship of hearing impairment to dementia and cognitive dysfunction in older adults." *JAMA.*, 1989;262:1916-1919.

EXERCISE

News From the American Heart Association, "23-Year Study of Middle-Aged Men in Hawaii Confirms: Physical Activity Will Lower Risk of Heart Disease." June 13, 1994.

Astrand, P.O., "J.B. Wolffe Memorial Lecture. 'Why exercise?' " *Med Sci. Sports. Exerc.*, February 1992. Vol. 24(2);153-162.

Christensen, H., et al. "The association between mental, social and physical activity and cognitive performance in young and old subjects." *Age Ageing*, May, 1993. Vol. 22(3);175-182.

Emery, C.F., et al. "Long term effects on psychological functioning in older men and women." *Journal of Gerontology*, November 1991. Vol. 46(6);352-361.

Evans, W.J. "What is sarcopenia?" *Journal Gerontol. A Bio. Sci Med. Sci.*, November, 1995;50 Spec:5-8

Kegel, Arnold. "The Physiologic Treatment of Poor Tone and Function of the Genital Muscles and of Urinary Stress Incontinence." *Western Journal of Surgery, Obstetrics and Gynecology*, 1949, Vol 57;527-35.

Raloff, Janet. "Vanishing Flesh: Muscle loss in the elderly finally gets some respect, *Science News*, August 10, 1996. Vol. 150(2); 90-91.

Sparrow, W.A., et al. "Effect of physical exercise on the performance of cognitive tasks." *Percept. Mot. Skills*, October, 1993. Vol.77;(2);675-679.

FERTILITY

Reuter's, *Today's News*, Feb 19, 1997. (Reporting on the February 1997 study in the *American Journal of Epidemiology* on caffeine and fertility study of 3,187 women in Denmark.)

Caplan, Arthur. "The Brave New World of Babymaking." *Life*. December, 1993;88-90.

Dowling, Claudia Glenn, et al. "Miraculous Babies." *Life*. December, 1993;75.

Joesoef, M.R., et al. "Are caffeinated beverages risk factor for delayed conception." *Lancet*, 1990;335:136-137.

Painter, Kim. "Doctors have prenatal tests for 450 genetic diseases." *USA Today*, August 15, 1997.

Wilcox, A., et al. "Caffeinated beverages and decreased fertility." *Lancet*, 1988;2:1453-1455.

HAIR

Cortois, M., et al. "Ageing and hair cycles." *British Journal of Dermatology*, Jan, 1995; 132(1): 86-89.

Legro, RS., et al. "Alterations in androgen conjugate levels in women and men with alopecia." *Fertil-Steril.*, October, 1994;62(4): 744-50.

Mielke, Howard, Ph.D., et al. "Lead Based Hair Products: Too Hazardous for Household Use"

Rhodes, L., et al. "The effects of finasteride on hair growth, hair cycle stage, and serum testosterone and dihydrotestosterone in adult male and female stumptail macaques." *Journal of Clinical Endocrinology and Metabolism*, October 1994; 79(4): 991-6.

Thorton, M.J., et al. "Differences in testosterone metabolism by beard and scalp hair follicle dermal papilla cells." *Clinical Endocrinology Oxford*, December, 1993;39(6): 633-9.

HEART

Cowley, Geoffrey. "The Heart Attackers." *Newsweek*, August 11, 1997;54-60.

Criqui, M.H., et al. "Does diet or alcohol explain the French paradox?" *The Lancet*, 1994;344 8939-8940): 1719-23.

Fackelmann, K.A., "Calcium Guards Against Hypertension." *Science News*, November 21, 1992. Vol. 142;340-341.

Gillman, M.W., et al. "Protective effects of fruits and vegetables on development of stroke in men." *JAMA.*, April 12, 1995;35: 316-318.

Mitchell, L.E., et al. "Evidence for an association between dehydroepiandrosterone sulfate and nonfatal, premature myocardial infarction in males." *Circulation*, January, 1994;89(1):89-93.

Olzewer, E. et al. "EDTA chelation therapy in chronic degenerative disease." *Medical Hypotheses*, 1988; 27: 41-49.

Rimm, E.B., et al. "Vitamin E consumption and the risk of coronary heart disease in men." *New England Journal of Medicine*, May 20, 1993;328(20): 1450-1456.

Sehub, J., et al. "Vitamin status and intake as primary determinants of homocysteinemia in an elderly population." *JAMA.*, December 8, 1993; Vol.270(2);2693-2698.

Stampfer, M., et al. "Vitamin E consumption and the risk of coronary heart disease in women." *New England Journal of Medicine*, May 20, 1993;328(20): 1444-1449.

Stephens, N.G., et al. "Randomized Controlled Trial of Vitamin E in Patients with Coronary Disease: Cambridge Heart Antioxidant Study (CHAOS)." *Lancet*, March 23, 1996;347:781-786.

Verschurten, W.M., et al. "Serum Cholesterol and long-term coronary heart disease mortality in different cultures." *JAMA*, July 12, 1995;74(2): 131-136.

Winslow, Ron. "Pricey Prescription" Powerful Medications For Cholesterol Pose A Paradox for HMO's." *Wall Street Journal*, December 6, 1996.

MEMORY

————. "Rescuing memories with age . . ." *Science News*, October 28, 1995; Vol.48;283.

Fackelmann, Kathleen. "Forecasting Alzheimer's Disease." *Science News*, May 18, 1996; Vol.149;312-3.

Fackelmann, Kathleen. "Forever Smart; Does estrogen enhance memory?" *Science News*, February 4, 1995;Vol. 147;74-75.

Hager, May, et al. "Battling Alzheimer's—can ibuprofen alleviate some symptoms?" *Newsweek*, March 24, 1997; 66.

Kanowski, S., et al. *Abstract from the Sixth Congress of the International Psychogeriatric Association*, September 10, 1993. Berlin.

Lindenbaum, J., et al. "Neuropsychiatric disorders caused by cobalamin deficiency in the absence of anemia or macrocytosis." *New England Journal Medicine*, June 30, 1988;318(26): 1720-1728.

Nasman, B. "Serum dehydroepiandrosterone sulfate in Alzheimer's disease and in multi-infarct dementia." *Biological Psychiatry*, 1991;30:684-690.

Murphy, Kate. "Taking Aim at Alzheimer's." *Business Week*, February 17, 1997;103-108.

Rauscher, F.H., et al. "Music and spatial task performance." *Nature*, 193;36.

Schrof, Joannie M. "Brainpower." *U.S. News & World Report*, November 28, 1994;89-97.

Socci, D.J., et al. "Chronic Antioxidant Treatment Improves the Cognitive Performance of Aged Rats." *Brain Research*, 1995;693:88-94.

Van Goor, L., et al. "Review: cobalamin deficiency and mental impairment in elderly people." *Ageing*, November 1995;24(6): 536-542.

MENOPAUSE

Alshuler, Lise, N.D. "Menopause: Easing the Change" *Nutrition Science News*, August, 1997; Vol.2, No.8; 398-402.

Barret, Connor E., et al. "A perspective study of dehydroepidandrosterone sulfate, mortality and cardiovascular disease. *New England Journal of Medicine*, December 11, 1986;315(24) 1519-1524.

Begley, S. "The mammogram war" *Newsweek*, Feb, 1997; 55-58.

Diamond, Jared. "Why women change." *Discover*, July 1996;130-137

Eddy, D.M., "The value of mammography screening in women under age 50 years." *JAMA.*, March 11, 1988;(10): 1512-1519.

Elmore, G., et al. "Variability in radiologists' interpretations of mammograms." *New England Journal of Medicine*, December 1, 1994;331(22): 1493-1499.

Feldman, Henry A., et al. "Impotence and Its Medical and Psychosocial Correlates: Results of the Massachusetts Male Aging Study." *Journal of Urology*, January, 1994;151: 54-61.

Matsumoto, Alvin M. M.D., full professor of gerontology, Veteran's Affairs Medical Center, Seattle, Washington. Personal Communication, February, 1997.

Morales, A.J., et al. "Effects of dehydroepiandrosterone in men and women of advancing age." *J. Clin. Endocrinol. Metab.*, 1994;78(6): 1360-1367.

Rice, Fay. "Menopause and the Working Boomer." *Fortune*, November 14, 1994.

Roy, J.A., et al. "Hormone replacement therapy in women with breast cancer. Do the risks outweigh the benefits?" March 1996;14(3):997-1006.

Rudman, D., et al. "Effects of human growth hormone in men over 60 years old." *New England Journal of Medicine*, July 5, 1990;323(1): 1-6.

Tenover, J. "Effects of testosterone supplementation in the aging male." *J. Clin. Endocr. and Metab.*, 1991;35 316-318.

Willis, Claudia. "The Estrogen Decision." *Time*, June 26, 1995;46-53.

NUTRITION

American Diabetes Association, "Diabetes Facts and Figures, 1997."

Avorn, J., et al. "Reduction of Bacteriuria and Pyuria After Ingestion of Cranberry Juice." *JAMA.*, 1994;271:751-754.

Condor, Bob. "Could milk (gulp) be dangerous?" *Chicago Tribune*, February 11, 1996.

Kilhama, Chris. "Kava For Anxiety and Insomnia" *Nutrition Science News*, May 1997; Vol.2(5);232-234.

Lecos, C. "Caffeine jitters: some safety questions remain." *FDA Consumer*. December 1987-January 1988; 21:22-27.

Palmer, J., et al. "Coffee Consumption and Myocardial Infarction in Women." *American Journal of Epidemiology*, April 1, 1995;141(8): 724-731.

Raloff, J. "Coffee: Brewing's link to cholesterol." *Science News*, September 16, 1995; Vol.18:182.

Salmeron, J. "Dietary fiber, glycemic load, and risk of non-insulin-dependent diabetes mellitus in women." *JAMA.*, February 12, 1997; 277:472-477.

Siesjo, B.K., "Glutamate, calcium, and free radicals as mediators of ischemic brain damage." *Annals of Thoracic Surgery*, May, 1995;59(5): 1316-20.

Silverman, K., et al. "Withdrawal Syndrome After the Double Blind Cessation of Caffeine Consumption." *New England Journal of Medicine*, October 15, 1992; 327 (16):1109-1114.

Walford, R.L., "The clinical promise of diet restriction." *Geriatrics*, 1990;45(4): 81-83, 86-87.

Weindruch, Richard. "Caloric Restriction and Aging" *Scientific American*, January, 1996;46

Ziegler, R.G. "Vegetables, Fruits, and Carotenoids and the Risk of Cancer." *American Journal of Clinical Nutrition*, 1991; 53: 251S-259S.

OSTEOPOROSIS

Bourgoin, B.P., et al. "Lead Content in 70 Brands of Calcium Supplements," *American Journal of Public Health*, August 1993; Vol.83.

Calcified Tissue International, February, 1997.

Lee, J.R. "Is natural progesterone the missing link in osteoporosis prevention and treatment?" *Medical Hypotheses*, 1991; 35: 316-318.

Massey, L.K. "Acute effects of dietary caffeine and sucrose on urinary mineral execretion in healthy adolescents." *Nutrition Research*, 1988; 8(9).

Nielson, Forrest H. "Studies on the Relationship Between Boron and Magnesium Which Possibly Affects the Formation and Maintenance of Bones." *Magnesium Trace Elements*, 1990;9: 61-19.

RETIREMENT

Greenfield, Stanley. "Financial Forum" *Dynamic Chiropractic*, July 31, 1995;13.

Del Prete, Dom. "Piecing Together Your Retirement Puzzle." *Fidelity Focus*, Spring, 1997;7-11.

Shute, Nancy. "A study for the Ages." *U.S. News & World Report*. June 9, 1997;67-103.

SKIN.

———. "Read This First" *U.S.News & World Report*, October 14, 1996;79-80.

Ehrlich, H., et al. "Inhibitory Effects on Vitamin E on Collagen Synthesis and Wound Repair." *Annals of Surgery*, 1972; 175:235-240.

Fisher, William J., M.D., board certified member of Plastic and Reconstructive Surgeons Association. Personal communication, January, 1997.

Ryan, F., et al. "Skin care, chemical face peeling, and skin rejuvenation" *Plastic Surgical Nursing*, Fall, 1995; 15(3):167-71.

Tanouye, Elyse, *The Wall Street Journal* February 10, 1997. "A Few Wrinkles Still Remain in Quest for Youthful Skin."

SLEEP

Capell, Kerry, (editor). *Business Week*, June 9, 1997. "Apnea: The Sleeper's Worst Nightmare"

Cowley, Geoffrey. "The Melatonin Craze." Cover Story: *Newsweek*, August 7, 1995;46-49.

Mace, J.W., et al. "Usefulness of Post-Sleep Human Growth Hormone Release as a Test of Physiologic Growth Hormone Secretion." *Journal of Clin. Endocrinol & Metabolism*, 1970. 31, 225-226.

Marquis, Mary Cole, R.PH., "Natural Sleep Remedies" *Nutrition Science News*, April 1997. Vol.2, No. 4;176-180.

STAYING YOUNG

Darrach, Brad. "The War on Aging" *Life*, October, 1992;33-43.

Jacobs, Tom. "Siegel ministers to body and soul." *Santa Barbara News-Press*, February 9, 1997.

Klatz, Donald. "Approaching Immortality" *Energy Times*, October, 1996;46-51,70.

Larsen, David. "Getting to Know the Oldest Old." *Los Angeles Times*, March 6, 1989.

Lehr, U. University of Heidelberg, Germany. "Health Aging: A Challenge in Our Time" *From the United Nations and World Health Organization First Joint Conference on Health Aging*. April 29-May 1, 1996. New York, NY.

Packer, L., University of California, Berkley. "Possible Factors Influencing Aging" *From The United Nations and World Health Organization First Joint Conference on Health Aging*, April 29-May 1, 1996. New York, NY.

Shapiro, Laura. "Is Fat That Bad?" *Newsweek*, April 21, 1997.

Shute, Nancy. "A Study For The Ages—Generations of volunteers are helping scientists to comprehend time's toll." *U.S. News & World Report*, June 9, 1997;67-78.

Stern, Caryl. "What We Can Learn From People Who Live To 100." *Parade Magazine*, January 26, 1996.

Rusting, Ricki L., "Why Do We Age?" *Scientific American*, December, 1992: 131-141.

Time: Special Issue Fall, 1996 "The Frontiers of Medicine"

U.S. Bureau of the Census 1994. "A Statistical Profile of Older Americans."

U.S. Department of Health and Human Services. "Elderaction: Action Ideas For Older Persons And Their Families, Fitness Facts For Older Americans."

STRESS

"Chronic Stress is Directly Linked to Premature Aging of the Brain." *National Institute on Aging, Research Bulletin*, October, 1991.

Weiss, Michael. "Something to Wish For: Time To Relax" *U.S. News & World Report.* November 11, 1996;17.

SELECTED BIBLIOGRAPHY

Barnard, Neal, M.D. *Eat Right Live Longer.* Crown Trade Paperbacks, New York, NY. 1995.

Bartlett, John. *Familiar Quotations, Fourteenth Edition.* Little, Brown and Company, Boston, MA. 1968.

Bloomfield, Harold H., M.D., et al. *Hypericum (St. John's Wort) and Depression.* Prelude Press, Santa Monica, CA. 1996.

Braverman, Eric R., M.D., et al. *The Healing Nutrients Within.* Keats Publishing, Inc., New Canaan, CT. 1987.

Casdorph. M.D., Ph.D., et al. *Toxic Metal Syndrome.* Avery Publishing Group, Garden City Park, NY. 1995.

Cox, James, D.C. *Low Back Pain.* Williams & Wilkins, Baltimore, MD. 1990.

Editors of, *Prevention Magazine Health Books, Age Erasers For Women.* Rodale Press, Emmaus PA. 1994;183-188, 597.

Erikson, Erik H. *A way of looking at things: Selected Papers from 1930 to 1980.* Edited by Stephen Schlein. Norton. New York, NY. 1986; 18-21, 24-33, 44-47, 175.

Estes, Clarissa Pinkola. *Women Who Run With The Wolves.* Ballantine Books, New York, NY. 1992;293.

Ford, Norman D. *18 Natural Ways To Stop Arthritis.* Keats Publishing, New Canaan, CT. 1997.

Guyton, Arthur C. *Textbook of Medical Physiology.* W.B. Saunders Co. Philadelphia PA. 1991; 209,441,643, 661,824,872.

Howard, Elliot J., M.D., et al. *Health Risks,* The Body Press, Tucson, AZ. 1986;66.

Kingma, Daphne Rose. *A Garland of Love.* Conari Press, Berkeley, CA. 1992.

Knoke, William. *Bold New World.* Kodansha International, New York, NY. 1996;309-10.

Landau, Carol, Ph.D., et al. *The Complete Book of Menopause.* The Berkeley Publishing Group, New York, NY. 1994.

Lark, Susan M., M.D., *The Estrogen Decision.* Westchester Publishing Company, Los Altos, CA. 1994.

Lee, John R., M.D. *What Your Doctor May Not Tell You About Menopause The Breakthrough Book on Natural Progesterone*. Warner Books, New York, NY. 1996;44,318.

Mahan, Kathleen, R.D., D., M.S., et al. *Krause's Food, Nutrition & Diet Therapy*. W.B. Saunders Company, Philadelphia, PA. 1992.

Masters, William and Johnson, Virginia, *Human Sexual Response*. Little Brown & Co. Boston, MA. 1966.

McCully, Kilmer, M.D. *The Homocystine Revolution*. Keats Publishing, New Canaan, CT. 1997.

Mindell, Earl, R.Ph., Ph.D., *Earl Mindell's Anti-Aging Bible*. Simon & Schuster, New York, NY. 1996.

Murray, M.T., *The Healing Power of Herbs*. Prima Publishing, Rocklin, Ca. 1995.

Olinekova, Gayle. *Go For It!* 1982. Simon & Schuster, New York, NY. 1982.

Oppenheim, Michael, M.D. *The Men's Health Book*. Prentice Hall, Englewood Cliffs, NJ. 1994.

Ornish, Dean, M.D. *Dr. Dean Ornish's Program For Reversing Heart Disease*. Ivy Books, New York, NY. 1996.

Pesman, Curtis. *How A Man Ages*. Esquire Press, New York, NY. 1984.

Peter, James and Thorpe, Nick. *Ancient Inventions*. Random House, New York, NY. 1994; 18-21,31,34-35, 46,175.

Physician's Desk Reference. Medical Economics Company, Montvale, NJ. 1996.

Pierpaoli, W., et al. *The Melatonin Miracle*. Simon & Schuster, New York, NY. 1995.

Reinisch, June, Ph.D., *The Kinsey Institute New Report on Sex*. St. Martin's Press, New York, NY. 1990.

Rosenthal, Saul H., M.D., *Sex Over 40*. G.P. Putnam's Sons, New York, NY. 1987.

Ryback, David, Ph.D., *Look Ten Years Younger Live Ten Years Longer*. Prentice Hall, Englewood Cliffs, NJ. 1995.

Sahelian, Ray, M.D. *DHEA A Practical Guide*. Avery Publishing Group, Garden City Park, NY. 1996.

Silverstone, Barbara, et al. *Growing Older Together*. Pantheon Books, New York, NY. 1992.

Stryer, Lubor. *Biochemistry. Third Edition*. W.H. Freeman and Company, New York, NY. 1988;422.

Taber, Clarence Wilbur, *Taber's Cyclopedic Medical Dictionary, edition 17*. F.A. Davis Co. Philadelphia, PA. 1989.

Tierney, Lawrence, M. Jr., MD, et al. *Current Medical Diagnosis & Treatment*. Appleton & Lange, Norwalk, CT. 1996.

Von Beltz, Heidi. *My Soul Purpose*. Random House, New York, NY. 1996.

Wade, Carole, and Tavris, Carol. *Psychology, Fourth Edition*. Harper Collins College Publishers. New York, NY. 1996; 521-530.

Watt, Bernice K., et al. *Composition of Foods*. United States Department of Agriculture, Washington, D.C. 1963.

Westheimer, Dr. Ruth, *Dr. Ruth's Guide to Good Sex*. Warner Books, New York, NY. 1983.

Whitaker, Julian, M.D. *29 Medically Proven Miracle Cures*. Phillips Publishing, Inc., Potamac, MD. 1995.

Winawer, Sidney J., M.D. Shike, Moshe et al. *Cancer Free*. Simon & Schuster, New York, NY. 1996; 81,181, 228.

Winters, Ruth. *A Consumer's Dictionary of Food Additives* Crown Publishers, Inc. New York, NY. 1984;107,205.

Winter, Ruth, M.S. *A Consumer's Dictionary of Cosmetic Ingredients*. Crown Trade Paperbacks, New York, NY. 1994.

WEBSITES/TOLL-FREE NUMBER REFERENCES

http://php.silverplatter.com. for *Medline*.

http://search.pbgc.gov and also www.dolgov are two sites for The Pension Director Search—a directory of the federal government to search for workers who have not received pension money due them.

http://www.adoptivefam.org for Adoptive Families of America or 1-800-372-300

www.nih.gov/nia/ for the National Institute on Aging—there are some wonderfully informative treatments on many topics.

http://www.veris-online.org for information on antioxidants.

Agency for Health Care Policy and Research (AHCPR) including the Center for Medical Effectiveness Research Publications Clearinghouse (800) 358-9295.

Answers to questions about noise, hearing loss and how to buy a hearing aid. American Speech-language-hearing Association, 1-800-638-TALK. (1-301-897-8682 in Maryland)

http://www.ama-assn.org Information on smoking and vision loss and other health news from the AMA's Science News Department.

www.cais.net/aca for information on chiropractic care, research and health news from the American Chiropractic Association

INDEX